GETTING OVER OCD

THE GUILFORD SELF-HELP WORKBOOK SERIES

Martin M. Antony, Series Editor

Workbooks in this series are crafted by respected scientists who are also seasoned therapists. Each volume addresses a specific psychological or emotional problem, putting powerful change strategies directly into the reader's hands. Special features include self-assessment tools, worksheets, skills-building exercises, and examples—plus the support and motivation readers need to achieve their goals.

The Anti-Anxiety Workbook: Proven Strategies to Overcome Worry, Phobias, Panic, and Obsessions

Martin M. Antony and Peter J. Norton

Getting Over OCD: A 10-Step Workbook for Taking Back Your Life

Jonathan S. Abramowitz

GETTING OVER OCD

A 10-Step Workbook for Taking Back Your Life

Jonathan S. Abramowitz, PhD

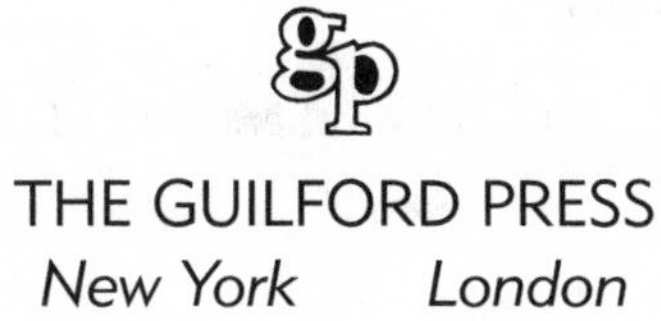

THE GUILFORD PRESS
New York London

A Division of Guilford Publications, Inc.
72 Spring Street, New York, NY 10012
www.guilford.com

Printed in the United States of America

This book is printed on acid-free paper.

Last digit is print number: 9 8 7 6 5 4 3 2 1

Library of Congress Cataloging-in-Publication Data

Abramowitz, Jonathan S.
Getting over OCD : a 10-step workbook for taking back your life / Jonathan S. Abramowitz. — 1st ed.
p. cm. — (Guilford self-help workbook series)
Includes bibliographical references and index.
ISBN 978-1-59385-999-2 (pbk : alk. paper)
1. Obsessive–compulsive disorder. 2. Cognitive therapy. I. Title.
RC533.A268 2009
616.85′227—dc22

2008054859

To my wife, Stacy,
and our daughters, Emily and Miriam,
with all my love

Contents

PART III

Your Treatment Program

Acknowledgments

No one walks alone, and when you are walking on the journey of life, just where do you start to thank those who joined you, walked beside you, and helped you along the way? I'm pleased to begin with my mother and father, Ferne and Les Abramowitz, who always knew what was best for me (even when I didn't) and continue to provide the unconditional love and support that has fueled my ambition and pushed me to achieve. Thanks to my most influential teachers—Kathy Harring, Joel Wade, Arthur Houts, Edna Foa, Marty Franklin, and Michael Kozak—who taught me to appreciate clinical psychology as a science and to understand the often misunderstood and secretive symptoms of obsessive–compulsive disorder (OCD). Your insights are to be found weaving in and out of the pages of this book.

I also want to thank all of the men and women with OCD that I've been fortunate to work with over the years. As they inspire me to work hard in my clinical and research endeavors, they've motivated me to make this workbook as comprehensive as possible. Without knowing it, they've also contributed a tremendous amount to its content.

Readers seldom realize that editors are the real workhorses of the publishing business. They read manuscripts line by line, word by word, and get almost as involved with the subjects as the writer. My editor, Chris Benton, cared so much about her work and this topic that she became my conscience as I worked on much of this book. She honed my language and presentation with the perfect blend of constructive feedback and positive reinforcement. Thanks also to Kitty Moore and Sawitree Somburanakul of The Guilford Press and Martin M. Antony, the series editor, who encouraged me to write this workbook.

Last, but certainly not least, I thank my lucky stars for my adoring wife and best friend, Stacy, and our wonderful girls, Emily and Miriam, who have been so patient as I worked on this project. It's not easy to write a book, maintain a clinical practice, hold a university faculty position and run a research lab, be associate editor of two professional journals, serve as associate chair of a psychology department, *and* be a good father and husband. Although I've always prided myself on my ability to put first things first, we'll all recall a few times when you (appropriately) questioned my judgment. Still, thank you for your understanding and sacrifices while I worked on this project. There is nothing in the world more important and more meaningful to me than your love and happiness—it's what I live for.

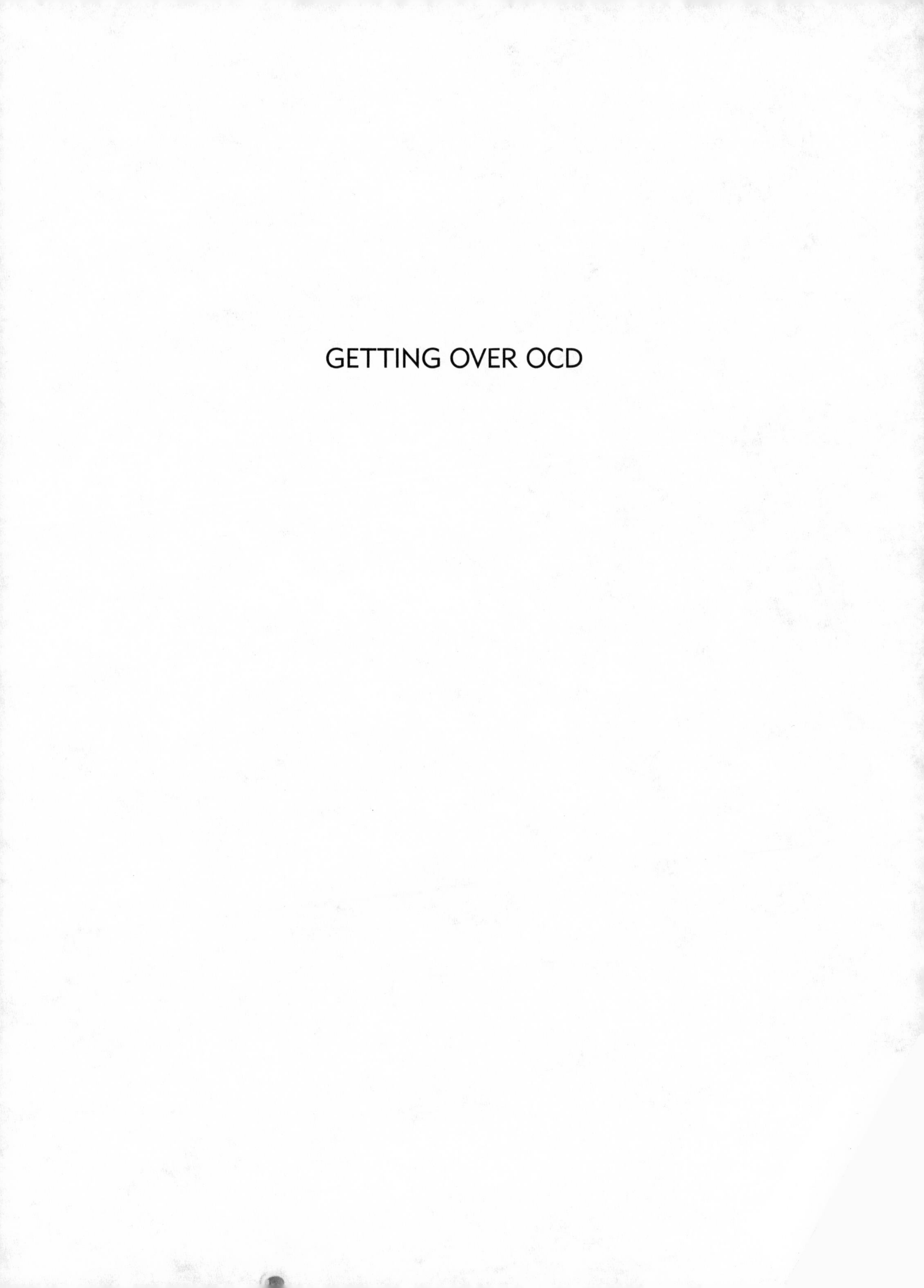

GETTING OVER OCD

Introduction

Are obsessions and compulsions stopping you?

Maybe you've never thought about it in exactly this way. After all, your life probably hasn't come to a complete halt. But the fact that you're reading these words says that in some way obsessive–compulsive disorder (OCD) *is* stopping you, whether it's keeping you from going where you want to go, preventing you from doing what you want to do, taking up time you'd rather spend on something else, or just causing you discomfort.

The way to stop obsessions and compulsions from stopping you is to work your way through the steps in this book.

Welcome to what I hope will be both a rewarding and challenging journey for you. *Rewarding* because it is likely you will gain tremendous improvement from practicing the skills you'll learn in this book. Just imagine: No more terrifying obsessional fear. No more need to avoid certain situations. No more relying on compulsive behaviors to cope. Fewer restrictions on your day-to-day life. Sounds nice, doesn't it?

Challenging because learning to use skills that will help you overcome OCD requires practice and (gulp) some hard work. Have you tried to get help before? Maybe treatment didn't work out. Are you currently seeing a therapist? Maybe it's difficult to find a professional who knows how to properly treat OCD. Maybe you've thought about getting help but have never done so. Most people who have OCD never get help from a mental or behavioral health professional—which is one of the main reasons I've written this book. This may be your first attempt to do anything about your OCD symptoms. Whatever the case may be, by selecting this workbook you've chosen a program that has half a century of scientific research to back it up. I have conducted some of this research and have also worked with hundreds (if not a thousand) people with OCD. So I understand this problem and how to treat it. In writing this book I've drawn on my scientific knowledge as well as my clinical expertise to make the most effective treatment for OCD—cognitive-behavioral therapy (CBT)—accessible to you in the most user-friendly format available.

Unlike many other books available on this subject, the techniques I describe here have all been researched extensively in well-designed clinical trials. It's a scientific fact that when the methods described in this book are put to use in a therapeutic way, people generally experience a significant decrease in their OCD symptoms. Basically, I have taken the strategies that are proven to be useful in therapy and adapted them in a self-help format for you. I will be your coach—teaching you all the tricks of the trade to help you overcome this problem. I will also be your cheerleader—giving you the encouragement you need to persevere in your battle against OCD.

How serious is your problem? Perhaps OCD is a "sometime thing" for you, getting in your way only in certain situations: you have to use a public restroom; you're the last person to leave work and responsible for locking up; you see a knife, a baseball bat, or a police officer's gun that triggers some horrible unwanted thought about violence. Or perhaps obsessions and compulsions are constant companions that interfere with relationships, family, your religious or spiritual life, work, and other areas of life: you have persistent unwanted sexual thoughts or fears that you've committed a sin or made a terrible mistake; you have an ever-present worry that you're responsible for something tragic; things never seem to be "just right," and you feel the need to order or arrange them more perfectly. Regardless of how often you experience trouble with obsessions and compulsions, I hope you will join me in this 10-step journey toward health and freedom. I think you'll find it worthwhile every step of the way.

Who Am I?

My first exposure to OCD came in 1994 as a PhD student in clinical psychology at the University of Memphis. As a therapist in training I was assigned to work with a very sweet and gentle woman who was afraid she would go berserk and murder her family in their sleep. She kept all the knives locked away and constantly prayed for God to keep her from acting on her senseless thoughts. Sure, I had read books and research papers about OCD, but nothing had prepared me to hear about this problem firsthand and to see how much this woman was suffering. Under the supervision of my professors, I eventually helped her overcome her obsessions using a form of CBT called "exposure and response prevention." My interest in OCD was piqued, and I decided to learn more by conducting my own research and gaining more clinical experience.

I was fortunate to finish my doctoral training and begin my professional career at the Center for Treatment and Study of Anxiety in Philadelphia (now part of the University of Pennsylvania) under the mentorship and supervision of Drs. Edna Foa, Michael Kozak, and Martin Franklin, some of the world's leading experts on OCD and CBT. The 4 years I spent learning about this problem by evaluating, treating, and studying people who suffered with it were invaluable to my career as a clinician and scientist.

In 2000 I moved to the Mayo Clinic in Rochester, Minnesota, and founded the Mayo OCD and Anxiety Disorders Clinic—a treatment and research program with a staff of dedicated psychiatrists and psychologists. People with OCD came to Mayo from across the

United States and around the world. I personally consulted with and treated hundreds of patients and trained and supervised numerous therapists wanting to learn how to help their clients with OCD. I also wrote and edited my first three OCD books (for professionals) while at Mayo, putting what I had learned though my research, training, and clinical work in print for others to benefit from.

In 2006, I moved to the University of North Carolina (UNC) at Chapel Hill, where I am professor and associate chair of the psychology department. I direct the UNC Anxiety and Stress Disorders Clinic, which is an outpatient clinic that primarily serves people with OCD and related problems with anxiety. My role is to train and supervise PhD students—the psychologists of tomorrow—in how to understand, study, and use CBT techniques to help people with OCD. Our team is working hard conducting research on the prevention and treatment of OCD so that we can minimize the suffering associated with this problem. In addition, I have a small private practice, which I devote almost exclusively to treating people with OCD who come to Chapel Hill from across the region for my services.

To put it simply, I love my work. I appreciate people's stories and enjoy the challenge of trying to understand each new individual's obsessions and compulsions. What's most rewarding to me, though, is helping people like you apply the principles of CBT (exposure and response prevention) to get relief from obsessive thoughts and fears, senseless rituals, and painful anxiety. Given my interest in and love of this work, and the extraordinary training and experience I've been so fortunate to have as a clinician and a scientist, writing a workbook for people with OCD seemed like the best thing I could do for all the people that I can't work with face to face. I hope you'll find that this book contains everything that science and art have to offer.

How Can This Workbook Help You?

Experts in the field of psychology and psychiatry agree that CBT is the most effective form of treatment for OCD. It has been studied with thousands of patients in centers around the world. The probability that you will get at least some improvement from CBT is 60–70%; if you complete a course of CBT, you are likely to get a 50–70% decrease in your OCD symptoms. This usually translates to significant reductions in obsessional anxiety and compulsive rituals and substantial improvements in your quality of life. While I can't offer you a guarantee of success, I can say that if you work hard, it's a good bet you'll benefit from CBT.

In my work with patients and in my research, one thing has become very clear about how best to overcome OCD: it's a step-by-step process. The exposure and response prevention form of CBT that is so effective in eliminating obsessions and compulsions succeeds precisely because you build on your own successes as you work your way through the therapy. This is why this workbook, unlike others you'll find in your local bookstore, is written in a step-by-step format, with the 10 steps corresponding to the stages of CBT treatment. At each step you'll be doing exercises and practices designed to teach you basic strategies for overcoming problems with obsessions and compulsions. I encourage you to have a pencil or pen handy as you read and to make copies of the blank worksheets and forms for your personal use so you can continue to use them in the coming months.

This is a self-help book—meaning it's designed for you to use on your own—but it's not intended to *replace* treatment by a qualified mental health practitioner should you need professional help. You can use this book in any of these ways:

- *As a supplement to working with a therapist.* In fact, one of my motives for writing this book was to have a good resource for my own patients and clients to use as they progress through treatment. If you've tried therapy without much success, it may be that your therapist is not a specialist in the treatment of OCD. If you've found a clinician that you like and trust—a critical ingredient in effective therapy—you may want to share this book with him or her to enrich the therapeutic relationship, giving you and your therapist a common language for talking about problems with OCD. As a companion to your treatment, this workbook can move your therapy forward and give it some structure.
- *For help with OCD symptoms that do not require ongoing professional care.* One reason that many people do not get professional help for obsessions and compulsions is that they have what we call a "subclinical" form of the disorder, meaning their problems are not severe enough to qualify for an official diagnosis of OCD. That doesn't mean, however, that their lives aren't impaired—or that they could not benefit from improvement. In Step 1 I'll help you get a feel for whether your problems may be more serious than you had thought and whether you should see a mental health professional for a diagnostic evaluation. If not, self-directed CBT with this workbook may very well be appropriate for you. If you're feeling depressed (which is common among people with OCD), or having thoughts about suicide, of course you should see a doctor right away.
- *If you have problems with OCD and are looking for additional emotional support.* The stories and examples you will read here—composites of real people, real symptoms, and real victories I have witnessed—will help you see that you are not alone in your struggle to find your way out of OCD. The people I counsel often feel ashamed of the symptoms that plague them, *despite the fact that they are not to blame for the intrusion of obsessions and compulsions in their lives*. Shame and guilt are obstacles to improvement that get swept away the more you see that OCD comes uninvited into innocent people's lives.
- *To facilitate your support network.* This workbook can help your friends, family members, and mental health professionals gain a fuller knowledge of OCD, better understand what you are going through, and learn some tools for helping you manage your problems.

If you are one of the many people with OCD who never get to see a mental or behavioral health professional—much less a professional with the degree of training and experience needed to successfully help people with OCD—I am pleased to have the opportunity to teach you about OCD and start you on your journey to recovery. If you are using this book while also working with a therapist, thank you for including me in your treatment. I am delighted to lend a helping hand. If you are a therapist who doesn't have a lot of experience with OCD, it is my pleasure to serve as a guide. I hope this book will be helpful in your work.

What's Inside?

It's normal to have all sorts of different feelings about starting a new treatment program. On the one hand, you feel stuck; but on the other hand, change can produce anxiety. You'd love to leave OCD in the dust, but what will it take to get there? With all of these mixed emotions, you might be feeling confused and vulnerable. The treatment program in this book will empower you by helping you understand your feelings better. It will also help you get beyond the fear and anxiety that are probably keeping you stuck right now.

This workbook is divided into three parts. Part I, which contains Steps 1, 2, and 3, will help you learn about the symptoms of OCD, their causes, and the available treatments. There are several different *types* of obsessions and compulsions; in Part I, I will help you learn more about your particular subtype(s) so that you can tailor the CBT techniques to meet your specific needs. Finally, you will learn how to think about your problems with OCD from a cognitive-behavioral perspective. These first three steps will lay the groundwork for understanding your symptoms in a way that will help you get the most out of the treatment strategies you'll use in later steps.

In Part II you will prepare yourself for using strategies to defeat OCD problems. Specifically, in Step 4 you'll develop a plan of action for battling your obsessions and compulsive rituals. In Step 5, you'll complete some exercises to help yourself stay motivated to do the challenging work of CBT.

Part III is the heart and soul of the workbook. In Steps 6, 7, 8, and 9, I will give you step-by-step instructions to help you apply the CBT techniques that are so effective in the treatment of OCD. These techniques will help you change the thinking, feelings, and behavioral patterns that keep OCD alive. In Step 10 I will help you develop plans for maintaining your improvement over the long term so that you can put your problems with OCD behind you for good. The illustrative examples, worksheets, and forms I provide will help you get the most out of this program. Each step in the workbook builds on the previous ones. So, for example, the self-analysis you conduct in Step 2 will be used in Steps 3, 4, 5, and 6 as you design and implement your treatment program. For this reason, I strongly recommend reading and working through the steps in order.

So, now that you know what lies ahead, let's get on with the program. Step 1 begins your journey toward a better, richer life—one with less fear and anxiety and more time for working, playing, and just being you.

PART I

Getting to Know Your Enemy

STEP 1

OCD 101

Learning about the Symptoms, Causes, and Treatments

Let's get one thing perfectly straight right up front: OCD is a real psychological disorder that can be truly debilitating to its sufferers and their loved ones. It's not something you're making up or indulging yourself in. You didn't ask for it—although how you respond to this "enemy" is definitely the key to getting it out of your life.

The best way of thinking about the symptoms of OCD is as a set of unwanted thinking, feeling, and behaving patterns that are very stressful, unproductive, and difficult to control without help. The thinking patterns involve senseless, unwanted, and often very unpleasant thoughts, images, and impulses—called *obsessions*—that intrude into your mind even though you don't want them there. These kinds of mental intrusions provoke feelings of anxiety or discomfort, along with fear and uncertainty that something bad or harmful might happen. In turn, the anxious feeling patterns trigger the urge to do something to reduce the anxiety and deal with the obsessional thoughts. *Rituals* (sometimes called *compulsive rituals*) and *avoidance* strategies are the kinds of behavior patterns people with OCD get into to try to cope with obsessional thoughts, restore a sense of safety and certainty, and reduce anxiety.

There are two critical take-home messages here:

1. *Obsessions* **provoke** anxiety.
2. *Compulsive rituals and avoidance are attempts to* **reduce** anxiety.

Although compulsive rituals and avoidance behaviors occasionally succeed in reducing obsessional fear and uncertainty *in the short term*, these strategies tend to backfire *in the*

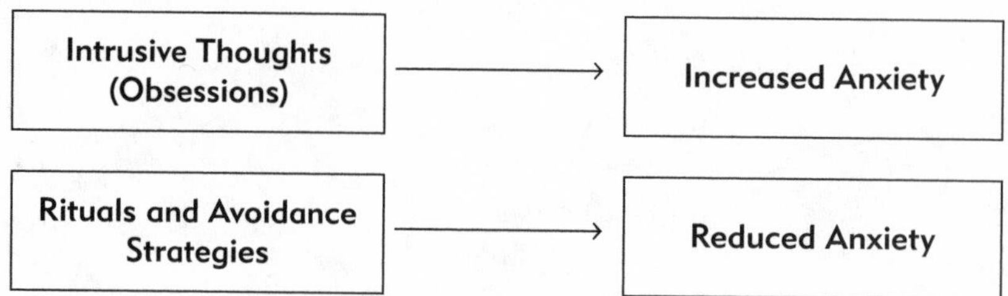

long run. This is because obsessions always return; so you just find yourself doing more and more of the same rituals and avoidance behaviors. Over time, these thinking, feeling, and behaving patterns intensify to the point that people end up spending too much energy on avoidance and rituals (which backfire anyway) so that their work, school, social, and leisure activities get disrupted.

Have you noticed this disruptive pattern in your own life?

According to the American Psychiatric Association's *Diagnostic and Statistical Manual of Mental Disorders*, now in its fourth edition (DSM-IV-TR), OCD is classified as an *anxiety disorder*, defined by the presence of recurrent obsessions or compulsive rituals that are severe enough to be time-consuming—taking up at least 1 hour a day—and that cause significant personal distress or interference with daily activities. Other psychological problems classified as anxiety disorders include phobias (irrational fears of things like animals, storms, the dark, and enclosed spaces), social anxiety disorder (fear of social embarrassment and speaking in front of groups), panic disorder (recurrent attacks of intense fear and dread), agoraphobia (fear of going out by yourself into crowds), posttraumatic stress disorder (PTSD; anxiety, flashbacks, and nightmares about traumatic personal events), and generalized anxiety disorder (excessive worrying about everyday matters such as relationships, finances, work, school, and health). Although these other problems often occur along with OCD, they are not the topic of this workbook.[1]

What Is *Not* OCD?

The treatment strategies in this workbook are very effective for OCD, but they are designed specifically to help with the problems that fit the description you just read. Unfortunately, many people (including some professionals) confuse other disorders that involve repetitive thinking and behavior with OCD. So, in addition to learning what OCD *is*, it is important to learn about what it *isn't*. If you think you might have either of the following types of disorders instead of OCD, this is not the workbook for you.

Obsessive–Compulsive Spectrum Disorders

Check off any of the following "obsessive" and "compulsive" problems that you have trouble with:

[1]Another workbook in this series may help you if you think you have one of these other anxiety disorders: *The Anti-Anxiety Workbook*, by Martin M. Antony, PhD, and Peter Norton, PhD (Guilford, 2008).

- ☐ Repetitive hair pulling (for example, trichotillomania)
- ☐ Tics or Tourette's syndrome (for example, sudden facial movements such as eye blinking, unwanted vocalizations such as throat clearing or grunting, sudden muscle movements in different parts of the body)
- ☐ Repetitive skin picking or nail biting
- ☐ Compulsive gambling
- ☐ Compulsive sexual behavior (for example, excessive pornography use or masturbation that interferes with relationships or functioning)
- ☐ Compulsive stealing
- ☐ Self-injury behavior (for example, cutting)
- ☐ Compulsive shopping, buying, and hoarding
- ☐ Unnecessary fixation with a part of your appearance (for example, body dysmorphic disorder)
- ☐ Excessive preoccupation with having a serious illness (for example, hypochondriasis/health anxiety)

If one or more of these are a problem for you, then you might have a so-called *obsessive–compulsive spectrum disorder*. These spectrum disorders have some overlapping features with OCD—thoughts that are repetitious and behaviors that are difficult to resist—yet they do not involve the same thinking, feeling, and behaving patterns shown in the diagram on the facing page. Therefore they require their own treatment approach. I recommend consulting with a mental health professional if your symptoms seem to fit better into this category.

Could you have an obsessive-compulsive **spectrum** disorder rather than OCD?

Obsessive–Compulsive Personality Disorder

Place a check mark next to any of the personality traits in this list that describe you:

- ☐ I am preoccupied with details and rules.
- ☐ I insist that people do things my way, and I can get angry or very upset if they don't.
- ☐ My perfectionism interferes with my getting things done.
- ☐ I am stingy and not very generous; I have a hard time sharing my things with other people.
- ☐ I am excessively devoted to work and productivity.
- ☐ I am generally rigid and stubborn.
- ☐ I am overly conscientious and rigid when it comes to ethics and morality.
- ☐ I cannot throw away even worthless or worn-out things such as clothes, books, or papers.

Is it possible that you have obsessive-compulsive **personality** disorder instead of OCD?

If you're like most people, you probably checked a few of those boxes. But if you have at least four of these characteristics, and they cause difficulties in your life, you might have a problem called *obsessive–compulsive personality disorder* or OCPD. OCPD is different from OCD (I always tell my patients and students that it's a shame the two conditions have such similar names). It doesn't share the same thinking, feelings, and behaving patterns as OCD, nor does it respond to the treatment techniques used in this workbook.

What Is It Like to Have OCD?

OCD is a very heterogeneous disorder. What it's like to have OCD for one person can be very different from what it's like for another, as the following four individuals illustrate. Underlying their widely variable symptoms, however, you'll undoubtedly begin to spot the thinking, feeling, and behavior patterns just described. Can you recognize how these patterns are related to one another in the following stories?

Brittain: The Mistakes That Were Never Made

"My symptoms began soon after I started college and began living away from home for the first time. Whenever I would finish a paper for class, or had to pay a bill, or fill out an important form, I would get these doubts in my head that maybe I had made a mistake—a serious one. For example, 'What if I underpaid my telephone bill?' or 'What if I copied the invoice number incorrectly from the statement?' Thoughts of my telephone service being cut off kept running through my mind. I also had images of collection agencies showing up at my door and coming after me.

"So, to make sure I never made any mistakes, I made myself reread everything I wrote before handing or sending it in. But my rechecking got out of hand after a while. I would get stuck reading over my bank checks to make sure the amount and invoice numbers were correct. Even after checking them several times over, I still had doubts. Sometimes, after I had finally put the check into the envelope, sealed it, and was on my way to the mailbox, I would have to reopen the envelope just to make sure I didn't make any mistakes. The whole process would start again. Of course, my rational mind knew this was completely senseless—I never made any of the mistakes I was so scared of. Still, checking gave me reassurance. I felt like I would go on obsessing forever unless I had a guarantee that everything would be okay."

Mike: The Fastidious Cable Guy

"As a cable TV installer, I was always going into different people's homes. That's when I started thinking that I could be spreading germs and other dangerous contaminants throughout the town where I live. Suppose I got germs from someone living on Elm Street and then spread them to a family on Maple Street later that day? It would be my fault if an innocent person—a child perhaps—got some terrible disease. I also worried that maybe I had stepped in dog poop or grass that had been sprayed with poisonous pesticides or fertilizer. What if I tracked that into someone's home? What if a baby

lived there and crawled where I had walked? I couldn't get these obsessive thoughts out of my head. They seemed to be with me every waking moment, and they made me very worried.

"To deal with these thoughts and fears, I carefully watched where I stepped and avoided walking on grassy areas. I also scrubbed my hands and washed down my shoes with wipes before going into people's homes. Even still, I had the feeling I might be spreading contamination without realizing it. At one point, I thought of calling all the homes I had visited to make sure everyone was okay. That's when I started arranging my route so I could go home, shower, and wash my uniform in between houses. Of course, my work was suffering; but I was so scared of causing innocent people to get sick. Needless to say, I ended up losing my job at the cable company."

Stephanie: Postpartum OCD

"It all started when my son, Tyler, was born. I had always been a worrier, but having a tiny and helpless infant to take care of made me absolutely terrified! To make matters worse, I couldn't stop thinking the most awful thoughts about the worst possible things I could do to this defenseless, innocent baby. I find it hard to even talk about these thoughts, but when he would cry, I would find myself thinking about wildly shaking him. Although I knew these thoughts were senseless, they were so frightening. Sometimes when Tyler was sleeping, I would check on him just to make sure I hadn't lost control and shaken him to death.

"Changing Tyler's diaper made me have all sorts of awful sexual thoughts. The word 'penis' would come into my head every time I changed him, and I had thoughts of touching him sexually. I wondered whether he was getting sexually aroused by me changing him. Even though I was trying hard to get rid of these thoughts, they just kept coming back. I tried thinking about nice things instead, but the bad thoughts always won out. Why? Was I secretly a pedophile? A pervert? Was it just a matter of time before I acted on these awful ideas? I ended up having to avoid changing Tyler—my husband did it all. The poor child had to sit in dirty clothes until my husband came home from work. I also constantly asked my husband if he thought I was a bad person because of my thoughts. He would reassure me that I was still a good person. I thought becoming a parent would be a wonderful thing. Instead, it was turning out to be a terrible nightmare."

Steve: "Not Just Right" OCD

"Since my early teen years, my days have been consumed with the need to make sure that things are 'even,' 'balanced,' and 'in order.' My brain thinks about this all the time—like it's on autopilot. Even though I hate it and wish I didn't think this way, I can't seem to ignore it or put it aside. For example, odd numbers are a problem for me because I think they're unbalanced. If I come across an odd number, I have to do something in order to 'even it out.' Like, if I know I've received 23 e-mail messages today, I'll have to send myself one more just to make it 24. Balance is also a big thing. If I touch something with my left side, I have to turn around and brush up against it with my right side (with the same amount of pressure) to 'balance it out.' If I don't, I won't feel 'balanced.' My bedroom at home also has to be ordered and arranged just right. The clothes in my drawers have a certain alignment. Items on

my desk must be placed a certain way. Even the way I put on clothes, shoes, eat my food, wash myself, and comb my hair has to be done just so. It's not that anything bad is going to happen if things aren't perfect, balanced, or even, but there's this overwhelming sense that things are 'not just right.' And it seems like that feeling would just go on forever and ever, and that I will lose my mind thinking about it. So, in order to get rid of that feeling, I just take the time to do these rituals. Unfortunately, they take up so much time that I can hardly get anything else done."

What similarities did you notice between these people and yourself?

Did you recognize the thinking, feeling, and behaving patterns of OCD in these stories? Since the aim of CBT is to weaken these OCD patterns, an important first step is to learn how to spot the patterns in your own thoughts, emotions, and actions.

Are You Alone in This?

Anxiety disorders are the most common mental health problems. About 20% of adults—*that's one in five*—will have clinically severe anxiety at some point in their life. As for OCD, it affects 2–3% of the adult population—*about one in every 40 people, or over six million adults in the Unites States alone.* And that doesn't even count millions more people who experience occasional obsessions and rituals that don't fully meet the criteria for OCD. As we'll see, *most* people have obsessions and rituals at some point in their lives. You probably know other people with anxiety or OCD problems even if you don't realize it. So if you suffer from OCD, you are not alone.

Most people start to develop OCD in their late teens or early 20s, when people in many societies are becoming more independent and are faced with greater responsibilities. As you might have noticed from reading the preceding stories, responsibilities often play a role in OCD. It can be hard to pinpoint when problems with OCD begin, and it doesn't really matter if you don't remember when you first had obsessions and compulsions. What's more important to understand is that once OCD patterns develop, they're hard to get rid of on your own. So the sooner you get started, the better. And the way to start is to be aware of the kinds of thoughts, feelings, and behaviors you're experiencing that are part of OCD.

What Kinds of Ideas Does OCD Put in Your Head?

Your best friend may claim to be "obsessed" with a new car. Your son may be "obsessed" with a sports hero. Your coworker might be "obsessed" with a musical group. You might remember at one time being "obsessed" with jealousy over a new love. But these uses of the term "obsession" trivialize the thinking patterns of OCD and how they affect you. To a psychologist, obsessions and obsessional thinking are much more than just thinking a lot about something. *In OCD, obsessions are persistent unwanted thoughts, impulses, doubts, or images that seem intrusive, inappropriate, senseless, and distressing.* For those with OCD, obsessions are not manifestations of intense interest in something. On the contrary, they are:

- Thoughts and doubts that you *don't* want to have,
- That you try to *ignore* or *resist* (often unsuccessfully), and
- That make you feel *uncomfortable, anxious*, or *unsafe*.

An obsession is *not* an intense interest in something.

This is entirely different from daydreaming about a new car.

This workbook is designed to be helpful for OCD-related obsessions. You, however, might experience other kinds of repetitive negative thoughts that suggest a different problem is present—one that may require different treatment approaches. Excessive *worrying*, for example, is often a sign of generalized anxiety disorder (GAD). Worries, which are different from obsessions, concern real-life issues such as work and school, relationships, decisions, health, and finances (for example, "What if I lose my job and end up on the street?"). *Ruminating* is another form of repetitious negative thinking often mistaken for obsessing. Ruminations are signs of depression and involve repetitive thoughts about an actual negative event such as a setback, loss, or other type of problem that you can't seem to get over. If your negative thoughts seem to fit better into the categories of worry or rumination, rather than obsession, I recommend seeking a professional evaluation to determine whether you have OCD or one of these other problems.

Types of Obsessions

Which obsessions do you typically have?

The obsessions that are part of OCD typically concern danger, violence, morality, or responsibility for harm. They often (but not always) fall into the following broad categories: (1) responsibility for harm or mistakes, (2) contamination, (3) symmetry and order, (4) violence and aggression, (5) sex, and (6) religion and morality. The most common obsessions in each of these categories are listed next. As you read through the list, place a check mark next to any obsessions that seem to get stuck in your mind, cause you a great deal of anxiety or distress, or get in the way of your daily routine.

1. Responsibility for harm or mistakes

Intense anxiety or concerns about:

- ☒ Making mistakes that would result in harm to other people
- ☐ Harming someone else because of your own carelessness
- ☐ Being responsible for disasters (for example, fire, burglary, other tragedy)
- ☐ Not doing enough to prevent something bad or awful from happening
- ☐ Hitting someone with your car
- ☐ Numbers or words associated with bad luck or disasters (for example, "9–11," "13")

2. Contamination

Intense anxiety or concerns about:

- ☐ Bodily waste or bodily fluids (for example, blood, saliva, urine)
- ☐ Dirt or germs

- ☐ Toxic chemicals and other materials (for example, pesticides, fertilizers, asbestos, cleaning fluids)
- ☐ Certain places or contact with certain people
- ☐ Germs from animals or insects
- ☐ Becoming ill because of contamination
- ☐ Spreading contamination to others (this is a contamination *and* a responsibility obsession)
- ☐ How disgusting it *feels* to be contaminated (rather than being afraid of illness)

3. *Order and symmetry*

Preoccupation with:

- ☐ Order and exactness
- ☐ Ideas that something is not arranged just right
- ☐ The need for left–right balance or symmetry
- ☐ Even or odd numbers

4. *Violence and aggression*

Unwanted thoughts, images, impulses, and intense fears of:

- ☐ Hurting or killing people you don't want to hurt (for example, loved ones)
- ☐ Violent images or thoughts
- ☐ Words associated with violence (for example, *death, murder, gun*)
- ☐ Harming yourself even though you don't want to (*not* suicidal thoughts)
- ☐ Obscenities, racial slurs, insults, and curse words—perhaps the impulse to say or yell offensive things at someone you don't want to hurt
- ☐ Upsetting thoughts and urges to act on unwanted, aggressive impulses

5. *Sex*

Unwanted thoughts, images, impulses, and intense fears related to:

- ☐ Forbidden or perverse sexual topics (for example, masturbation, pornography, adultery)
- ☐ Homosexuality (if you are straight) or heterosexuality (if you are gay)
- ☐ Molesting children, committing incest, or having sex with animals
- ☐ Becoming a pervert
- ☐ Aggressive sexual behavior (for example, rape)

6. *Religion and morality (scrupulosity)*

Unwanted thoughts, images, doubts, and intense fears related to:

- ☐ Blasphemy and sacrilege
- ☐ Whether you're following the teachings of your religion well enough
- ☐ Your relationship with God

- ☐ Sin, hell, and punishment
- ☐ Morality, and right and wrong
- ☐ Other unwanted or immoral topics (for example, thoughts of curse words)

7. *Miscellaneous obsessions*

Extreme fears and preoccupation with:

- ☐ Having, or being diagnosed with, a serious medical illness (for example, cancer)
- ☐ Having something else rather than OCD (for example, schizophrenia)
- ☐ Aspects of your physical appearance

Even within these different types of obsessions, the particular content varies from person to person. The table on the next page shows examples of specific obsessions within each category. Don't worry if your obsessions don't fall neatly into one of these categories: everyone's are a little different, and this will not affect your ability to benefit from this workbook.

But obsessions can be even more bizarre or senseless than those listed in the table. Here are some less common ones that I have come across:

- Rhona feared becoming contaminated by a certain geographic area—the Pocono Mountains in Pennsylvania.
- Ronnie had an obsessional doubt that crumbs from the communion wafer might have fallen into his underwear, and therefore he had had sex with Jesus Christ.
- Scott experienced the recurring senseless thought that *he* might become pregnant.
- Shari had an obsession that she might have accidentally cheated on her husband by having sex with a total stranger *without realizing it*.

What theme(s) do your obsessions belong to? What *forms* do they take? Obsessional *images* are troubling mental pictures—for example, a recurrent image of a loved one smashed to smithereens in a car accident. Obsessional *impulses* are unwanted urges or notions to do things that would be harmful or inappropriate—for example, the urge to yell a racial slur or beat up on someone you love. Obsessional *doubts* are characterized by persistent uncertainty about something you feel it's important to know for sure—for example, whether you were exposed to mercury when you changed the lightbulb, whether you committed an awful deed by mistake, whether you're really gay or straight, and whether you're going to heaven or to hell when you die. Other sorts of obsessions can involve unwanted words, numbers, tunes, or other thoughts and fears that you find distressing, but that you have difficulty dismissing from your mind.

Use the worksheet at the bottom of the next page to identify your top three obsessions—the ones we'll target first in your treatment program. If you need help deciding on your top three, ask yourself which obsessions bother you the most or cause you the most anxiety? Which ones are you most eager to get rid of? Which ones come up most often? Which ones lead you to do the most time-consuming, disruptive rituals?

Category	Examples of obsessions
Responsibility for harm or mistakes	• What if I dropped my pills on the floor and a child took them? • I could be responsible for causing a fire in my house. • I might injure someone with my car and not realize it. • The number 13 could bring bad luck to someone I love.
Contamination, germs, sickness, poison, and disgust	• Thoughts that germs from the doorknob are on me. • What if I shook hands with someone who didn't wash after using the bathroom? • If I touch the baby, I will contaminate her with my germs. • Was I exposed to a harmful chemical?
Order and symmetry	• Thoughts about the desk being messy. • Thoughts about odd numbers. • Need to feel things are "just right."
Obsessions concerned with violence, sex, morality, and religion	• Thoughts of curse words, nasty comments, or racial slurs. • Thoughts about harming or killing someone I love. • What if I lose control and do something terrible? • Images of my grandparents having sex. • Urge to stare at someone's genital area. • Am I absolutely sure that I am not a child molester? • Ideas of having inappropriate sexual relations. • Unwanted blasphemous images, such as the image of Jesus with an erection on the cross. • Doubts such as "What if I committed a sin without realizing it and God is very upset with me?"

My Top Three Obsessions

1. CHECKING
2. __________
3. __________

Obsessions: Hitting You Where It Hurts

To further explore your obsessions, think about the most important things in your life—the things you value most. Answers I typically hear from my patients include their health, family, religion and God, work or school, money, relationships, and their reputation. In the worksheet at the bottom of the page, make a list of what you value most. Next, look back at the list of your top three obsessions and think about how these obsessions are related to the things you value most in life. Describe this relationship in the worksheet below.

Most people say that their obsessional thoughts, images, and doubts are tied to whatever they consider most important—the things they value or treasure the most. This explains why obsessions seem so personally distressing and why they make you feel so uncomfortable, anxious, or unsafe. After all, when constantly bombarded by upsetting thoughts about the most important areas in one's life, who wouldn't feel this way? Consider some general patterns I've observed in my own experience working with many OCD sufferers:

- Obsessional doubts about responsibility for making mistakes are frequently found among people who consider themselves very sensible and cautious, or who are in positions of responsibility.
- Obsessions about germs and contamination are often reported by people who value cleanliness and maintaining their (and their loved ones') good health.
- Violent and aggressive obsessions are often found among people who consider themselves sensitive, caring, and gentle.
- Obsessions about hurting family members are usually found in people who have strong family ties and who love and care about their relatives very much.
- Religious obsessions mostly occur in people who take religion and their relationship with God very seriously.
- Sexual obsessions are often found in people who consider themselves highly moral, or whose sexuality plays an important role in how they view themselves.

What are the things you value most in your life? MY JOB

How are your obsessions related to what you value most in life? FAILING TO SECURE THINGS PROPERLY COULD COST ME MY JOB.

What Does OCD Make You Do to Feel Better?

Like the term *obsession*, people overuse the words *compulsion* and *compulsive*—usually when talking about repetitious problematic behaviors, such as "compulsive" gambling, shopping, or sexual behaviors. Clinically speaking, however, compulsive rituals in OCD are responses to the feelings of threat, anxiety, uncertainty, and distress that accompany obsessions. No one likes feeling anxious or worried, so people with OCD naturally try to get rid of the obsession and reduce the unpleasant feelings by performing some kind of behavior that reduces anxiety and makes them feel safer. When such a "safety-seeking" behavior is repeated over and over to excess, and often according to certain self-prescribed rules, it is called a *compulsive ritual*. Recall this pattern from the OCD sufferers you met earlier:

- Brittain performed compulsive checking rituals in response to her obsessional fears of making mistakes when paying bills. The checking served to guard against mistakes.
- Mike washed and cleaned in response to his fears of spreading germs and contamination. He thought this was the only way to keep him and others safe.
- Steve performed balancing and ordering rituals in response to the obsessional thought that things were "not just right." He felt that if he did not put things in order, his feelings of discomfort would make him "go crazy."

You're probably familiar with this type of strategy, but maybe it's not the only thing you do to cope with obsessions and anxiety. You might also use other strategies that are not so repetitive or rule-driven—that is, they are not *compulsive*. We call these "mini-rituals"—for example, quickly wiping your hands on your pants to remove contamination, or gripping the steering wheel more firmly if you have a thought of driving into oncoming traffic.

Do you perform any little safety-seeking actions without much thought?

Perhaps you perform some (or all) of your compulsive and mini-rituals in your mind—what are called "mental rituals." Stephanie used mental rituals (thinking *nice* thoughts) along with other compulsive rituals in response to sexual and harm-related obsessions about her infant.

You might also try to reduce obsessional discomfort and make yourself feel safer by seeking reassurance that everything is all right. Reassurance seeking can be compulsive, such as if you ask a relative the same questions over and over (for example, "Are you sure you locked the door? Are you sure? Are you really sure . . . ?"), or reviewing a website about harmful chemicals over and over. Reassurance seeking can also occur mentally, such as if you review the information from the website over and over in your mind, or if you go over in your mind all of your conversations to make sure you didn't use any curse words, racial slurs, or act inappropriately.

Reassurance is a very important, yet often overlooked, ritual in OCD, so we'll set it apart from other rituals in this program to make sure it's addressed.

Despite the differences in how these rituals look, they all serve the same purposes: to reduce obsessional anxiety and make you feel safe. As you read about these different types of rituals in more detail below, think about the kinds of rituals you use and how they help you try to cope with your obsessions.

Compulsive Rituals

Compulsive rituals are behaviors you perform repetitively to reduce obsessional anxiety and restore a sense of safety. Of course, these rituals are clearly excessive and unrealistic in relation to the obsessional fears they are designed to quell. Most compulsive rituals fall into several general categories, including (1) checking, (2) decontamination, (3) repeating actions, and (4) ordering and arranging. The table below lists some of the most common ones. After you read through the table, go through the list of different types of rituals and check the boxes next to those that cause problems for you—those that take up too much time, are difficult to resist, and get in the way of your life.

1. *Checking*

Irresistible urges to check and recheck (more than just once or twice) that:

- ☑ Doors, water faucets, windows, and appliances are locked, off, or unplugged
- ☑ Something isn't lost or missing (for example, your wallet)
- ☐ You didn't make a terrible mistake
- ☐ Loved ones are safe
- ☐ Disasters didn't happen
- ☐ You didn't cause a negative event or disaster

Category	Common compulsive rituals
Checking	• Going back to the door, window, or stove to make sure it is locked or off • Checking the news to make sure there were no car accidents that you could have caused • Reopening envelopes to make sure you paid the bills correctly
Decontamination	• Ritualistically washing hands • Taking a shower after every time you urinate or defecate • Washing all store-bought groceries before they enter the house
Repeating routine actions	• Rewriting bank checks so that the handwriting is perfect • Flicking a light switch on and off several times • Going back and forth through a doorway several times
Ordering/arranging	• Arranging clothes in your closet a certain way • Brushing the *left* side of your body up against the wall because you had touched the wall with your *right* side

- [x] Asking others for reassurance
- [x] Counting while checking

2. Decontamination

Excessive washing or cleaning that might be according to certain rules, involving:

- [ ] Hand washing
- [ ] Showering, bathing, grooming, or tooth brushing
- [ ] Special toilet routines (for example, when wiping)
- [ ] Changing clothes
- [ ] Cleaning inanimate objects (the mail, items from a store, laundry)
- [ ] Using hand gels or other sanitizers
- [ ] Other means of preventing or removing contamination (for example, using gloves)
- [ ] Counting while washing or cleaning

3. Repeating

Performing the following types of actions repeatedly:

- [ ] Routine activities such as going through a doorway, going up or down steps, turning light switches on and off, getting up from a chair, and so on
- [x] Rereading or rewriting
- [x] Touching or tapping
- [x] Counting while repeating
- [x] Repeating these pointless behaviors until unwanted thoughts or images go away
- [ ] Repeating these behaviors to prevent disastrous consequences (for example, bad luck, death)

4. Ordering and arranging

- [ ] Arranging items in a certain order (for example, clothes, books)
- [x] Counting to an even number to neutralize an odd number
- [ ] Trying to achieve balance (for example, left and right)
- [x] Other ways of making things seem "just right"

Mini-Rituals

In contrast to compulsions, which are often drawn out, *mini-rituals* are brief and can be very subtle and discreet. In fact, you might not even recognize them as a part of your problems with OCD. When Jerry was driving with his family he would experience obsessional thoughts of killing everyone by steering the car into a tree. To counteract his obsessions, he used a mini-ritual in which he gripped the steering wheel more tightly to make sure he didn't lose control of the car. Elaine, who had obsessional thoughts of harming her husband, played loud music to distract herself from her upsetting ideas. She didn't recognize this distraction as part of her OCD; but it can be a mini-ritual if you use distraction to cope with an obsession. George had obsessional fears of contamination triggered by contact with things that other people routinely touched: public door handles, elevator buttons, and the like. If he came into contact with feared surfaces, George quickly wiped his hand on his pants or shirt to "rub off the germs" and reduce his fears of contamination.

Do your problems with OCD include mini-rituals? Review the list below and place a check mark next to those brief strategies you use to cope with or reduce obsessional anxiety.

- ☐ Quickly rubbing or shaking your hands or clothes to get rid of germs
- ☑ Performing some other kind of brief action to reduce obsessional anxiety or the feeling that something bad might happen

  My mini-ritual action(s):

  ____

  ____

- ☐ Trying to distract yourself from the obsession or situation with some other activity

  My distraction activities(s):

  ____

  ____

Mental Rituals

Brooks had obsessional thoughts about family members dying. Whenever these thoughts were triggered (such as by seeing the word *death*), Brooks had to repeat the word *life* 10 times to himself. This ritual "canceled out" or "neutralized" his death obsessions. Connie had obsessional doubts about whether she had sinned by being "too proud." To reduce her anxiety, she silently repeated prayers over and over until she felt God would not punish her. Laurie was preoccupied with the idea that she might have been unfaithful to her husband without realizing it. As a result, she felt compelled to mentally review (over and over) each and every activity she had done that day to be absolutely sure that she had not committed adultery. She also spent a great deal of time trying to analyze what her thoughts meant—if she was happily married, why would she have these kinds of thoughts?

We need to pay special attention to these kinds of rituals in this program. Mental rituals that go unrecognized and unaddressed can stand in the way of successful treatment—sort of the way a computer virus can end up destroying your computer unless you get rid of *all* of the infected files so the virus doesn't have a chance to spread. Like a computer virus, mental rituals are easy to miss because they're *thoughts* rather than outward *behaviors*. This means no one except you knows they are there. To make matters worse, mental rituals can be confused with obsessions (even *professionals* sometimes have difficulty telling them apart).

Following is a list of types of mental rituals. Place a check mark next to those mental acts you use to cope with obsessions:

- ☐ Thinking special words, sayings, images, or phrases to neutralize obsessions and anxiety
- ☐ Saying prayers over and over (in your head) a certain number of times or in a special way
- ☐ Constantly repeating lists (for example, to-do lists) to yourself
- ☐ Reviewing other matters (conversations, activities) over and over in your mind or until it is done "perfectly"
- ☐ Trying to stop or suppress unwanted thoughts
- ☐ Spending excessive time trying to rationalize or think through or "figure out" an obsessional situation or thought (for example, could this really be true?)

Ask yourself:

- *Is this an intentional thought that reduces my anxiety?* If so, it's a mental ritual
- *Or is this an unwanted thought that provokes my anxiety?* If so, it's an obsession.

Reassurance-Seeking Rituals

Many infectious disease experts had told Jack that he would probably not get AIDS by using a public toilet. Yet he continued to seek information and get blood tests for this disease just to be *absolutely* sure. Marcia called her pastor on the phone several times each week to ask him whether she was going to heaven or hell ("If people did ___________, could they still get into heaven?"). She had obsessions about hell and worried she was not a "good enough Christian." Marvin had obsessional doubts about whether he had "concentrated enough" at his wedding (which had occurred nearly 10 years earlier), and if not, whether his wedding vows really "counted." To reassure himself, he repeatedly asked his wife and other people who attended the wedding (including the priest who performed the ceremony) whether he had looked "attentive" during the ceremony. He even reviewed the videotape of the wedding to see if he looked "attentive enough."

"Do you think God loves me?"
"Are you sure the iron is off?"
"What are the chances I will get sick?"
"Will I act on my thoughts of harming someone?"
"Am I a pervert if I think about sex too much?"

If you find yourself persistently asking questions like these, you experience an often overlooked and unnoticed part of OCD called *reassurance seeking*. You might recognize that you're seeking reassurance about things you already know the answer to, as in Jack's example. Like Marcia, you might seek a definitive solution to supernatural, existential, or philosophical questions that we can only answer based on *faith*, rather than having absolute guarantees. In cases like Marvin's, the question you seek reassurance about might not even have an answer. Maybe you don't come right out and ask reassurance-seeking questions over and over, but rather pose them without being too obvious. Maybe you try to get reassurance simply by confessing your thoughts or observing how other people react in certain situations. Wanting to be discreet is understandable, but to overcome your problems with OCD, you will have to recognize these strategies as rituals and target them in treatment.

Elliott was afraid of pesticides. He worried that exposure to these chemicals would cause him to develop cancer someday. Aside from compulsive washing and cleaning, Elliott engaged in endless question asking. When very anxious, he would visit local stores and corner a clerk to ask dozens of questions about the risks associated with pesticides: "Is it safe to walk somewhere that has been sprayed with pesticides in the last week?" "How long should I wait to walk where the ground was sprayed?" "Can using this product lead to cancer?" "If I can smell the pesticides, does it mean I'm too close?" The interesting thing is that Elliott already knew the answers to his reassurance-seeking questions! He'd asked many people the same questions over and over. So the aim of reassurance seeking isn't to get new information. Rather, it is to reduce anxiety by hearing someone else confirm what you're already reasonably sure about, but can't be 100% certain of. Other ways of seeking reassurance include repeating tests (such as medical tests), and checking reference books and websites for information to reduce uncertainty. Do you have a problem with compulsive reassurance seeking? Check off the strategies you use to get reassurance about your obsessional fears:

- ☑ Asking people the same (or similar) types of questions over and over
- ☑ Looking up information on the Internet excessively
- ☐ Rereading books, labels, or other sources of information about your obsessive fears
- ☐ Excessively watching other people to see what happens before you do something similar
- ☐ Having someone else be with you as a form of reassurance (for example, while driving)
- ☐ Apologizing for or confessing to the same thing (or thought) over and over

Your Top Three Rituals

Before moving on, review the checklists of compulsive, mini-, and mental rituals and consider any reassurance-seeking strategies you use. Which of these take up the most time for you? Which get in the way of your life the most? Which should we target in your treatment program? Briefly describe these in the "My Main Rituals" worksheet on the following page. In Step 2, I'll help you analyze these behaviors more carefully so we can understand and reduce them.

Different Types of OCD

As I said earlier, OCD is heterogeneous—like ice cream, it comes in many different "flavors." Obsessions can involve different themes, and rituals can take different forms. Certain obsessions, however, tend to occur along with certain types of rituals (almost like how

My Main Rituals

____

____

____

____

____

certain flavors of ice cream seem to taste good together), and these pairings break down into four major "subtypes" of OCD. Knowing which one or ones you have is important because you'll apply the treatment techniques described in Part III differently depending on the subtype you're tackling.

Responsibility Obsessions and Checking Rituals

If you obsess over making mistakes; causing accidents, fires, burglaries, or bad luck; or being responsible for hurting people in other ways (such as hurting their feelings by mistake), you probably belong in this subtype—as does Brittain, whom you read about earlier. Often, responsibility obsessions take the form of doubts that you can't erase from your mind ("*What if* I didn't unplug the iron?" or "*What if* I hit someone with my car and didn't realize it?"). You might also have obsessional fears of "unlucky" words, numbers, or colors that you associate with awful consequences (such as that the number 13 will cause bad luck).

If you have obsessional fears of causing harm, it makes sense that you'd take precautions such as compulsively checking the situation to ensure that no harm or damage occurs, or to reassure yourself that everything (and every*one*) is safe. You might check doors, windows, lights, and electrical appliances (especially before leaving home or going to bed) if you are afraid of robberies or fires. You might check the rearview mirror in your car, or even the news for information about accidents, if you were afraid you'd caused one without realizing it. Excessively checking paperwork for mistakes, seeking information from the Internet, and asking others for reassurance are also common rituals for people within this subtype. Finally, you might use superstitious behaviors like repeating actions (for example, going back and forth through a doorway) or conjuring up a "safe" thought or image (for example, of a lucky number) to make you feel safer.

Contamination Obsessions and Decontamination Rituals

This form of OCD usually involves fears of bodily fluids (urine, feces, or semen), dirt, germs, or toxic chemicals and substances. You might also obsess about contaminating other people (loved ones, strangers), as Mike did. Perhaps you're afraid of the feared contaminant because you think it will make you (or others) very sick; or maybe the contaminant merely triggers a sense of *disgust* rather than a fear of illness. Regardless, you probably try to avoid situations and objects that you believe are sources of contamination (doorknobs, bathrooms, hospitals, certain people, places, parts of the body) or that remind you of contaminants (for example, if anything red makes you think of blood). Even when you have not come directly into contact with a feared object or contaminant, you might worry whether there *could* have been contact or whether you were "close enough" to become contaminated. It might seem as if the contamination can be "spread" from one object to another very easily, such as through coincidental contact.

Do your obsessive thoughts often start with "what if"?

To make you feel safe from contamination and any feared sicknesses, you probably avoid your feared contaminants. When you can't avoid, you might engage in excessive cleaning and washing rituals, including ritualized showering, bathing, bathroom routines, and excessive use of wipes or disinfectant hand gels. Maybe you have to perform these rituals in a particular way, such as counting while you wash your hands or scrubbing in a set routine.

Do your obsessions often involve a feeling of disgust?

Symmetry ("Just Right") Obsessions and Ordering/Arranging Rituals

If you have this symptom combination (sometimes called "incompleteness" or "just right" OCD), your obsessional anxiety is focused on the need for precision and you try to avoid the distressing idea that something is "not just right." Steve (from page 13) experienced this pattern, and maybe you do too. You might have to order or arrange objects in certain ways, make sure to avoid odd numbers, and try to make things seem symmetrical and "balanced." Your compulsive arranging rituals might serve to reduce feelings of incompleteness or imperfection—for example, tapping twice with your right foot and twice with your left. Or you might feel as if your ordering rituals serve to prevent disastrous consequences—for example, if you don't arrange the clothes in a certain order, a loved one will die in a plane crash.

Are you plagued by the sense that things just aren't the way they should be?

Violent, Sexual, and Religious Obsessions and Mental, Mini-, and Reassurance-Seeking Rituals

If your problems with OCD are mainly *obsessional*—that is, if you *don't* have the classic checking, washing, or ordering compulsions—chances are you fit into this category. At one time, this symptom subtype was called "pure obsessions" (or "pure O") because of the lack of compulsive rituals. Now we know that most people do have compulsions even if they are not overt or "classic." They may, in fact, not even be recognized by you as rituals because they are subtle mental rituals, mini-rituals, and reassurance-seeking behaviors. Violent, sexual, and religious obsessions are grouped together in this subtype because they often occur together and have several overlapping characteristics. Specifically, you can experience all of them as thoughts, images, impulses, or doubts; they all tend to represent the exact opposite of your normal moral or spiritual character; you often have them at the most awful times (for example, when you're with your family or trying to pray); and you try to deal with them using mental rituals, mini-rituals, and/or reassurance seeking.

Violent Obsessions

These are aggressive thoughts and images of injury or death that you find utterly repugnant; ideas of physically or verbally attacking people you care about—often innocent people or those who can't defend themselves (such as infants and the elderly); and impulses to do something self-destructive like reaching for a police officer's gun or driving your car into a tree. You look at your son and can't stop thinking about murdering him. You see a knife and think of stabbing the person seated next to you. You think of racial slurs when you see a person of a different ethnic or racial background. You have an impulse to open the emergency exit of a plane while in flight.

I'd be willing to bet anything that you've never acted on these obsessions. You're probably even afraid to *think about* such actions. To reduce your anxiety, you most likely carry out mental rituals that involve trying to dismiss the obsession or replace it with "good" thoughts ("Everyone is okay"). Perhaps you repeat what you were doing when the thought occurred (for example, putting on a piece of clothing) until you can finish the activity without its being "ruined" by having the obsessional thought. You might also use a variety of other more subtle (and noncompulsive) strategies for dealing with violent obsessions, including telling (warning) others about your violent thoughts and asking for reassurance that the obsessions are *just* thoughts, rather than a sign that you are actually dangerous or evil. You might also have tried "testing" yourself somehow to see if you'd really act on the impulse.

Sexual Obsessions

You just got married, but have *unwelcome* thoughts of cheating on your spouse. You have *unacceptable* images of your grandparents, or, like Stephanie, your *child* engaged in sexual behavior. You have *unwanted* impulses to glance at someone's crotch as she walks by. You worry that you're turned on sexually by children or by people of the same sex as you. I am not talking about sexual *fantasies* that lead to actually becoming aroused or to actual sexual behavior. Quite the opposite; in OCD your sexual obsessions provoke *anxiety* and *distress*. You do *not* enjoy thinking this way, but try as you might, you can't control these thoughts.

Your fight to control these forbidden and scary sexual obsessions may involve mental rituals to dismiss or replace them with more acceptable thoughts. You might also turn to prayer or to overanalyzing what the obsession might mean (for example, is it a sign of perversion?). One form of overanalyzing is a ritual in which you "test" yourself to see if the unwanted sexual thought provokes a sexual response (a form of mental checking). Rituals involving confessing and asking others for reassurance about what the thoughts mean ("Do you think I'm a pervert?") are also common.

Religious Obsessions (Scrupulosity)

These are *unwanted* blasphemous thoughts (against God), unholy images (having sex with a priest), and impulses to do sacrilegious things (defiling a place of worship). You might also have fears and doubts about whether you committed a sin or violated a religious or moral commandment (scrupulosity). You may worry that God will punish you and have obsessional doubts about whether you're truly faithful and devoted to your religion. If you have these kinds of obsessions, you might pray or confess excessively, engage in compulsive reassurance seeking (for example, from religious authorities), and perform other mental rituals (for example, overanalyzing, repeating certain phrases like "God is good") to reduce your anxiety.

What's Your OCD Subtype?

Most likely, your problems with obsessions and rituals fit into at least one of these subtype categories; perhaps they fit more than one. Mike, for example, had contamination obsessions and washing and cleaning rituals, but he also had obsessions concerning responsibility for harming others. Think about which subtypes your symptoms fit into and place a check mark in the appropriate box below (check as many as necessary):

- ☐ Responsibility obsessions and checking rituals
- ☐ Contamination obsessions and decontamination rituals
- ☐ Symmetry obsessions and ordering/arranging rituals
- ☐ Unacceptable obsessions and mental, mini-, and reassurance-seeking rituals
  - ☐ Violence obsessions
  - ☐ Sexual obsessions
  - ☐ Religious obsessions (scrupulosity)

How Did You End Up with Symptoms of OCD?

How does a town end up in the middle of a blizzard? A blizzard occurs when several ingredients come together in the same place: moisture, very cold air, and certain wind conditions. Any of these circumstances by themselves cannot produce a blizzard—they must all be present in the right amounts. Most likely OCD is similar in that it's caused by a complex combination of biological, genetic, learning, and circumstantial factors. My best guess from the available research is that genetic and biological factors make you vulnerable to developing problems with anxiety, while learning and environmental factors dictate the particular sorts of obsessions and rituals you have. Following is a quick summary of what we know (and don't know) and what it means to your chances of eliminating OCD from your life. But first, let me make something perfectly clear: *having OCD is not your (or anyone else's) fault*. You are not responsible for your biological makeup. You didn't ask to have certain experiences or to be exposed to other environmental factors. As you'll see, though, that doesn't mean you can't do anything to help yourself.

Depression: A Reason to Get Help Before Tackling OCD

At one point or another you have probably felt ashamed of your problems with OCD. Maybe you've tried to hide your obsessions and rituals from other people. Perhaps, like many people with OCD, you've experienced extended periods of time when you've felt sad, worthless, or hopeless about the future. Although these feelings are entirely understandable—after all, OCD is a depressing problem to have—extreme levels of sadness and hopelessness can interfere with your being able to benefit from this workbook. Take a look at this list of common signs of depression. If you've been experiencing one or more of these problems for 2 weeks or more, I recommend getting help for depression. In addition to improving your mood, treatment for depression will increase your ability to benefit from the strategies described in this workbook.

- Feeling sad, down, or irritable most of the time for 2 weeks or longer
- Feeling shame, hopelessness, worthlessness, or guilt
- Diminished interest or pleasure in your typical activities or hobbies
- Increased crying
- Trouble getting things done
- Feeling tired and out of energy despite not being as active as usual
- Significantly increased or decreased appetite and corresponding changes in weight
- Trouble sleeping—not being able to fall asleep *or* sleeping more than usual
- Feeling slowed down, having trouble making decisions, and difficulty concentrating
- Feeling that life is not worth living, or having thoughts of death and suicide

Is OCD a Brain Disease?

One widely held view is that OCD is a medical or biological disorder caused by a disease or problem with the brain, such as an "imbalance" of *serotonin*. Serotonin is a chemical messenger that operates in the brain and all over the body and might be linked to depression and anxiety. However, many biological studies have not supported the serotonin imbalance view of OCD. That is, lots of people with OCD have perfectly functioning serotonin systems. So, although it is a very *popular* theory, experts agree that the serotonin imbalance view is not a proven fact.

Some brain-imaging studies have suggested that certain structures in the brain—the frontal cortex, cingulate, caudate nucleus, and thalamus—are malfunctioning in people with OCD. Although it is fascinating to know about what might be occurring in the brain when someone has obsessions and rituals, the results of these imaging studies have been very mixed. Consider also that even the scientists conducting this research cannot tell whether the apparent malfunction in certain areas of the brain is the cause of OCD or simply a reflection of the fact that the person has OCD. There are interesting studies showing that when someone without OCD becomes very anxious, his or her brain looks a lot like the brain of someone with OCD.

Do you have close relatives with OCD or with other types of anxiety problems? Many people do. Since OCD tends to run in families, some researchers have labeled it as a genetic disorder. Yet despite over a decade of research, no one has found an "OCD gene." That's because there probably isn't one. Instead, it's the tendency to easily become anxious that seems to be genetic. So "anxiety-proneness" genes likely interact with other factors to cause OCD. You should also consider that just because OCD runs in families does not necessarily mean it is a genetic problem. It's equally likely that we can inadvertently *learn* OCD tendencies (just as we learn many other things) from our family (and other influential people in our lives). This is good news because it means that rather than viewing OCD as genetically determined and permanent, you can see it as something you could change.

If there is a learned component to OCD, you might be able to *unlearn* it. This is an important concept behind the power of CBT.

Learning Theories

Learning theories propose that obsessional fears and rituals can be acquired in a number of ways. For example, they could be learned by observing others. If your close relative has a fear of the number 13 or washes her hands excessively, you might follow this example. You might also learn OCD tendencies through sources such as the media, teachers, and other influential people in your life. For example, you might learn to fear germs if you're repeatedly told that "germs are everywhere." Traumatic events can also lead to OCD. Like some people I have worked with, your problems with obsessions and rituals might have started following a tragedy that made you think twice about your own safety.

You might also have been exposed to certain circumstances during your formative years that could be linked to OCD. For example, as a young person, perhaps you found yourself in a position of responsibility, such as having to care for a younger sibling because your parents were unable to do so. Maybe you were raised in a family with extremely strict rules that were very hard, if not impossible, to follow; and perhaps you were also threatened with serious consequences for not abiding by these rules. For example, Andrew's parents were both doctors and repeatedly warned Andrew that he must keep his hands perfectly clean and free of germs, or else he would become seriously ill. Because germs are invisible, Andrew worried that he wasn't doing a good enough job of cleaning and he developed a compulsive washing ritual to be *sure* he was perfectly clean.

Finally, coincidences where it appears that your thoughts or behaviors may have led to a negative event could play a role in acquiring OCD. For example, Richie had been thinking that his grandfather was an old man and would probably die soon. Coincidentally, within a week, his grandfather passed away from a heart attack. Unfortunately, Richie attributed his grandfather's death to the "bad thoughts" he had earlier that week. From that point, Richie developed mental rituals to "cancel out" bad thoughts, which he used every time negative thoughts about family members came to mind.

As with biological theories, these learning theories have not yet been proven as fact. Nonetheless, many of my patients and clients report these types of learning experiences, which might have influenced the development of their OCD. Can you identify any in your own past? Record them on the worksheet on the following page.

Understanding what might have contributed to causing your OCD symptoms can help you see that there are routes to improvement. It can also relieve any anxiety you may feel about having somehow caused your own problems. But don't get sidetracked by the search for a cause. OCD is not like a sore throat caused by bacteria—kill the bacteria with antibiotics and you eliminate the sore throat. As I said, we don't know precisely what combination of factors causes any individual's OCD symptoms. The treatment that forms the basis for the program described in this workbook requires a keen understanding of the *symptoms* of OCD, but not the *cause*. And, thanks to over a quarter century of psychological research, we understand these symptoms extremely well. In Steps 2 and 3 I will help you become an expert on your OCD symptoms so that you can get the greatest possible benefit out of this program.

My Learning Experiences That Could Lead to Obsessions and Rituals

Traumatic events: LEAVING A CLASSIFIED DOOR OPEN

Observations:

Influential sources (for example, media, teachers, parents):

Experiences:

CBT: Your Weapon against the Enemy You Know

At the time of this writing, CBT and certain medications known as *selective serotonin reuptake inhibitors* (SSRIs) are the only two types of treatment shown in clinical studies to be safe and effective for OCD. Which mode of therapy is best for you? In 2007, the American Psychiatric Association published practice guidelines for the treatment of patients with OCD and made the following recommendations:

- CBT alone is recommended if you are willing to do the work that is required and are not severely depressed.
- CBT combined with medication is recommended if you are trying CBT, but are not responding as well as you would like, and if you have problems with severe depression or other anxiety disorders.
- If you are currently taking a medication, CBT is recommended if you continue to have problems with OCD, and if you would like to be able to stop using the medication you are on.

Should you combine CBT and medicine?

- If you have tried CBT but found it overwhelming and are unwilling to try it again, medication alone is the recommended treatment.

The practice guidelines refer to CBT *with a trained therapist*—not self-help CBT that is done completely on your own. This workbook contains a self-help version of these CBT techniques that can make a real difference in your life even without a therapist, especially if your OCD is mild to moderate in severity and not complicated by other problems. In most cases, however, using this book along with the aid of a trained therapist who can help you correctly implement the strategies will produce greater improvement than going it alone.

Unlearning Obsessions and Rituals

In CBT, you learn and practice skills that reduce the two connections in OCD: the one between obsessions and increased anxiety and the one between rituals and anxiety reduction. The first part of CBT involves learning about your obsessions, anxiety, and rituals to help you better understand how these problems are related. You've already started this by completing Step 1. Steps 2 and 3 are also part of this process. The second component of CBT involves developing an individualized plan or road map for treatment. This plan helps you take aim at the specific obsessions and rituals you will weaken with the CBT strategies. You'll develop your own treatment plan in Step 4.

Like most people, you probably have some mixed feelings about change. Thus, an important part of CBT (which is covered in Step 5) involves thinking about your readiness to begin treatment and work hard toward the goal of breaking free of OCD. The fourth component of CBT is called *cognitive therapy*. The term *cognition* refers to thinking, and cognitive therapy (covered in Step 6) includes a set of strategies for helping you identify and correct the problematic thinking patterns that keep obsessions and rituals alive. Cognitive therapy helps set the stage for the main ingredients in CBT as described next.

The most potent tools in CBT are *exposure* and *response prevention* techniques. Exposure therapy, which I cover in Steps 7 and 8, involves confronting the situations and thoughts that trigger your obsessions in a gradual and therapeutic way. When you practice gradually facing the things that you fear and avoid, you'll weaken their connection with obsessional fear and they'll no longer make you anxious. When you get to Step 9, I'll help you use response prevention techniques to resist urges to ritualize and seek reassurance. By ending these behavioral patterns, you'll learn that you don't need to rely on rituals to keep you safe, prevent disasters, or reduce obsessional fear. Simply put, response prevention weakens the connection between rituals and anxiety reduction.

CBT programs conclude with learning some strategies that will help you maintain your progress over the long term. For example, by incorporating CBT techniques into your lifestyle, you'll solidify what you've done in the program and be able to achieve long-term improvement. In Step 10, I'll give you suggestions for how to prevent OCD from creeping back in.

As you've probably guessed by now, doing CBT means you'll have to put forth a great deal of effort whether you work with a therapist or use this workbook by yourself. You'll need to muster up the courage to face situations you have been avoiding and work hard

Medications for OCD

The SSRI medications are safe and can also be effective treatments for OCD, but they tend to be less effective overall when compared to CBT. You have about a 50% chance of responding to a medication, and are most likely to see a 20–40% reduction in your obsessions and rituals if you do respond. These medicines can be prescribed by most psychiatrists who are knowledgeable about OCD. The SSRIs currently approved by the U.S. Food and Drug Administration for treating OCD include:

- Paxil (paroxetine)
- Prozac (fluoxetine)
- Luvox (fluvoxamine)
- Zoloft (sertraline)
- Anafranil (clomipramine)
- Celexa (citalopram)

It is hard to say which SSRI is *best* for OCD, and even more difficult to predict how helpful these drugs might be for you. But they are a convenient form of treatment. There are no regular therapy sessions and no exposure and response prevention—the pill does all of its work inside your body. But this convenience comes with a price. Even if SSRIs help, they probably won't completely get rid of OCD symptoms by themselves. Also, you'll need to keep taking the medication to sustain any improvement, or risk relapse if you stop—even if you've been taking the medication for a long time. Another drawback is that SSRIs can produce unpleasant side effects such as dry mouth, sleep changes, constipation, headaches, weight gain, and sexual difficulties. It's hard to predict the kinds of side effects you might have since everyone responds to medication a little differently.

How to Identify a Qualified CBT Therapist

Unfortunately, CBT is not widely available. Not every mental health professional is well trained to use these techniques for OCD. The people who are most likely to receive the proper training in CBT for OCD are clinical psychologists (with a PhD, PsyD, or Master's degree), psychiatrists (with an MD), and social workers. You should ask your potential therapist where he or she received training in CBT for OCD, how much experience (how many patients) he or she has, and what form of treatment he or she uses. Listen carefully for how the therapist answers this last question. If he or she describes the techniques of exposure and response prevention, chances are you are on the right track. If not, you might ask whether the person would be open to helping you work your way through this book.

You must invest anxiety up front in order to have a calmer future.

resisting urges to do rituals you have been relying on for a long time. But as difficult as this seems, CBT gets easier with time and practice. The greatest advantage of CBT is that it's the safest and most effective way to reduce your OCD symptoms. The effects of CBT are also long lasting, so once you've learned and practiced the CBT techniques, no one can ever take them away from you.

STEP 2

Analyzing Your Own OCD Symptoms

As you learned in Step 1, OCD symptoms can take many different forms. In fact, there are probably no two people with exactly the same obsessional fears, avoidance patterns, and ritualistic behaviors. That's because people who have OCD all have their own way of thinking about situations that seem frightening to them and their own way of developing strategies for avoiding disasters and making themselves feel safe. In other words, your obsessions and rituals are driven by a certain type of "OCD logic" that is all your own.

Jessica, for example, has hand-washing rituals that are triggered by contact with toilets, toothbrushes, shampoo bottles, bath towels—anything associated with bathrooms—which she fears have germs that will make her very ill unless she washes. Maurice also feels compelled to wash his hands. He washes to dispel his anxiety over touching things that people often touch—money, doorknobs, railings, and so on—which makes him think about other people's germs. But Maurice doesn't worry about getting sick; he's just afraid his feelings of anxiety and disgust will go on forever if he doesn't wash his hands. Sumi also has hand-washing rituals, although hers are triggered by unwanted thoughts of having sexual relations with anyone but her current partner. For Sumi, hand washing erases anxiety over feeling "morally dirty" and represents a symbolic cleansing of her mind. As you can see in these three examples, the links between obsessions and rituals are very individualized.

How are your obsessions linked with your rituals and avoidance strategies?

It's essential to understand these highly individualized obsession–ritual links because it's those links that keep you trapped by OCD. Identifying the details of your obsessions and how your fears are linked to your rituals is also the key to designing an effective CBT program. Remember, CBT is not a "one size fits all" treatment. Together we'll shape your program so that it's just right for you. Think about it this way: If your clothes don't fit quite right, you take them to a tailor. But the tailor needs to measure you before making alterations. It's similar with CBT. Before we can target your obsessions and rituals, we need to understand the details of these problems. In this step, therefore, I'll help you analyze your OCD symptoms and gather in-depth information about your obsessions, rituals, and other aspects of your OCD so that you can begin putting together your personally tailored treatment plan. This self-analysis will require a lot of thought on your part; I recommend allowing yourself a few hours to do a good job. It's also sometimes helpful to walk through one or more "OCD episodes" before you begin. So, before you start your self-analysis, take a moment right now to identify a situation in which you started obsessing or got stuck ritualizing. Ask yourself these questions:

- What was the first sign of trouble?
- What were you feeling and thinking?
- What happened next?
- How anxious did you become?
- What did you do to reduce this anxiety (for example, compulsive rituals, avoidance)?
- How did this make you feel better?

Try to recognize how your obsessions *increased* distress or anxiety and how rituals and avoidance *reduced* the distress or anxiety.

A cautionary note: Because conducting a self-analysis forces you to think about upsetting or shameful thoughts and behaviors, it's common to feel distressed during this process. Be assured that this is normal. If you become anxious during your self-analysis, it's okay to pause and take your mind off your problems with OCD by doing something else like exercising, watching a movie, or spending time on a hobby that you enjoy. Then, when you're feeling better, try returning to your self-analysis. Also, keep in mind that the distress you feel is temporary. It will dissipate with time; and it will also get less and less intense as you practice confronting (as opposed to *avoiding*) thinking about your symptoms. As you progress through the 10 steps in this workbook, you'll find that focusing on OCD-related thoughts and behaviors becomes easier.

If analyzing your obsessions and compulsions causes you distress, don't give up. Just take a break: distract yourself for a short while with exercise, a movie, or a hobby and then get back to it.

Analyzing Your Obsessions

The Anatomy of Obsessions

Mitch has obsessions about contamination from environmental toxins and is particularly fearful of mercury exposure from fluorescent lightbulbs. Such bulbs actually do contain small amounts of mercury, but they pose only a very slight risk of harm—even if the bulb is broken. For Mitch, however, being in a room with a fluorescent bulb serves as a *trigger* for obsessional anxiety, especially if the bulb is flickering or appears not to be working properly. He tries to avoid these situations. When he finds himself near a flickering bulb, however, he experiences unwanted thoughts, such as "That bulb could be broken, and I could be exposed to mercury." He also begins to worry about awful things that might happen to him as a result of mercury contamination, such as "I could be permanently brain-damaged" and "I will lose my mind." These feared consequences create urges to leave the room, take a shower, and wash his clothes.

In Step 1 I defined obsessions as intrusive thoughts, images, and impulses that cause anxiety. But there's more to an obsession than meets the eye. In fact, obsessions have three parts, or *components*. Understanding these components will be very important to shutting down your obsessions:

1. **The *trigger* is the situation or object that, when confronted, triggers or prompts anxiety and distress.**
2. **The *obsessional intrusion* includes one or more unwanted thoughts, images, and impulses that cause anxiety, guilt, uncertainty, doubt, and other distressing feelings.**
3. **The *feared consequence* is the dreadful outcome or tragedy you predict (and fear) will happen if you don't do something to deal with the obsession, such as protecting yourself or others by doing rituals, seeking reassurance, or avoiding certain situations altogether.**

Can you pick out the three components of Mitch's obsession?

1. Mitch's *trigger*: being in a room with fluorescent lighting
2. Mitch's *obsessional intrusions*: thoughts about the bulb being broken and possible contamination
3. Mitch's *feared consequences*: becoming brain damaged

Here's another example: Tina has harming obsessions that occur whenever she drives past someone walking on the side of the road (*trigger*). This situation evokes anxiety and intrusive thoughts and images (*obsessional intrusions*), such as "Maybe I wasn't paying enough attention to the road just then" and "I could have accidentally struck that person with my car and not even realized it." The intrusive image of a person lying injured by the side of the road also comes to mind. She worries she's responsible for committing a crime and leaving the scene of an accident and wonders if anyone else might have seen the (mythical) accident and will turn her in (*feared consequences*). These feared consequences lead Tina to go back and check the roadside for bodies over and over again to reassure herself that she couldn't have hurt anyone.

You will use the OCD Analysis Worksheet on the facing page to record what you learn about your own OCD symptoms as you analyze them in this step. To begin with, turn back

What Triggers Your Obsessions?

Once you've listed your top three obsessions, you can start clarifying the situations, objects, and other stimuli in your surroundings that trigger each of these obsessions. The questions in the worksheet below are designed to help you. After you've considered these questions, go back to the OCD Analysis Worksheet and fill in the column marked "Triggers" by listing the objects, situations, and other things that consistently provoke each of your obsessions. Examples of Mitch's and Tina's triggers appear on the facing page.

Do your obsessions just seem to pop up out of nowhere, and suddenly you find yourself caught up in a ritual to make them stop?

If you have a mental block and can't think of all your triggers right now, that's fine. This exercise may get you thinking about what triggers the obsessions that seem to come out of the blue, and you can always come back and add to your OCD Analysis Worksheet as

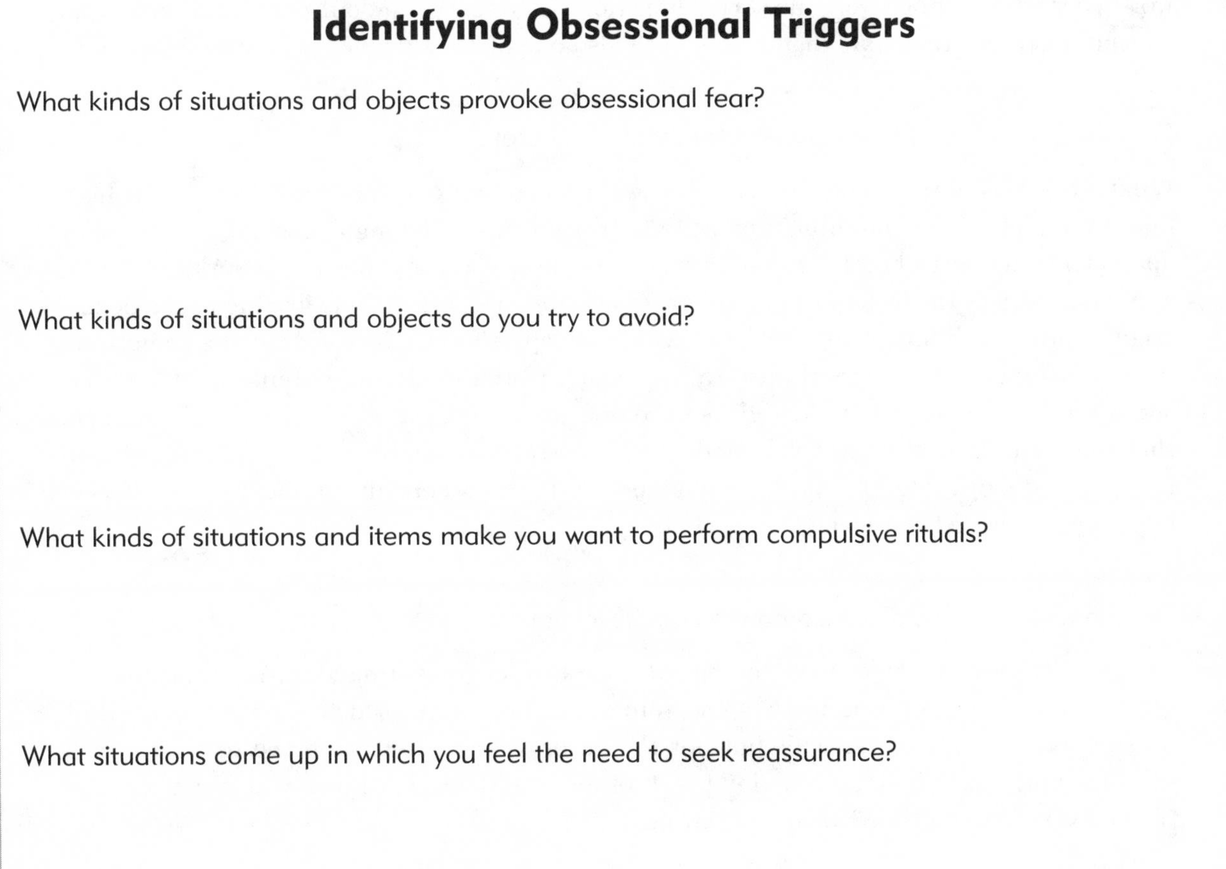

Identifying Obsessional Triggers

What kinds of situations and objects provoke obsessional fear?

What kinds of situations and objects do you try to avoid?

What kinds of situations and items make you want to perform compulsive rituals?

What situations come up in which you feel the need to seek reassurance?

you become aware of new ones. Meanwhile, these examples of common triggers might jog your memory.

Common Situations and Objects That Trigger Obsessions

For Contamination Obsessions

What would make you want to wash or clean? Perhaps your triggers include contact (or possible contact) with bodily waste and fluids such as urine, feces, blood, sweat, semen, or saliva. Maybe you're afraid to touch dirty laundry or certain parts of the body (genitals, anus). Garbage cans, bathrooms, floors, doorknobs, railings, and other things (like pens and pencils) that lots of people touch might also be triggers. Additional ones include chemicals such as cleaning agents and pesticides, dirt, animals, and dead bodies (in funeral homes or cemeteries). Perhaps there are specific people and places that trigger contamination obsessions for you. These need to be included on your list too. For example, Rosa's fear of contamination was triggered by being near anyone who had a cold sore on his or her mouth. Joe considered his wife (who worked as a nurse) a trigger until she had taken a shower after work (her work clothes were also triggers). He was concerned about contamination from "hospital germs." Hospitals themselves were also one of Joe's triggers.

For Obsessions about Responsibility for Harm or Mistakes

What situations always seem to make you want to go and check because you might have made a mistake, left something undone, or not been careful enough? Leaving the house or apartment? Going to bed for the night? Doing schoolwork or other paperwork? Using an appliance such as the iron or the oven? Other possible triggers include driving past a pedestrian or hitting a bump in the road, throwing old papers away (if you fear losing something important), putting an important letter or check in the mail, and potentially dangerous situations such as seeing broken glass or ice on the floor. One person I worked with said that the mere sight of a fire truck made him obsess about whether his house might be on fire because maybe he had left an appliance on. Perhaps certain numbers or words also trigger your obsessional fear.

For Symmetry, Order, and Incompleteness Obsessions

Common triggers include books arranged out of order, messy handwriting, and finding one's clothes not folded perfectly. One woman became distressed if she was touched or brushed on one side of her body but not the other. Odd numbers (on the odometer or a sales receipt) might be triggers, along with other situations that make you feel a sense of "asymmetry," "imbalance," or "disorderliness."

For Violent Obsessions

Violent obsessions might be triggered by the sight of potential weapons such as knives, hammers, guns, or baseball bats. Other triggers include horror movies, Halloween, cemeteries, and words associated with violence, such as *kill* and *stab*. Seeing or being with a vulnerable person (an infant or an elderly person) or being in a potentially dangerous situation (such as on a train platform) may also trigger these types of obsessions.

For Sexual Obsessions

If you have sexual obsessions, these might be triggered by seeing small children (that could be molested), relatives (incest obsessions), and people or other triggers associated with homosexuality—for example, passing by a gay bar or seeing an attractive member of the same sex at the pool or health club or pictured in a magazine. Your obsessions might even be triggered just by going to the gym. Sexual words, suggestive shapes, and erotic sounds might also trigger these obsessions.

For Religious Obsessions

Religious obsessions might be triggered by religious icons, Bibles, places of worship, saying prayers, doing religious rituals, or reminders of the devil. One person I treated had religious obsessions that were triggered by anything associated with the New Jersey Devils hockey team. He even avoided everything having to do with the state of New Jersey (maps, postcards, license plates).

Identifying Your Obsessional Intrusions

Next, identify the obsessional intrusions that are part of your obsessions. These are the unwelcome, senseless, or unacceptable thoughts, ideas, images, impulses, and doubts that evoke distress in the form of anxiety, fear, shame, horror, embarrassment, and the like—for example, the idea of raping or murdering a member of your family or a doubt about whether you have germs on your hands. Your intrusions might be provoked by one (or more) of the triggers you just identified, or perhaps they occur unexpectedly or "spontaneously." The worksheet on the following page contains questions to help you identify your intrusions. Think through how you would answer these questions for each of your top obsessions. Then complete the column in the OCD Analysis Worksheet labeled "Obsessional Intrusions" by listing yours. Use Mitch's and Tina's examples to help you.

Common Obsessional Intrusions

Here are some examples of common obsessional intrusions so that you have some idea of the kinds of thoughts and images you should record.

> Does trying to name your obsessional intrusions make you uncomfortable? That's a sign that you need to include them on your list so you can work at eliminating them.

For Contamination Obsessions

If you have contamination obsessions, you might have intrusive thoughts and images of germs and illnesses—for example, the

Identifying Obsessional Intrusions

What unpleasant or senseless thoughts do you have that provoke anxiety or distress?

What unwanted thoughts or images do you have that you feel you should try to control or resist?

What kinds of immoral, deviant, or aggressive thoughts do you have that make you feel unsure of who you really are?

What unwanted thoughts do you have that make you feel afraid of acting in ways you don't really want to act?

What upsetting thoughts, images, or ideas do you have that you would prefer not to tell other people about?

image of germs crawling all over your hands. You might also have doubts about whether you came close enough to the feared contaminant to be harmed—for example, "When I walked past the biochemistry lab, could I have inhaled any toxic fumes?" Psychologist Jack Rachman has described a different type of contamination obsession he calls *mental pollution* in which the person feels an "inner dirtiness" because of thoughts and memories of traumatic events, unwanted sexual thoughts, or humiliation.

For Obsessions about Responsibility for Harm or Mistakes

If you have obsessions concerning responsibility for harm or mistakes, chances are you experience intrusive doubts, such as "Did I remember to be careful enough?" or "Am I sure I turned the iron off, unplugged the toaster, locked the doors, signed the check?" or "What if I offended my friends [or boss], hit a pedestrian with my car, or caused my family to have an accident?" Images of misfortune are also common, such as visions of accidents, fires, injuries, and death involving loved ones. Some people, including those with scrupulosity, have obsessional doubts for which it is difficult to obtain a guarantee of certainty, such as "Does God think I was acting too proud?" and "Am I sure I won't regret this decision?"

For Violent Obsessions

You probably experience upsetting images, ideas, and impulses that represent the exact opposite of who you really are: the unwanted idea or image of hurting someone you love or the thought to attack a vulnerable or helpless person such as a baby or someone who is sleeping or otherwise unable to defend him- or herself. You might even experience unwanted impulses to act violently (for example, to hit your dog with a hammer) that seem very real and make you wonder whether you really *want* to do such things.

For Sexual Obsessions

Sexual obsessions can take several forms, including unwanted and distressing images of engaging in personally unacceptable sexual behaviors such as having sex with children, members of the same sex, relatives, or otherwise inappropriate people (for example, someone other than your partner or spouse). Sexual impulses might include thoughts or urges to do "dirty" or "perverse" things such as glance at other people's crotch or chest and touch a baby's genitals while changing a diaper. Remember that sexual fantasies that you find arousing do not count as obsessions since they are not anxiety-provoking.

For Religious Obsessions

Religious obsessions typically include blasphemous images, impulses to act in ways that are against God, and thoughts or doubts questioning your faith and the basis of your religion. Finally, people with religious scrupulosity often have obsessional doubts that they have committed a sin or violation of a religious commandment.

For Symmetry, Ordering, and Incompleteness Obsessions

Some people with these obsessions have the kinds of intrusions described above—usually those related to harm, violence, and religious or moral issues—but others don't have such intrusions. If you can't identify any intrusions, perhaps you have obsessional ideas that things are "incomplete" or "not just right." You might also have images of yourself "going crazy" or "losing control" if things are not orderly or balanced.

Identifying Your Feared Consequences

The third component of an obsession is the feared disaster or other negative outcome you anticipate. For example, "I'll be responsible for causing a fire because I left the iron on" or "I'll have an accident because I saw the number 13." Your feared consequences might be tied to the failure to perform a protective ritual, such as "I'll get sick *if I don't wash my hands*," "A loved one will get hurt *if I don't repeat a behavior again*," or "God will be upset with me *if I don't say my prayers perfectly*." You might also be afraid of negative consequences as a result of thinking obsessional thoughts: "If I think too much about hurting the baby, I'll lose control and act on my thoughts" or "Thinking sacrilegious thoughts means my faith in God is slipping." These *feared consequences* represent the "logic" of OCD—the glue that binds obsessions and rituals together. By identifying your feared consequences, you'll be putting yourself in an excellent position to weaken your OCD symptoms when you begin your CBT program.

Do your fears center on not knowing for sure whether the worst will happen?

Perhaps your obsessions involve short-term feared consequences, such as "If I don't wash my hands, I'll come down with an illness *soon*." But you might be obsessed with disasters that wouldn't happen for many years, such as "If I'm exposed to pesticides, I'll get cancer *in 40 years*." Most likely your feared consequences also include *not knowing for sure* whether the worst will happen. This is an important point that we'll return to in Step 3.

Now that you've read some examples, you're ready to identify the feared consequences that are part of your top three obsessions. What do you think would happen if you were confronted with an obsessional trigger but didn't do any rituals to protect yourself or others? The worksheet on the facing page contains some questions to help you pinpoint these fears. Ask yourself these questions for each of your obsessions and then record one or two feared consequences for each obsession in the appropriate box on the OCD Analysis Worksheet (page 39). The examples of feared consequences that appear below might help you further identify your own.

Research my colleagues and I have conducted clearly shows that an intolerance for uncertainty and doubt plays a major role in obsessions and rituals.

Common Feared Consequences

For Contamination Obsessions

As explained in Chapter 1, people with contamination obsessions generally fear that they or someone else will get sick because of contaminants. You might worry that contact with blood or urine will lead to a terrible disease unless you wash your hands for a specified period of time. Or you're afraid that traces of the detergent you used earlier are still on your hands and will make your family ill when they eat the meal you've prepared. Or the consequence you want to avoid might simply be feeling "contaminated" or having to tolerate the sense that germs are spreading.

Identifying Feared Consequences

What is the worst thing that might happen if you faced your triggers and didn't/couldn't do any rituals?

Why are your triggers so dangerous?

Why is it a problem if you confront a trigger without doing rituals?

Why do you feel like you have to avoid your obsessional triggers?

What is bad or dangerous for you about thinking your intrusive obsessional thoughts?

What might happen if you think certain thoughts and don't do anything about them?

For Obsessions about Responsibility for Harm or Mistakes

You're probably afraid of getting hurt or being responsible for causing harm or for failing to prevent harm to someone else. For example, if you don't check the oven, it will be your fault if a fire wipes out the entire house and burns all the family's precious keepsakes. People with "hit-and-run" obsessions have urges to check the road for fear they might have hit someone, left the victim for dead, and will be found and charged with leaving the scene of an accident. Perhaps you worry someone in your family will have bad luck if you encounter the number 13, that someone you love will be hurt if you don't ritualize, and it will be your fault.

For Symmetry, Ordering, and Incompleteness Obsessions

Generally, you either fear that failing to arrange items in a certain way will cause harm or bad luck to befall people you care about or that if things aren't "just right" you'll never shake the sense of incompleteness and will go crazy or have a panic attack. With these obsessions, your fear that things are "not just right" can extend to more and more aspects of your environment as time goes on.

For Violent Obsessions

You might worry about losing control and accidentally acting on your thoughts: "*I'll go crazy and drown the baby* unless I pray to God to stop me from doing this" or "*I'll murder my partner in her sleep*, so I must sleep in a separate room and lock the knives away." You might also be afraid that because you can't stop thinking violent thoughts (despite trying to dismiss them), you must *want* to be violent, or *want* someone you love to be hurt, or just that deep down you're actually a violent, coldhearted person.

For Sexual Obsessions

As with violent obsessions, it's common to fear acting on sexual obsessions—"I'll turn gay" or "I won't be able to stop myself from molesting children"—or that the obsessions reveal a core truth about you: "This thought means I really want to have sex with an animal" or "Because I think about molesting children, I must really *want* to try it." Fears of sin, punishment from God, and hell are also common.

For Religious Obsessions

You probably fear violating religious rules, angering God, and perhaps even being damned to hell—and/or that your obsessions mean you are truly turning against your religion or that deep down you hate God and love Satan.

Keep in mind that some feared consequences will concern disasters resulting from objects or situations—for example, getting sick if a "dirty-looking" person bags your groceries and you don't wipe them down afterward, or causing the electricity to be shut off because you made a mistake when paying the bill and didn't check. Others will concern disastrous consequences resulting from intrusive thoughts—for example, that too many sexual thoughts will cause you to commit rape or that a family member will die because you imagined that person having an accident but didn't ritualize. Still other feared consequences might seem like they will happen if you don't perform rituals—for example, God will be angry with me if I don't say the prayers six times, or I will have bad luck if I don't drive around the block again and arrange the pictures on the wall just right.

Not everyone with OCD has specific fears of disasters. Perhaps your triggers and intrusions evoke a vague sense that "something bad will happen" or that you will "feel anxious forever" unless you perform a ritual. In the latter case, call the feared consequence "harm from experiencing long-term anxiety" (perhaps losing control, "going crazy," having a heart attack or stroke). Putting some label on feared consequences is important, because it will help you design your treatment plan in Step 4.

Analyzing Your Avoidance Behavior

The way many people deal with obsessional fear is to avoid the situations or activities they know are triggers. Because of his fear of mercury, Mitch won't change a fluorescent lightbulb, walk near a display of these bulbs in a hardware store, or, when possible, go into a room lit by fluorescent bulbs. Because of her obsessions about hitting pedestrians, Tina avoids driving in parking lots, business districts, family neighborhoods, and schoolyards—wherever a lot of people are likely to be walking around. Notice the OCD logic of these avoidance strategies: steering clear of these triggers seems to safeguard Mitch and Tina from their feared consequences.

Are you spending a lot of time avoiding whatever triggers your obsessions—and still find they keep coming back?

It's only natural to avoid what seems dangerous, so you may have your own avoidance strategies. If you're afraid of germs, you might avoid touching doorknobs, railings, and other surfaces you associate with germs so that you don't get sick. If cemeteries or funeral homes trigger obsessional thoughts and fears of death, you might avoid these places. But avoidance only temporarily makes you feel safe. It doesn't permanently reduce obsessional fear. Not only that, but avoidance patterns are self-perpetuating: they tend to balloon over time, leaving you stuck using this ineffective coping strategy more and more. In later steps you'll learn strategies for reducing your avoidance patterns and practicing more helpful strategies for dealing with obsessions. So it's important to identify what you avoid, using the worksheet on the following page.

Now use the worksheet to generate a list of the main things you avoid for each of your top three obsessions and enter this information in the appropriate box in the Avoidance column on the OCD Analysis Worksheet. Mitch's and Tina's examples are provided on page 40. As with the rest of the worksheet, be as specific as possible. The more you zero in on exactly

Is it **all** bathrooms or odd numbers or "sinful" images that you avoid—or just certain ones?

Analyzing Avoidance Strategies

Name the things you avoid because of your obsessional fears:

Situations (for example, being alone with a child, watching certain movies or shows):

Places (for example, hospitals, funeral homes, public bathrooms):

People (for example, with disabilities, with AIDS):

Objects (for example, pornographic magazines, knives, floors):

Activities (for example, driving past schools, touching parts of your body):

Thoughts (for example, about violence, sex, the devil):

Other:

what you avoid, the easier it will be to identify targets for intervention and avoid a lot of discouraging trial and error. If only *certain* bathrooms are off limits, or if you avoid driving only in *certain* areas (as with Tina), make sure you note this on the worksheet. If you're having trouble identifying your avoidance strategies, try looking over your list of triggers. You probably avoid many of the things that trigger your obsessional distress. The following thoughts might also help stimulate your memory.

Common Avoidance Patterns

For Contamination Obsessions

You might avoid shoes, floors, public restrooms (including certain *parts* of the restroom, such as the toilet or sink), trash cans, dumpsters, and other surfaces touched by lots of people (for example, elevator call buttons). You might avoid certain clothes, stores (and other places), and even people or animals you fear are "contaminated." One man feared being poisoned by lawn chemicals such as fertilizer. During the springtime he couldn't leave his home. Because he worried that people and items from outside might bring in traces of harmful lawn chemicals, he established "safety zones" in his house where items (and people) from outside were not allowed unless they had been thoroughly washed first. All other "contaminated" parts of his home were avoided.

For Obsessions about Responsibility for Harm or Mistakes

Do you avoid certain activities that could *possibly* lead to accidents, mistakes, harm, or other negative circumstances—driving, using the oven, cooking for other people, doing important paperwork? Maybe you avoid situations that make you think about misfortune, such as certain words, bad luck numbers (for example, 13), and reading about disasters or illnesses. Other things you might avoid include being in charge of pets, locking up the house or workplace, and being responsible for confidential material. Be sure to also list subtle forms of avoidance, such as not driving near school buses for fear of hitting children and not listening to music while completing important paperwork for fear of being distracted and making serious mistakes.

For Symmetry, Ordering, and Incompleteness Obsessions

You might avoid having things disorganized or imbalanced. You might also steer clear of certain places, knowing that going there would evoke distress and the need to spend lots of time rearranging objects, creating "balance," and performing counting rituals.

For Violent Obsessions

Maybe you avoid triggers that spark anxiety and upsetting violent thoughts and impulses: knives, guns, baseball bats, potential victims of your violence (loved ones, babies, the elderly), police officers, words associated with violence (*blood, murder*), and activities, places, pictures, movies, or newscasts associated with harm or violence. Situations that seem to increase the chances of acting on unwanted thoughts may also be avoided, such as being *left alone* with someone you're afraid of harming. Remember that your particular avoidance patterns might be highly individualized.

For Sexual Obsessions

In sexual obsessions, common avoidance patterns include erotically charged images or movies; sexually provocative people (of either sex) or places (for example, gay bars, gyms, swimming pools, and locker rooms); changing diapers; looking at certain parts of people's bodies; shows or newscasts about pedophiles or rapists; and words like *rape, penis*, or *bestiality*. Some sufferers avoid masturbation or other sexual activity because it triggers unwanted sexual thoughts.

For Religious Obsessions

If you have religious obsessions, you might avoid places of worship for fear of committing blasphemy, or religious objects for fear of offending God. Words such as *hell, devil, Satan*, or curse words may also be avoided. One person I worked with avoided sermons about how to serve God because they triggered obsessive doubting about whether she was doing enough. Obsessions about sin often result in excessive avoidance of activities associated with particular offenses. For example, a religious woman with obsessional fears that she would unintentionally have an abortion (or influence others to do so) avoided using the word *choice* because of the connection with the pro-choice slogan of the abortion rights movement. She also avoided watching movies made in Hollywood because she associated Hollywood with promoting godlessness and thought God would be upset if she supported such things.

Analyzing Your Rituals

Try as you might to avoid fear-evoking obsessional thoughts and situations, some of your triggers might be inescapable. A car with your unlucky number on its license plate pulls in front of you. A police officer walks by and you see his gun. You drop something important on the floor that you must pick up. You hear someone make a sexual comment. When you can't avoid feared situations altogether, it seems like the next best strategy is to perform a ritual to reduce anxiety and protect yourself from feared consequences. If Mitch couldn't avoid fluorescent lightbulbs, he showered as soon as he could to remove possible mercury contamination. If Tina couldn't avoid passing a pedestrian, she compulsively checked her rearview mirror or turned her car around to make sure she hadn't hurt anyone. Rituals—including compulsive rituals, mini-rituals, mental rituals, and reassurance seeking—are all ways of reducing obsessional fears that have already been triggered. They are basically ways of escaping from anxiety and making you feel safer, as if you've prevented a disaster or "put things right."

But, as with avoidance, rituals are not good long-term solutions for dealing with obsessional fears. Although they might give you an immediate feeling of relative safety, it's only a temporary reprieve. Eventually your obsessions come back, which only leads to more and more ritualizing. So you need to learn how to stop these behavior patterns and develop healthier strategies for managing obsessional triggers and thoughts. Doing so first requires that you be familiar with your rituals. In this section, I'll help you analyze them, with the particular goal of recognizing the relationship between your obsessions and your rituals.

How long does the relief you get from rituals last?

Compulsive Rituals

Compulsive rituals are the most common types of rituals and often the easiest to notice. Most of the time, you're probably well aware (perhaps *painfully* aware) of when you perform these rituals. But some compulsions may have become so ingrained—so automatic—that you complete them without much conscious thought. You might also be so ashamed of your compulsive behaviors that you overlook them or pretend they aren't there. Because your analysis needs to be as accurate and thorough as possible, it's important to identify and acknowledge all of your compulsive rituals. You'll also have an easier time stopping these rituals when you understand how they're related to your obsessions.

To begin your analysis, review the checklist of compulsive rituals you completed in Step 1 (pages 21–22). Do any of these appear on your list of "Main Rituals" (page 26)? Next, use the questions in the worksheet on the next page to help you analyze these compulsions.

The far right column of the OCD Analysis Worksheet contains space for recording the compulsive rituals (and other rituals) you use in response to each of your top three obsessions. List the compulsive rituals you use in the appropriate boxes. You might consult Mitch's and Tina's examples on page 40, and the tips and hints below, for help.

Tips for Analyzing Compulsive Rituals

As you read in Chapter 1, certain types of compulsive rituals tend to go along with certain types of obsessions. Obsessions about contamination are often associated with decontamination rituals; checking is often associated with obsessions about responsibility for harm and mistakes; repeating and ordering rituals are often used to reduce fears of harm or bad luck. The box on page 55 contains more hints for identifying and describing compulsive rituals. Be sure to include all the details you can think of.

Mini-Rituals

Recall that mini-rituals are *nonrepetitive* acts you perform in response to obsessions. Did you identify any that you do in the checklist on page 23 in Step 1? These rituals are more subtle than compulsions and therefore can be more difficult to spot. When Mitch is around fluorescent lighting, he takes shallow breaths because he believes this will prevent him from inhaling too much mercury. He didn't realize this strategy is part of his problems with OCD until he learned more about his obsessions and rituals by completing a symptom analysis. Perhaps you've also been using mini-rituals to deal with obsessional situations, but never labeled them as rituals. Because mini-rituals are also ineffective ways of coping with obsessions, you need to include them in your OCD symptom analysis and target them in your treatment program. Use the questions in the worksheet on page 56 to help you examine your mini-rituals more closely. Then briefly describe these strategies in the appropriate box of the far right column in the OCD Analysis Worksheet (as Mitch did on page 40).

Analyzing Compulsive Rituals

What situations, objects, actions, places, people, or obsessional thoughts (or other cues) *trigger* the urge to perform compulsive rituals?

How much do you try to *resist* your urges to perform compulsive rituals?

When you try to resist performing compulsive rituals, how *successful* are you? In what situations can you resist?

In what situations can you *not* resist?

How much do compulsive rituals reduce anxiety, relieve discomfort, or make you feel safe?

Tips for Analyzing Mini-Rituals

Mini-rituals can be brief and automatic—which makes them difficult to spot and tough to gain control over. But if you can think of these strategies as similar to compulsive rituals, only less repetitive (more subtle), you're on the right track to being able to pick them out in your own repertoire of rituals—we'll deal with how to control them in Step 9. In the meantime, here's some help for identifying your own mini-rituals.

Hints for Analyzing Compulsive Rituals

Washing and cleaning rituals

- Do you have to follow a specific routine?
- Do you have to wash or clean a certain number of times?
- Do you have to use certain cleaning agents such as hand gels or detergents?
- Do you ask others to help you with your compulsive washing or cleaning?

Checking rituals

- Do you do special routines when checking (for example, flipping a light switch several times)?
- Do you have to touch the objects you are checking?
- Do you ask others to check for you or if they're sure that *you* checked?

Ordering, arranging, counting, and repeating rituals

- Do you have to arrange things or put them in order over and over?
- Do you count (perhaps up to a certain number) when ritualizing?
- Do you repeat behaviors such as going through doorways, putting on clothes, and so on?

Look for hidden, subtle, or quick actions you take to prevent a feared consequence—for example, tightly gripping your knife or moving it farther away from a "potential victim" so that you don't accidentally lose control or act on any thoughts about harming someone. Other common examples are quickly wiping your hands or other objects to get rid of contaminants (quickly wiping your hand before you touch someone else to prevent spreading germs) and glancing quickly to make sure a situation appears safe (which is similar to checking, only not in a compulsive way). Any brief action performed in response to an obsession that is aimed at making you or someone else safer can be considered a mini-ritual.

The fact that you don't feel compelled to do it over and over doesn't mean it's not a ritual.

Mental Rituals

Mental rituals are special thoughts, sayings, prayers, numbers, images, and other strategies that you perform entirely (or almost entirely) *in your mind* (as opposed to outwardly) to counteract, dismiss, or prevent obsessional thoughts and anxiety. As you can see from Tina's OCD Analysis Worksheet, she ritualistically reanalyzed her doubts about car accidents. This means that whenever she had an obsessional doubt, she had to carefully think through whether she felt any bumps, heard any strange noises, or remembered hitting anyone while driving. She also had to mentally analyze the question "Would I know it if I'd hit someone with my car?" Other examples of mental rituals include saying a prayer three

Analyzing Mini-Rituals

What brief actions or strategies do you use to reduce anxiety or to make you feel safer?

What situations, objects, actions, places, people, or obsessional thoughts (or other cues) *trigger* the urge to perform mini-rituals?

How much do you try to *resist* your urges to perform mini-rituals?

When you try to resist performing mini-rituals, how *successful* are you? In what situations can you resist? In what situations can you *not* resist?

How much do your mini-rituals reduce anxiety, relieve discomfort, or make you feel safe?

times in your head to prevent bad luck, repeating the word *safe* over and over in your mind to counteract thoughts of harm, and analyzing (trying to figure out) what an obsessional thought "really" means.

Did you identify any mental rituals in Step 1 (page 24)? As you've probably guessed by now, mental rituals are problematic in the same ways that compulsive and mini-rituals are: they might reduce your anxiety in the short term, but they don't keep obsessional anxiety

Analyzing Mental Rituals

What mental strategies (special words, phrases, prayers, and so on) do you use to try to control obsessional thoughts or to reduce anxiety and make you feel safer?

Do you try to push certain thoughts away or analyze (figure out) what they mean?

What situations, objects, actions, places, people, or obsessional thoughts (or other cues) *trigger* the urge to perform mental rituals?

How much do you try to *resist* your urges to perform mental rituals?

When you try to resist performing mental rituals, how *successful* are you? In what situations can you resist? In what situations can you *not* resist?

How much do your mental rituals help you control your unwanted thoughts, reduce anxiety, or make you feel safer?

from coming back. In fact, mental rituals develop into patterns that become stronger and difficult to stop on your own. Therefore, you must recognize and understand any mental rituals you're using to deal with obsessions so that you can learn strategies for stopping them as part of CBT. Use the questions in the worksheet on page 57 to help you learn more about your mental rituals. Then add them to your lists of rituals in the far right column in your OCD Analysis Worksheet.

Tips for Analyzing Mental Rituals

It might be difficult to put your finger on mental rituals since they tend to occur exclusively in your mind. So, let me offer a few hints about what falls into this category. You might use mental rituals if you have distressing violent, sexual, and religious obsessions that you feel you've got to control or else face some dreaded consequence. Rich, for example, was bothered by unwanted obsessional images of the devil and hell. He had mental rituals of "undoing" or "canceling out" his obsessions by conjuring up and holding in his mind "good" or "holy" images of Jesus or a crucifix. He also repeated prayers, biblical verses, and phrases such as "God knows I love Him" over and over to make him feel more comfortable.

Are your obsessions violent, sexual, or religious? If so, you probably have mental rituals.

If you have obsessions about responsibility for harm or mistakes, you—like Tina—might have mental reviewing rituals. Another woman I treated some time ago had obsessional fears that she could have poisoned someone by mistake at her pizza parlor, so after closing every night she went through all of her receipts and tried to remember adding each ingredient to each pizza to reassure herself that she hadn't poisoned anyone. Of course, she was never completely satisfied with the vividness of her memory, so the ritual didn't work very well. Nevertheless, she performed it for up to an hour every day of her life.

Reassurance-Seeking Rituals

Ritualistic responses to obsessional fear often include reassurance seeking. Maybe you call a friend or relative *over and over* to ask if he or she was offended by something you said. Or you *can't stop* asking religious authorities if they think you've offended God. You might search *many different* websites to find out whether a certain kind of soap is strong enough to kill a particular type of germ. Or you *repeatedly* consult with an infectious disease specialist about the risk of becoming infected. Notice that I'm *not* talking about innocently asking questions to learn about something new for the first time. Reassurance seeking is an OCD symptom if it's repetitive (asking similar questions again and again), if it interferes with interpersonal relationships, or if you're asking questions when you already have a good idea of what the answer is. When she cooked, Hope ritualistically read and reread food labels out loud (such as "extra virgin olive oil," "brown sugar," and "low-fat milk") to reassure herself that she wasn't putting any poisonous materials in her family's food.

When you ask others for assurances, do you already know what the answer will be?

As with other types of rituals, reassurance seeking sometimes results in an immediate reduction in anxiety and doubt; but in time, OCD either ends up convincing you that you didn't get enough reassurance or it throws a new obsessional doubt your way, which makes you feel like you need more reassurance. Hope, for example, still worried about serving her family food she had cooked. She had to continually ask if anyone felt sick.

Like many other types of rituals, reassurance seeking usually doesn't eliminate obsessions in the long run but instead leads to more and more reassurance seeking.

The questions in the worksheet on page 60 can help you analyze your reassurance-seeking strategies more closely. After answering them, record your reassurance-seeking strategies in the appropriate box(es) in the far right column of the OCD Analysis Worksheet. Notice that Mitch's obsessions about contamination from fluorescent lighting lead him to seek reassurance by continually looking up information on the Internet about mercury poisoning from such lights.

Using Your Completed OCD Analysis Worksheet

Your symptom analysis provides us with critical information about how OCD operates. Your completed OCD Analysis Worksheet is a sort of quick reference guide to OCD's game plan. Review this worksheet and note the relationships between your obsessions, intrusive thoughts, feared consequences, avoidance strategies, and rituals. In Step 3, I'll help you get a better sense of how these problems fit together. Understanding these connections will turn you into an OCD expert, which will help you develop the best possible treatment program for you.

Your OCD Analysis Worksheet is a work in progress. Adding to it as your self-knowledge increases improves your odds of beating OCD.

But don't worry if you couldn't answer all of the questions in this chapter's worksheets on the first try. You'll refer back to the OCD Analysis Worksheet regularly as you work your way through the 10 steps and can add to all your worksheets as you learn more about your OCD symptoms. It's a good idea to think of your self-analysis as an ongoing process.

Measuring the Severity of Your OCD Symptoms

The final part of your symptom analysis involves measuring the *severity* of your problems with OCD. It's important to figure out how much anxiety and discomfort your symptoms cause now because seeing that discomfort decrease is the way you know you're beating OCD during the active phase of the program (Part III). I'll give you the opportunity to measure the severity of your symptoms again at the end of the program (in Step 10) so you have the satisfaction of seeing how far you've come—sort of like looking at "before" and "after" photos of yourself after a new diet and exercise program—which will in turn help you maintain your improvements.

We use the Target Symptom Rating Form on page 62 in our clinic to measure problems with obsessional fear (Part 1), avoidance (Part 2), and rituals (Part 3). To complete the form and determine the severity of your symptoms, begin by choosing up to three "target"

Analyzing Reassurance-Seeking Rituals

What do you seek reassurance about?

SECURING DOORS & UNPLUGGING & TURNING OFF LIGHTS

From where do you try to get this reassurance?

People (for example, list specific relatives, clergy):

- What do you ask these people when you're trying to get assurance?

- How do other people respond to you when you ask for reassurance?

The media (for example, web pages, television):

- What, specifically, are you looking to find out?

Other sources (for example, books, labels on cans):

- What, specifically, are you looking to find out?

How much does getting the reassurance reduce anxiety or make you feel more comfortable?

triggers *or* obsessional intrusions from your OCD Analysis Worksheet (page 39)—the targets you'd most like to focus on in treatment. Feel free to select these triggers from across your top three obsessions. Then record the triggers or intrusions in the column marked "Feared trigger or intrusive thoughts" in Part 1 of the form. Next, use the 0 (no fear) to 8 (extreme fear) rating scale to indicate how afraid you are of each trigger or thought. Mitch's and Tina's forms are provided as examples on pages 63 and 64.

To complete Part 2 of the form, look at the Avoidance column of your OCD Analysis Worksheet and choose up to three situations, objects, people, and so on that you avoid because of obsessional fears. Again, try to choose avoidance strategies that create the most problems for you, those that you wish to target in your treatment program. You might find that your target avoidances are similar to (or the same as) your target obsessional fears—that's fine. When you've written your avoided items in the rating form, indicate how often you have been avoiding these stimuli using the 0 to 8 rating scale.

Finally, for Part 3, review the rituals you recorded in your OCD Analysis Worksheet and decide on up to three target compulsive, mini-, mental, or reassurance-seeking rituals. These should be the rituals that take up the most time, cause the most interference with your life, or that you would most like to gain control over. List these in the column marked "Rituals" in Part 3 of the Target Symptoms Rating Form. Then use the rating scale provided to indicate how often (each day) you are performing these rituals. You can use Mitch's and Tina's rating forms to help guide you through the process.

Answering questions about OCD symptoms can be difficult since your ratings of fear, avoidance, and time spent ritualizing sometimes depend on many different factors. For example, your rating of how much time you spent checking might depend on such things as what you did that day, whether you were alone, or whether you were on vacation, among other factors. I suggest you handle these difficult questions by trying to estimate your response based on a *typical* or *average* day over the last week or two. So, if on some days you spend only 1 hour doing rituals, and on other days you spend 3 hours, you might decide on 2 hours because it's the average. Another solution, if you prefer, is to consider the *range*, such as 1–3 hours.

Now take a look at your form. If your fear ratings are in the 0 to 2 range, it means you've chosen one or more targets that don't provoke much obsessional distress. Are there other triggers or intrusive thoughts that are more frightening for you? If so, perhaps you should make these your treatment targets since they seem to create more of a problem. Fear ratings between 3 and 5 suggest moderate levels of distress. Those of 6 or higher indicate your most challenging triggers and obsessional thoughts. We'll be working in Part III of the book to reduce these fears, and I hope that this will show up when you assess yourself at the end of your program. You can see that Mitch's greatest fear is fluorescent lightbulbs themselves, with rooms lit by these lightbulbs, and any flickering bulbs not falling too far behind. Tina's target triggers are driving past a pedestrian on the road and intrusive images of her feared accident victim lying by the side of the road. Both of these triggers evoke very strong fear reactions.

Now look over your avoidance ratings. Ratings of 0 to 2 mean you're not avoiding so much, although you might be performing more rituals to compensate. If your ratings are 6 or above, it means avoidance is a severe problem for you. When you begin doing exposure

Target Symptom Rating Form (Baseline Version)

Part I. Obsessional Fears

Rate how much you are afraid of each target trigger/intrusion using the scale from 0 (no fear) to 8 (extreme fear).

0	1	2	3	4	5	6	7	8
None		Mild		Moderate		Strong		Extreme

	Feared trigger or intrusive thought	Fear rating
a.		
b.		
c.		

Part 2. Avoidance

Rate how much you avoid each item.

0	1	2	3	4	5	6	7	8
Never		Rarely		Sometimes		Often		Always
0%				50%				100%

	Feared item, situation, or intrusive thought	Rating
a.		
b.		
c.		

Part 3. Time Spent Ritualizing

Rate how much time per day you spend doing each ritual.

0	1	2	3	4	5	6	7	8
Never		Rarely		Sometimes		Often		Always

	Ritual	Rating
a.		
b.		
c.		

Mitch's Target Symptom Rating Form

Part I. Obsessional Fears

Rate how much you are afraid of each target trigger/intrusion using the scale from 0 (no fear) to 8 (extreme fear).

0	1	2	3	4	5	6	7	8
None		Mild		Moderate		Strong		Extreme

	Feared trigger or intrusive thought	Fear rating
a.	*Fluorescent lightbulbs*	*8*
b.	*Rooms with fluorescent lighting*	*7*
c.	*Flickering lightbulbs*	*6*

Part 2. Avoidance

Rate how much you avoid each item.

0	1	2	3	4	5	6	7	8
Never 0%		Rarely		Sometimes 50%		Often		Always 100%

	Feared item, situation, or intrusive thought	Rating
a.	*Rooms with fluorescent bulbs in use*	*4*
b.	*Changing lightbulbs*	*8*
c.	*Hardware stores with fluorescent bulbs*	*6*

Part 3. Time Spent Ritualizing

Rate how much time per day you spend doing each ritual.

0	1	2	3	4	5	6	7	8
Never		Rarely		Sometimes		Often		Always

	Ritual	Rating
a.	*Looking up information about lightbulbs (reassurance seeking)*	*7*
b.	*Showering*	*6*
c.	*Washing clothes*	*4*

Tina's Target Symptom Rating Form

Part I. Obsessional Fears

Rate how much you are afraid of each target trigger/intrusion using the scale from 0 (no fear) to 8 (extreme fear).

0	1	2	3	4	5	6	7	8
None		Mild		Moderate		Strong		Extreme

	Feared trigger or intrusive thought	Fear rating
a.	*Driving past someone walking on the road*	7
b.	*Image of a person lying on the roadside*	7
c.		

Part 2. Avoidance

Rate how much you avoid each item.

0	1	2	3	4	5	6	7	8
Never		Rarely		Sometimes		Often		Always
0%				50%				100%

	Feared item, situation, or intrusive thought	Rating
a.	*Driving where there are lots of pedestrians walking around*	7
b.	*Listening to the radio while driving*	8
c.		

Part 3. Time Spent Ritualizing

Rate how much time per day you spend doing each ritual.

0	1	2	3	4	5	6	7	8
Never		Rarely		Sometimes		Often		Always

	Ritual	Rating
a.	*Checking the rearview mirror*	8
b.	*Turning the car around and checking the roadside*	5
c.	*Analyzing and trying to remember (mental ritual)*	6

therapy in Steps 7 and 8, you'll be targeting your avoidance behavior. Mitch, despite his fear of rooms with fluorescent lights, avoids these situations only sometimes. He's more likely to avoid changing these bulbs (which he avoids without fail) and hardware stores that sell fluorescent bulbs. Tina can't avoid driving altogether, but she very often avoids areas where there are lots of pedestrians, such as busy parking lots and business districts. She completely avoids listening to music when she drives because of the fear of distraction.

Finally, look at your ratings for how much you're ritualizing. If your avoidance is high, you might have fewer rituals, and vice versa. Ratings below 3 indicate minor problems with rituals, and those above 6 suggest much more severe rituals. We'll target your rituals in response prevention, which you'll learn about in Step 9. Look at Mitch's ritual ratings: his most time-consuming behavior is looking up information about the dangers of exposure to mercury in lightbulbs. He also compulsively showers fairly often. Less of a problem is excessively washing his clothes. As for Tina, she constantly checks mirrors when she drives and occasionally turns the car around to check for injured people. She also often engages in mentally analyzing her doubts about whether she actually hit anyone.

Moving On to Step 3

When I begin therapy with someone suffering from OCD, my first step is always to learn about the specifics of the person's problems using the same techniques that you've used in this step. Without those details, I know that the treatment I offer won't be as effective as it could be because it won't be based on a full understanding of the individual's strengths and weaknesses. Now that you have a good grasp of your own individualized OCD symptoms, it's time to scout your opponent and learn OCD's strengths and weaknesses. In Step 3, you'll learn why obsessions keep replaying themselves over and over in your mind and why you just can't seem to get enough of ritualizing. When you know OCD's battle plan, you can use your own weapons most effectively.

STEP 3

Understanding OCD's Battle Plan

There's no way to defeat an enemy that's a total mystery to you. And you can't expect to repair a computer, TV, or car unless you know how the machine operates. The same is true for OCD. To beat a problem this complex, you need to understand its workings. At the most fundamental level, the key components of your problems with OCD form a vicious cycle, and that's why you feel trapped by obsessions and rituals. In this step you'll learn about the intricacies of these components and the various factors that keep the vicious cycle going. Once you're familiar with OCD's battle plan, you'll see where this enemy is most vulnerable and where we need to focus our attack. The vicious cycle begins with unpleasant intrusive thoughts, so let's start there.

Intrusive Thoughts: The Seeds of Obsessions

Have you ever had any of these (or similar) kinds of thoughts?

Harm/death-related thoughts

- ☐ Thought of jumping off a bridge onto the highway below
- ☐ Thought of running the car off the road or into oncoming traffic
- ☐ Thought of poking something into your eyes
- ☐ Impulse to jump on train tracks as the train comes into the station
- ☐ Idea and image of hurting someone you love
- ☐ Idea of doing something mean to a defenseless or undeserving person
- ☐ Thought of pushing someone in front of a train
- ☐ Wishing a person would die
- ☐ Impulse to be violent toward small children
- ☐ Thought of putting a person or animal in the oven or microwave

- ☐ Thinking about your spouse or partner dying
- ☐ Image of a loved one being injured or killed
- ☐ Thought of receiving news of a loved one's death
- ☐ Image of your funeral, or that of someone you love
- ☐ Imagining what it would be like if a loved one died
- ☐ Image of your family being tortured in front of you
- ☐ Thought of being forced to choose between being killed and watching a loved one be killed
- ☐ Image of your family being killed in a car crash
- ☐ Thought of a plane crashing with friends/family in it

Thoughts about being responsible for harm or disasters

- ☐ Thought of causing an accident or mishap
- ☐ Thought that something will go wrong because of your own error
- ☐ Thought of getting into an accident while driving with children
- ☐ Thought of accidentally hitting someone with your car
- ☐ Thought that someone you love might die and you never said good-bye
- ☐ Thought that you've forgotten something important

Thoughts about contamination

- ☐ Thought of catching diseases from various places
- ☐ Thought of having a life-threatening disease
- ☐ Thought that using a public bathroom will cause you harm
- ☐ Thoughts that you may have caught a disease from touching a toilet seat
- ☐ Thought of dirt and germs always being on your hands
- ☐ Thought of contracting a disease from contact with another person
- ☐ Thought of your hands being contaminated after using the toilet
- ☐ Thought of getting germs from someone you shake hands with
- ☐ Thought of passing germs or illness to another person

Thoughts about acting inappropriately

- ☐ Idea of insulting/abusing family/friends for no apparent reason
- ☐ Thought of swearing or screaming rudely at your family
- ☐ Thought that you might have ruined a relationship with a friend
- ☐ Impulse to call your spouse or partner and break up for no reason
- ☐ Impulse to say something nasty and damning to someone
- ☐ Impulse to push your children away

Thoughts about safety

- ☐ Thought that you left a door unlocked
- ☐ Thought that you haven't locked the house up properly
- ☐ Thought of your house getting broken into while you're not home

- ☐ Thought that you left an electrical appliance on and caused a fire
- ☐ Thought that your house has burned down and you've lost everything you own
- ☐ Thought that someone will break in and hurt you or your family

Thoughts related to morality and religion

- ☐ Thought of doing something morally wrong
- ☐ Thought that God doesn't really exist
- ☐ Doubt or uncertainty about whether you've prayed to God or to the devil
- ☐ Idea of not being nice all the time to everyone
- ☐ Hopes that someone won't succeed
- ☐ Wondering about whether you have committed sins
- ☐ Doubts about whether you'll go to heaven or hell
- ☐ Doubts about whether you're being faithful enough to God

Thoughts of acting impulsively

- ☐ Thoughts of smashing a table full of crafts (at a market, for example) made of glass
- ☐ Thought of doing something dramatic like rob a bank

Generally negative thoughts

- ☐ Thought of past embarrassment, humiliation, or failure
- ☐ Thought of a previous upsetting incident
- ☐ Thought of disappointing your friends

Thoughts related to sex

- ☐ Thoughts of acts of violence in sex
- ☐ Sexual impulse toward an attractive person, known and unknown
- ☐ Thoughts of engaging in "unnatural" sexual acts
- ☐ Image involving sex with inappropriate partners
- ☐ Images or thoughts about someone else's genitals

Thoughts related to symmetry

- ☐ Thought about objects not arranged perfectly
- ☐ Thoughts about not liking odd numbers
- ☐ Thoughts of rooms or places being "unbalanced" to the right or left

You say you *have* had some of these types of thoughts?

Well, guess what? So has almost everyone else, *whether they have OCD or not*. In fact, research has revealed that 90–99% of the entire population experiences strange "intrusive" (meaning "unwanted" or "disturbing") thoughts from time to time. This shouldn't be too surprising when you consider that the average person has about 4,000 distinct thoughts each day. Naturally, some of these thoughts are going to be random, senseless, unpleasant, useless, and contrary to your typical nature or personality. In fact, the list you just read is made up of intrusive thoughts reported by people in the general population—people *without* OCD problems. I compiled this list with the help of a large group of friends, relatives, and colleagues—and, I'll admit, even some of my own experiences with strange thoughts.

In a famous research study, psychologists Jack Rachman and Padmal deSilva gave experienced therapists a similar list of intrusive thoughts from people *without* OCD, as well as a list of clinical obsessions from people *with* OCD. Interestingly, when asked to guess where each thought came from, the therapists couldn't identify which ones were reported by people with OCD and which ones were reported by people without OCD. What this study and several others like it show is that abhorrent, dirty, senseless, naughty, bizarre, offensive, violent, and otherwise upsetting thoughts—just like your obsessional intrusions—are a universal experience.

The average person has about 4,000 separate thoughts a day, and for almost everyone—*OCD or no OCD*—some of them are intrusive.

Of course, there is an unspoken "don't ask, don't tell" dynamic with these kinds of thoughts. So don't expect anyone to walk up to you and just reveal thoughts like the ones on the list. Unfortunately, this discretion might make you feel like you're the only person in the world who has these kinds of thoughts and that having them makes you abnormal, dangerous, perverted, or immoral. But now you know that just about everyone—your parents, your children, teachers, religious leaders, friends, coworkers, doctors, civil servants, siblings—has them from time to time.

Since the 1970s, scientists have been very interested in learning about intrusive thoughts and have studied them in people of all ages, nationalities, races, religions, and occupations. It turns out that people's most unpleasant, unwanted thoughts typically concern harm and violence; vulgarity and sexuality; religion and blasphemy; contamination, health, and disease; and mistakes and dishonesty. They may also involve order, symmetry, and minor or unimportant details. Furthermore, these kinds of thoughts sometimes seem to come out of nowhere, although they're often triggered by cues in the environment. For example, you might touch a doorknob and think about germs; you might see the number 666 and think of being possessed by the devil. I'll admit that when I see a dog with its head sticking out a car window, I have unpleasant thoughts about the dog being decapitated.

Do you assume that other people never have outrageous thoughts just because they don't tell you about them?

The obvious next question is "*Why?*" Experts in the fields of biology, psychology, and philosophy haven't been able to come up with a definitive answer but there are two explanations that make the best sense. The first is the "thought generator hypothesis," which suggests that these thoughts are just part of the human mind's natural creative abilities. Our minds are highly developed, allowing us to solve problems efficiently and protect ourselves from harm. So it's useful for us to be able to imagine and anticipate all sorts of scenarios—some pleasant and some unpleasant. Just as we sometimes daydream about positive and happy events (such as what it would be like to win the Superbowl or have a lot of money), the "thought generator" in our brains sometimes produces negative ideas and images we would rather not think about.

If your mind wasn't capable of conjuring up all kinds of cause-and-effect scenarios, how good would you be at planning, surviving a crisis, or solving the tough problems of life?

The second explanation is the "mental noise" hypothesis. Some researchers agree that negative intrusive thoughts might have no real importance and are simply harmless pieces of driftwood that float through the mind. To illustrate this idea, you might think of the human brain as similar to other complex machines such as a computer or a refrigerator. These machines, when working properly, often make strange noises such as clicking, whirring, buzzing, screeching, and so on. But these noises aren't anything to be concerned about—they sound worse than they are. Similarly, even a healthy human brain produces all sorts of bizarre and senseless thoughts from time to time—some of which might seem worse than they are.

Good news! Your obsessions come from normal thoughts. It's a scientifically proven fact that the content of your obsessions is similar to the intrusive thoughts reported by just about everyone.

If the *content* of your obsessions is no different from the upsetting intrusive thoughts reported by most people in the population at large, how *are* your obsessions different from normal intrusive thoughts? The main differences are:

- Your obsessions *occur more often* than normal intrusive thoughts.
- Your obsessions *last longer* than normal intrusive thoughts.
- Your obsessions are *more distressing* to you than normal intrusive thoughts are to people without OCD problems.
- You interpret your obsessional thoughts as *more important* than other people interpret their normal intrusive thoughts.
- You put *more effort* into trying to deal with or fight your obsessions than people experiencing normal intrusive thoughts.

If having intrusive thoughts is unavoidable, is trying to eliminate them the best way to beat OCD?

I'm giving you all this information because it has ramifications for what you should expect from your CBT program. You probably wish you could simply eliminate all obsessional thoughts from your head. But if intrusive thoughts similar to your obsessions are a normal and universal experience, there is no use trying to banish obsessional thoughts from your mind forever (if you've tried this strategy, you already know it doesn't work very well). Instead, the goal of CBT is to help you change your *reactions* to these thoughts by changing the importance you give to them and the strategies you use to deal with them. As you'll learn in the next section, reacting to normal intrusive thoughts as if they are very important makes them snowball into chronic obsessions. So, when you learn to change how you react, you reverse this process and your obsessional thoughts occur less often, take up less time, and become less distressing.

How Does an Intrusive Thought Become an Obsession?

If everyone has intrusive, unpleasant thoughts from time to time, why do only *some* people have problems with obsessions?

Jennifer and Erica: Different Reactions to the Same Thought

Let's take Jennifer and Erica—two healthy women (who don't even know each other) who have both recently given birth to healthy baby boys. While giving her infant a bath, Jennifer has a thought about drowning him in the tub. She then says to herself, "Yikes, what a strange thought! I've heard stories about mothers who drowned their children, but *I'm* not the kind of person who would do this. It's probably just a senseless thought—my mind's playing tricks on me again." Erica, who has the very same thought while bathing her baby, thinks, "Oh no! I've got to understand why I'm having this thought. Maybe deep down I'm really a murderer! What if I really kill the baby? I'd better not let myself think about this again—I might lose control and do something awful! I'm a terrible person and an awful mother for even thinking such a dreadful thing. Maybe I'm too dangerous to be left alone with the baby."

For Jennifer, this unpleasant thought is nothing but a fleeting annoyance, whereas Erica is very anxious and fearful about it. While Jennifer will probably continue bathing her child and then move on to other activities without any concerns about the thought, Erica will likely become more and more troubled by it. She might try to recall past experiences, looking for reassurance that she's not an evil or murderous person below the surface; but the more she does this, the *less* self-assured she'll feel because she'll realize that her memory isn't perfect or that there's no way to absolutely prove or disprove what she's trying to find out. The more she thinks about the thought, though, the more she's likely to think about it when she's with her baby—and this will seem to validate her worst fear. The baby will become a trigger for thinking the unwanted thought—which is now an obsession.

Erica may then begin to avoid being alone with her baby. She might use mental rituals to fight or "neutralize" the thought by trying to think a "good" thought instead. She might pray to God to keep her from committing murder or ask family members for reassurance that she's not an evil person. Her avoidance might prevent Erica from having to experience her obsession. Her rituals may temporarily relieve the distress she feels. As a result, Erica will resort to avoidance and rituals more and more often.

Beliefs and Interpretations Make All the Difference

Jennifer and Erica had the same (or a very similar) thought, but their *beliefs* and *interpretations* about why the thought comes to mind and what it means are anything but similar. As you've already learned, there's scientific proof that Jennifer's interpretation is accurate—the intrusion is probably just "mental noise"—while Erica's (mis)interpretation is based on a misunderstanding of how the human mind works. Indeed, gentle and conscientious people sometimes have thoughts about acting violently. Careful and diligent people sometimes have doubts about whether they've made awful mistakes. Very faithful and moral people sometimes experience perverse or sacrilegious thoughts. The tidiest, cleanest, most health-conscious, and orderly people also sometimes think about germs, illness, and disorderliness. But these kinds of renegade thoughts don't tell us much about a person's character. In the same way, Jennifer's and Erica's unwanted thoughts don't imply that they're awful, violent people at heart.

Obsessions develop when intrusive thoughts are misinterpreted in ways that lead to becoming anxious and scared of these thoughts.

Here's another example that shows how a senseless intrusive thought can develop into a time-consuming and distressing obsession if you interpret the thought as very significant and meaningful:

While checking out from the grocery store, Don has the intrusive thought that the cashier might have used the bathroom without washing his hands. He jokes to himself, "Could you imagine if everyone took this idea to heart? We'd all wear gloves to the grocery store. How silly!" But Linda, who has the same thought as she's checking out, says to herself, "Uh-oh! My groceries could be contaminated with germs from the cashier. I can't take that chance. I've got to do something to be sure I don't bring any germs into my house. What if I got sick or made my family sick because of this?"

Because of his interpretation, Don will probably forget all about the intrusive thought within a few minutes. Linda, however, will struggle with it because she interprets it as a threat. She might analyze the situation by trying to figure out how long germs can live on a food container or whether the cashier looked like the "kind of person" who washes his hands after going to the bathroom. The more analyzing she does, the more negative thoughts she'll have and the less confident she'll feel. Finally, she might decide to wipe down the groceries before bringing them into the house as a way of guaranteeing that she and her family remain healthy. Further, she may begin scrutinizing anyone with whom she has contact (especially cashiers) and avoid those who look "filthy" or "unclean." Because these behaviors reduce her germ anxiety and make her feel safer, she'll use them more and more (that is, compulsively).

Like Don, Linda, Erica, and Jennifer, we all have internal dialogues in which we interpret what we see, hear, smell, taste, and experience in the world. You see someone you haven't seen in a long time and think to yourself, "Wow, she looks great for her age." As you scan a restaurant menu, you say to yourself, "I bet the pork tenderloin is good—but mmm, I can just taste the salmon." We also constantly evaluate *internal* experiences. You feel pain in your stomach and say to yourself, "I must have gas" or, perhaps, "Oh no, what if my appendix just burst!?" Likewise, we all interpret our intrusive thoughts, ideas, and impulses, such as "My mind is playing tricks on me again" or "This thought must be an omen." Hundreds of times each day all of us interpret thoughts that go through our mind, deciding whether each is useful or counterproductive, important or unimportant. Most of these interpretations are automatic, and you might not even realize they're occurring. But even so, some of these judgments play an important role in your problems with obsessions. Here's how:

We're constantly monitoring and judging the thoughts that go through our head, deciding whether each is good or bad, important or unimportant, safe or dangerous.

How Misinterpreting Thoughts Can Lead to Obsessions

Like Linda and Erica, when you misinterpret a normal intrusive thought (like the ones in the list on pages 66–68) as very important or threatening, you trick your body into reacting as if this normally occurring and harmless thought is actually very *dangerous*. Specifically, when you interpret the thought as a threat, it activates your *fight-or-flight* system—the human body's natural response system for dealing with dangerous situations. Controlled by a release of the hormone *adrenaline*, the fight-or-flight response prepares you to take action (attack or run) against potential threats, often by causing noticeable changes in your body such as:

- Increased breathing rate—this allows more oxygen into the body. Oxygen is converted to energy for use by your muscles.
- Racing heart—this pumps more blood, which carries oxygen and other nutrients, to your large muscles so you can use them to attack or run from the danger.
- Sweating—this keeps your body cool so you can attack or run for longer periods.
- Muscle tension—this keeps you alert and ready to react on a moment's notice.
- Stomach distress—your digestive system shuts down because the focus is on getting you to safety rather than digesting food.
- Other symptoms—light-headedness, trembling, hot or cold flashes, tingling in the extremities, and blurred vision are all effects of the fight-or-flight response.

These physical symptoms can be very intense, and sometimes they can seem scary. So the otherwise innocent thought becomes associated with all sorts of physical responses that put you on high alert. But rest assured that they are all just part of the fight-or-flight response. They, like the intrusive thoughts, are not harmful. In fact, these symptoms are all designed to *protect* you from harm. It wouldn't make sense for nature to design a system for keeping us out of harm's way that produces the symptoms that harm us!

Even if you don't experience intense physical symptoms when you have intrusive thoughts, another effect of the fight-or-flight response is that it causes us to pay attention—to become *preoccupied*—with whatever we perceive to be threatening. This is important because if you didn't pay attention to a dangerous situation, you could be taken by surprise. So, the fight-or-flight response can work in subtle ways to keep your mind focused on the threat and scanning for any possible danger. If you were in real danger—say, there was a tiger stalking you—this would come in very handy. It would probably keep you safe by making you aware of how close the tiger is to you. But in the case of an intrusive thought, this process only leads to focusing more and more on the otherwise normal thought, helping to turn it into an obsession that you can't get out of your mind. This starts a vicious cycle of feeling threatened, focusing more on the unwanted thought, feeling more threatened, focusing even more, and so on.

> Have you ever tried **not** to pay attention to a car speeding straight at you?
>
> Could you hear an explosion or suddenly smell smoke in your house without your heart starting to race?

If you trick your brain and body into thinking that an intrusive thought is very important or threatening, you'll automatically start focusing your attention on the thought, which will make it seem more and more threatening and ominous, making you even more preoccupied; in other words, the thought will become an obsession.

Common Beliefs and Misinterpretations in OCD

Researchers have found that people with OCD tend to hold certain inaccurate beliefs and attitudes that lead to misinterpreting intrusive thoughts as threatening or very significant, leading to this vicious cycle of obsessing. These "obsessional" beliefs and attitudes are listed in the table on the facing page. You'll need to be able to recognize them if you're going to reverse the obsessional process.

Holding these types of beliefs and attitudes sets you up for misinterpreting normal, harmless intrusive thoughts as significant and threatening. To help you identify the beliefs and attitudes that affect you, each of the following sections begins with three statements for you to consider. Decide whether you agree or disagree with each statement and check the appropriate box.

Threat Exaggeration

I believe the world is a dangerous place.

☒ Agree ☐ Disagree

Bad luck is more likely to happen to me than to other people.

☐ Agree ☒ Disagree

I am very vulnerable to disasters that I couldn't cope with.

☐ Agree ☒ Disagree

If you agreed with one or more of the statements above, you might jump to conclusions and assume your obsessional thoughts (the ones you identified in Step 2) are very realistic and your feared consequences are very likely to occur. You might also underestimate your ability to cope with the feared disasters you obsess about. For example, Carly, who worked in a library, had intrusive thoughts about germs being on the books she was handling. She misinterpreted these thoughts as realistic and became very fearful of catching terrible diseases. She even began using gloves to touch the library books and developed hand-washing rituals to reduce her anxiety and prevent illnesses.

Responsibility Exaggeration

If I don't try to *prevent* a disaster, it's just as bad as *causing* it.

☐ Agree ☒ Disagree

Obsessional Beliefs and Attitudes

Threat exaggeration: You overestimate the probability and severity of negative consequences.

Responsibility exaggeration: You overestimate how much influence or power you have to cause harm and to protect others from harm.

Importance of thoughts: You believe that intrusive thoughts reveal your true personality or moral character—who you *really* are deep down.

Thought-action fusion: You believe that thoughts are the equivalent of actions. An intrusive thought about a bad deed is just as bad as actually committing the bad deed.

Need to control thoughts: You believe that you *can* and *should* have complete control over your intrusive thoughts.

Need for absolute certainty: You believe it is possible and necessary to be completely certain that negative outcomes associated with your obsessional fears will *absolutely* not occur.

Not doing something to erase negative thoughts is the same as wanting the thought to come true.

☐ Agree ☐ Disagree

I often feel responsible for protecting people from the things I obsess about.

☐ Agree ☐ Disagree

While walking through the mall one day, Melissa dropped her purse and some medication spilled out, with the pills landing on the floor all around her. Later that day, she had an intrusive thought that perhaps she hadn't picked all the pills up off the floor—maybe she missed a few. She began thinking that a small child could have come along and eaten one of the pills off the floor thinking it was a piece of candy. "What if the child got sick or even died from the medication? It would be entirely my fault!" she thought to herself. Melissa felt very guilty and anxious over her "carelessness" in dropping her purse.

If you agreed with one or more of the statements in the box above, you—like Melissa—probably overestimate your degree of responsibility for causing and preventing harm. If so, when normal intrusive thoughts about harm occur, you'll misinterpret them as meaning that you could be the sole cause of some tragic event and that it's your responsibility to do whatever it takes to prevent the feared catastrophe. These kinds of beliefs and misinterpretations often lead to compulsive checking, reassurance seeking, and confessing (or warning others of potential harm) to gauge the probability and reduce the chances of feared disasters. Melissa, for example, called the mall security office several times to warn them about her mishap and to ask whether there had been any emergencies.

Personal Importance Exaggeration

If I have violent or immoral thoughts, it means I might be a violent or immoral person.

☐ Agree ☐ Disagree

I wouldn't have negative intrusive thoughts unless there was something real about them.

☐ Agree ☐ Disagree

If I have any blasphemous or sacrilegious thoughts, it means deep down I don't believe in God.

☐ Agree ☐ Disagree

If you agreed with one or more of the preceding statements, you probably overestimate the personal significance of your negative thoughts. You experience an intrusion that runs counter to your typical upstanding nature and believe that it reveals some deep-seated evil, dirty, perverted, or immoral side of you. You might think "Why would these thoughts occur if they weren't at least partially true?" An unwanted thought of harming a loved one means that deep down you're actually a cold-blooded murderer. An unacceptable sexual image or impulse automatically means you are a pervert or "sexual deviant." But as you've now learned, these beliefs and interpretations are incorrect: these intrusive thoughts probably don't mean anything important.

A television show about adults who solicit sex from minors over the Internet prompted Andrew to have unwanted thoughts about having sex with children. Believing that these thoughts meant he was actually a child molester deep down inside, Andrew became very anxious and started obsessing. Subsequently, he used mental rituals to try to dismiss the thoughts, and he made sure not to let anyone know about his "dirty little secrets." Margaret, who was very religious, had an intrusive doubt about whether God really exists. She exaggerated the significance of this *unwanted* thought and misinterpreted it as indicating that she was losing her faith in God and forsaking her religion. She compulsively sought reassurance from her faith counselor that God wasn't upset with her for doubting.

Thought–Action Fusion

It's best not to think about awful things because it might make them come true.

☐ Agree ☐ Disagree

If I think about doing something bad, I could lose control and end up acting on my thoughts.

☐ Agree ☐ Disagree

***Thinking about* doing something terrible is as bad as *actually doing* something terrible.**

☐ Agree ☐ Disagree

Thought–action fusion refers to two mistaken beliefs: (1) the belief that thinking about a negative event will make the event more likely to occur and (2) the belief that thinking of doing something bad is morally the same as actually doing the bad thing (or wanting it to happen). If you found yourself in agreement with one or more of the statements on the facing page, you might fall into these traps.

If you believe that just thinking about a disaster raises the probability that the disaster will happen, and then you happen to have an intrusive thought about your father having a car accident on his way to work, you might interpret it as follows: "Thinking about this is too risky. I'd better stop these thoughts before something terrible happens to Dad." Merek had an unwanted upsetting thought about stabbing her husband while he slept. She was horrified by this idea and did her best to keep it out of her head. "It's just not worth the risk—thinking about it too much could cause me to lose control and do something awful."

If you believe that thinking about something bad is morally equivalent to actually doing a bad deed, then you'll see yourself as an adulterer even if you merely have an unwanted or harmless sexual thought about a supermodel or a coworker. In addition to fears of acting on her stabbing obsession, Merek believed that it was immoral to even *think* of such things. In her mind, she was as bad as a murderer.

Need to Control Thoughts

I should be able to rid my mind of unwanted or upsetting thoughts.

☐ Agree ☐ Disagree

If I don't control my bad, impure, or immoral thoughts, something bad could happen.

☐ Agree ☐ Disagree

I would be a better person if I had better control over my thoughts.

☐ Agree ☐ Disagree

If you marked that you agreed with one or more of the statements above, you might hold the belief that it's possible and important to control unwanted or upsetting obsessional thoughts, images, and doubts. If you could just exercise enough willpower to control your mind, you'd be a better person. Dorothy, who was Jewish, sometimes found herself thinking that if she converted to Christianity, she would have more in common with her Christian friends. Although she didn't take these thoughts seriously—she was on the board of her synagogue and was considered a leader in the Jewish community—Dorothy told herself it was wrong to even *think about* converting: "It's immoral to allow myself to keep having this thought. I need to find a way to stop it." Robert was a truck driver

As you have read, there is no reason why you need to resist, fight, or control your obsessional thoughts. They're not harmful. In fact, trying to control your obsessions might actually be making things worse!

who experienced unwanted intrusive images of driving his truck into oncoming traffic. He believed (incorrectly) that his inability to control this thought meant that he was actually suicidal. Afraid that deep down he really wanted to kill himself, Robert gave up his job as a driver.

Need for Absolute Certainty

I should be 100% certain that everything is safe.

☒ Agree ☐ Disagree

If I'm not absolutely sure of the things I obsess about, I can't feel comfortable.

☒ Agree ☐ Disagree

I often try to get reassurance that my fears and obsessions are "just thoughts" or "nothing to worry about."

☒ Agree ☐ Disagree

After baking and delivering cookies to a new neighbor down the street, Cindy catches a glimpse of a shelf containing bottles of detergent, bleach, and other household chemicals. This triggers an intrusive and senseless doubt that by mistake she might have poisoned the cookies with these chemicals. She says to herself, "What if this really happened? I have to make sure I didn't hurt this nice family." She becomes very anxious and goes back to her neighbor's home to check to be *absolutely sure* no one has been poisoned. Of course, everything is fine.

Gloria, after using the bathroom, has intrusive images of "toilet germs" crawling on her arm. She thinks, "I can't take the *chance* that these germs are really there," and she rolls up her sleeve and scrubs her arm in a ritualistic way until she feels better.

When Graham sends e-mails to his friends, coworkers, and those in authority, he has intrusive thoughts of curse words and other foul language. Afterward, he obsesses over whether he just *imagined* typing these insults into his e-mail messages or actually did it. He spends hours reading and rereading his e-mails to reassure himself that he didn't write anything offensive.

If you agreed with one or more of the statements above, you might believe that it's necessary to have a *guarantee* of safety before you can feel comfortable about a feared situation. This, however, will lead to focusing on the remote *possibility* that your intrusive thoughts could be realistic, rather than the very strong *probability* that they're just thoughts. It can be distressing not to have a definitive guarantee of safety, which makes some intrusive thoughts particularly tough to handle. These include metaphysical thoughts ("God might not love me") and thoughts about events that took place in the distant past ("I might have hurt someone's feelings 15 years ago without realizing it") or that won't occur until the distant future ("I could get cancer in 40 years"). There are some uncertainties in life that we're just stuck with. We'll work on helping you deal with these uncertainties in later steps.

Are These Obsessional Beliefs and Interpretations Really Mistakes?

Yes! Remember that it's completely normal to have intrusive negative thoughts. Pretty much everyone has them from time to time. Your intrusive obsessional thoughts originate from normal mental processes, and they don't imply anything dangerous, perverse, deviant, immoral, or otherwise negative about you. In fact, you might have little control over when these thoughts occur and what you think about. These thoughts also can't make bad things happen any more than wishing to win the lottery or rooting for your favorite team to win a ball game can influence these events. Finally, your intrusive thoughts can't force you to do anything you don't already plan or wish to do. Acting—especially when it involves doing something against your will—requires planning and decision making, which are *deliberate* thought processes and very different from the automatic, intrusive, unwanted thoughts I'm talking about here. An important aim of CBT, as you'll see in Part III of this workbook, is to help you correct faulty beliefs and interpretations. Once you realize that your obsessional thoughts are normal and harmless, you'll no longer be bothered by them, and this will begin an *upward* spiral out of obsessing.

Normal intrusive, unwanted negative thoughts are transformed into persistent and distressing obsessions when you interpret these thoughts as threatening, personally significant, dangerous, and needing to be controlled. In CBT, you learn how to correct these faulty interpretations and stop being bothered by your intrusions.

If Obsessions Aren't Dangerous, Why Can't I Get Over Them?

It's quite a paradox: obsessions are distressing, time-consuming, and, what's more, they're really just normally occurring, senseless, intrusive thoughts on steroids. I would bet that your obsessional fears have rarely, if ever, come true. So why don't you realize all of this and just get over your obsessional fears? Obviously, it's not that simple, or you probably wouldn't need this book. There's something keeping you from changing your beliefs and interpretations on your own—something that prevents you from realizing that your obsessional fears *are* irrational. It turns out that the *something* is the very strategies—rituals and avoidance—that you use to try to reduce anxiety and make you feel safer when obsessional anxiety strikes. *Rituals and avoidance actually make OCD stronger.*

What's Wrong with Doing Something That Makes You Feel Better?

It seems to make perfect sense to use rituals as a coping strategy. When you experience an obsession, you feel distressed or anxious; and when you engage in compulsive rituals, mini- and mental rituals, and reassurance seeking, you usually end up feeling better. But for how long? Although they sometimes relieve obsessional anxiety in the short run, avoidance, compulsions, and other rituals backfire in the long run. Here's how rituals are self-defeating:

First, rituals prevent you from falsifying your mistaken beliefs and interpretations. They keep you from learning that obsessions are *just* senseless thoughts and that your feared consequences are unlikely to occur. Take Amalie, for example, who performed compulsive rituals—knocking on wood eight times and saying a prayer—in response to obsessional fears of bad luck from the number 13. These rituals kept her from being able to find out that the number 13 wouldn't really cause bad luck, that her obsessional thoughts and fears were senseless. That's because she attributed the fact that no bad luck materialized to her rituals ("If I hadn't ritualized, the number 13 would have caused something awful"). But since she never put her fears to the test by *consistently* not ritualizing, the number 13 remained frightening and she continued to have urges to ritualize.

A second problem with rituals is that, because they sometimes lead to an immediate reduction in anxiety (even if the anxiety reduction is slight or only temporary), you find yourself wanting to resort to these strategies over and over again ("compulsively"). They begin to seem like the only way out of obsessions. But this is a dirty trick that OCD plays to get you stuck using more and more self-defeating strategies. You resort to rituals more and more.

Third, because rituals generally expand and take up increasing time and effort, they often reach the point where they severely disrupt day-to-day life. So instead of providing temporary relief from anxiety, they become problems in their own right. For example, someone concerned with safety at home starts with checking doors and window locks, but then begins checking electrical appliances, and then the water faucets. Soon one round of checking doesn't do the job, and several rounds have to be made. This might go on and on to the point that the person is able to do little else beyond checking and seeking reassurance of safety.

Finally, rituals make OCD worse by serving as reminders of obsessions. That is, the more rituals you perform, the more opportunities you have to be reminded of your obsessional fears. This is similar to what happens if you look at your alarm clock when you're having trouble falling asleep. You may know that watching the clock is sometimes the worst thing you can do if you have insomnia because it only reminds you of how much sleep you're *not* getting. It makes you more stressed about trying to get to sleep, which makes you less likely to actually fall asleep. Similarly, as rituals grow over time, you might find yourself utterly preoccupied with your obsessions.

In Step 9, we'll work on changing these self-defeating behaviors and developing more helpful and healthy ways of dealing with obsessional thoughts.

Why Doesn't It Make Sense to Avoid What You Fear?

If you never confronted obsessional triggers, you wouldn't have to do any rituals. Wouldn't that be a good thing?

Remember Amalie? If she was assigned to a hotel room ending in 13 (for example, 413), she'd request a different room because of her obsessional fear. Carol suffered from sexual obsessions about children. Although she found the obsessional thoughts utterly repugnant, she worried she was becoming a child molester. As a result, she avoided schools and playgrounds. David had obsessive fears of contracting HIV from public bathrooms and went to

How Rituals Keep the Vicious Cycle Going

1. They keep you from discovering that your obsessional thoughts and fears are unrealistic and can be ignored the way most people shrug them off—that you won't get sick if you don't compulsively wash your hands, a burglar won't break in if you don't check all the doors and windows 12 times in a certain order, you won't feel worse and worse if you don't ask for reassurance or arrange things in a certain pattern, and so forth.
2. Because they may provide temporary relief from anxiety, you start to rely on your rituals more and more. In other words, rituals become stronger as time goes by.
3. But as they demand more of your time, rituals stop providing temporary relief from anxiety and become problems in their own right.
4. Rituals remind you of your obsessions and eventually can make you completely preoccupied by them.

---

great lengths to avoid them. This included not eating or drinking within hours of leaving the house, and never venturing more than a few miles from his home (so he could return in the event that nature called).

Rick had unwanted obsessional thoughts of insulting people he spoke with. He worried that he would just blurt out curse words, racial slurs, and other degrading comments that came to his mind (against his will) during conversations. As a result, Rick avoided using curse words and saying other nasty things—he even tried to avoid *thinking* these things. As his problem got worse, he avoided conversations with important people that he didn't want to offend, such as his boss, customers, clergy, and doctors.

Of course, avoiding situations or thoughts that you find upsetting or frightening is a normal response. Anyone concerned about getting sick from using a public bathroom would avoid public bathrooms. But, as with compulsive rituals, avoidance backfires in the long run. One problem with avoidance is that it's only temporarily helpful because eventually you probably will encounter a feared situation that you can't avoid, and it will trigger obsessions. For example, sooner or later Amalie will run into the number 13. So avoidance is futile.

A second problem with avoidance is that it maintains faulty obsessional beliefs. That is, by avoiding, you rob yourself of the opportunity to find out that the situation or object is not really that dangerous and that your intrusive thoughts are not harmful. For example, as long as Carol avoids small children, she'll never have the chance to see that she's not going to molest them. Therefore, she will go on believing she is a child molester who had better stay away from children. Avoidance keeps you from disproving your fears.

> Have you ever been amazed to find that the "ferocious" dog that got bigger and bigger in your mind the longer you avoided him was a big pussycat once you got close enough to pet him?

Third, because there are usually many situations that can trigger obsessional fears, trying to avoid them will end up severely restricting your lifestyle. For example, Rick's avoid-

How Avoidance Keeps the Vicious Cycle Going

1. Whether it's dirt, a certain number, a situation, an item, or a certain type of person, you're bound to come across the things that trigger obsessional thoughts eventually. When you do, the obsessions will come up again.
2. As with rituals, avoiding triggers of obsessions will prevent you from confronting them to find out they're not so dangerous after all. You'll stay fearful of the content of your obsessions.
3. Avoidance narrows your life and creates a problem of ever-expanding magnitude. If you're afraid of catching germs from dirt, you might start avoiding dirty-looking objects. But your obsessions will come up every time you can't avoid a dirty object, so your mind will tell you to step up your efforts, and the next thing you know you're avoiding all rooms that typically can be dirty (bathrooms, garages, attics), then entire buildings that strike you as dirty, whole neighborhoods, and so forth.

ance of having conversations started with a few individuals, but gradually expanded to more and more of the people he interacted with. After a while, he became extremely limited in whom we could speak with. As another example, consider Sarah, who was afraid of hitting pedestrians with her car. At first she avoided driving in crowded areas at night. Then this gradually expanded to all nighttime driving, driving during the day in crowded areas, and then all driving when alone. Many people with so-called "hit-and-run" obsessions stop driving altogether.

The Vicious Cycle of OCD and How to Stop It

As the diagram on the facing page shows, OCD's battle plan is to get you caught up in a self-perpetuating vicious cycle of thinking, feeling, and acting patterns (as indicated by the gray arrows in the diagram) that are difficult to stop on your own. Unpleasant intrusive thoughts are normal—just about everybody has them. They may be triggered by something you see or hear in the environment, or they may occur without an obvious trigger. But holding obsessional beliefs and interpreting normal intrusive thoughts in ways that make these thoughts seem important and threatening leads to feelings of anxiety and the fight-or-flight response. This, in turn, causes you to become even more preoccupied with the unwanted thought, which begins to take on a life of its own. To cope with the obsessional anxiety, you use rituals and avoidance strategies that sometimes seem effective in the short term but that end up making your problems with obsessions worse in the long run. But because you sometimes get immediate relief with these maladaptive strategies, you end up using them more and more.

Does this model imply that OCD is your (or anyone's) fault? As I said in the Introduction of this book, *absolutely not.* In fact, three parts of this vicious cycle are completely beyond your control: (1) the occurrence of unwanted negative intrusive thoughts, (2) the activation of anxiety and the fight-or-flight response when you detect a potential threat,

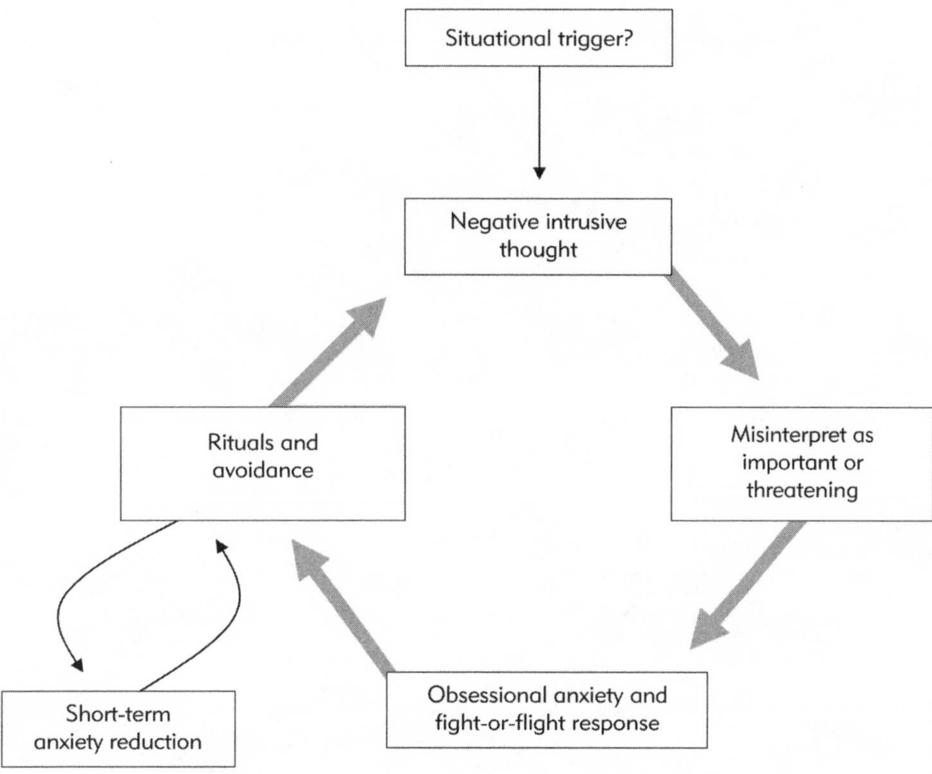

and (3) the fact that rituals and avoidance aimed at escaping from intrusive thoughts simply intensify these thoughts. These three effects are *involuntary*, and researchers, including me, have observed and studied them in people with *and without* OCD. Fortunately, two other parts of this vicious cycle probably seem automatic, but you could learn to bring them under your control: (1) the way you misinterpret your intrusive, unwanted negative thoughts and (2) using rituals and avoidance strategies in response to obsessional fear. These are *voluntary* parts of the vicious cycle because they can be controlled—albeit with lots of practice.

> **There are two parts of the vicious cycle that you can learn to bring under control to beat OCD:**
> - **Learning to interpret intrusive thoughts differently**
> - **Learning healthier long-term strategies other than rituals and avoidance for responding**

If you want to put a halt to this vicious cycle, you won't have much luck trying to change the involuntary parts. But you *can* intervene at the voluntary parts of the cycle. This is where OCD is most vulnerable—the chink in its armor. Specifically, you can learn and practice skills for changing how you think about and interpret triggers and intrusive unwanted thoughts. When you correctly interpret these as nonthreatening, your problems with obsessions and obsessional fear will begin to improve. You can also learn to change the behaviors you use to deal with obsessions and obsessional fear. Right now it might seem very difficult to change these thinking and acting patterns, but the goal of the CBT program in this workbook is to gradually help you do so. In Step 4, we'll get started by developing a plan for your treatment.

PART II

Getting Ready

STEP 4

Customizing Your Action Plan

In the first part of this workbook (Steps 1–3) you became an expert on OCD by learning how it operates and by analyzing your own obsessions, avoidance, and rituals. Understanding your enemy and its vulnerabilities has prepared you to weaken and defeat OCD. So Step 4 begins with an introduction to the strategies we know can help you win your battle. The more you know about how and why these strategies work, the better equipped you'll be to use them effectively. Then we'll begin devising an action plan for putting these tactics to work.

At the end of Step 3 you learned that you can break OCD's vicious cycle by changing how you interpret and respond to the intrusive thoughts and obsessional triggers you identified in Step 2. These are the places to intervene because your mental interpretations and your behavior are voluntary. You can learn to bring them under your control. The CBT techniques you'll be using in this book are aimed at helping you learn to control these responses to thwart OCD's battle plan. You'll use gradual *exposure* to situations and thoughts that provoke fear along with *response prevention*, which means abstaining from rituals and other fear-driven behaviors that seem to make you feel better in the short run but make OCD worse in the long run. Before you begin, though, we need to draw up a plan for how you'll adapt the exposure and response prevention exercises to your particular problems with obsessions and rituals.

Learning about CBT

I'd be foolish to expect you to expose yourself to the discomfort of facing your obsessional fears without making sure you understand what's in it for you. So, before we jump into planning your self-help program, let me explain how the various CBT techniques work. Understanding exactly how exposure and response prevention reduces OCD symptoms will help you see what a sensible way to defeat OCD CBT is. I want you to know that the anxiety you'll feel at first is not only something you need to get through to reap the benefits of treatment—like tolerating the discomfort of dental work to get that attractive, healthy smile—it's actually instrumental to the process of vanquishing OCD.

How could purposely facing your fears and stopping your rituals make you **less** scared and **less** miserable?

The History of CBT for OCD

CBT is one of the most stringently tested forms of psychotherapy available. There's clear and consistent scientific proof that it works *and works well.* These techniques were first applied and studied with OCD patients in the late 1960s and 1970s. Before then OCD was considered unresponsive to treatment (keep in mind that antidepressant medications such as Prozac, Anafranil, and Celexa had not been developed yet); most therapists were using psychoanalysis and other forms of talk therapy that were not scientifically based and did not work very well. Psychologist Victor Meyer, however, was a *behavior* therapist who worked in a psychiatric hospital in England. After watching patient after patient with OCD fail to improve after years and years of talk therapy, Dr. Meyer decided to try something considered drastic in his day: using his knowledge of the research on OCD, he helped his patients with contamination obsessions gradually confront the situations and touch the objects that provoked their fears (exposure therapy). But simply confronting these stimuli wasn't enough—after touching the feared objects the patients would go and wash away the "contamination" and thereby reinstate a sense of safety and cleanliness. So Dr. Meyer also had his patients refrain from any washing or cleaning rituals so that they stayed "contaminated" for long periods of time (response prevention).

Consider your anxiety a critical weapon. With it, you'll conquer OCD.

Of course, Dr. Meyer realized that his new therapy would initially make his patients feel very distressed, but he encouraged them to stick it out and see what happened when they remained in a "contaminated" state for longer than usual. As he had predicted, over a few hours, the patients' anxiety levels decreased—and so did their worries about contamination and germs. When this process was repeated daily over a few months, the obsessions about contamination and urges to wash and clean *were weakened and (in most cases) did not return.* Practicing repeated exposure and response prevention had taught these patients that they didn't have to be so worried about contamination and that the anxiety and distress they felt when first confronting these situations would not go on forever or spiral out of control.

When Dr. Meyer reported on the beneficial effects of this new behavioral treatment for OCD, clinics worldwide began using his approach and carefully studying it. Researchers in North America, Europe, Asia, Africa, and Australia worked to improve on this therapy and adapt it for all the different types of obsessions and rituals you read about in Part I. Today, as a result of over 40 years of research, we have a highly successful CBT treatment program that consists of four techniques: (1) actual exposure to the triggering situations, (2) exposure in imagination, (3) response prevention, and (4) cognitive therapy. The table on the facing page shows how each component of CBT addresses components of the OCD vicious

CBT technique	Aim or goal of the technique
Situational exposure	Reduce fear and avoidance of obsessional triggers
Imaginal exposure	Reduce fear and resistance to intrusive obsessional thoughts
Response prevention	Reduce urges to perform compulsive rituals and other rituals
Cognitive therapy	Help you get the most out of exposure and response prevention by correcting misinterpretations of normal intrusive thoughts

cycle that you read about in Step 3. The pages that follow provide a more in-depth overview of these techniques since we will use all four of them in this self-help program.

The Techniques of CBT

Situational Exposure

Think of a time when you faced something you were afraid of only to see that the situation wasn't so awful or scary after all. Remember how scared you were before you faced your fear? Recall how it felt as you came face to face with the dreaded situation? Then remember your feeling of relief and mastery ("I can do it!") once you realized the situation wasn't so bad in the end? That's a little like what happens during situational exposure. Situational exposure is a tool designed to help you reduce your fear and avoidance of situations, objects, and other stimuli that trigger obsessional fear.

Remember being flooded with relief when you faced a fear and found it wasn't so threatening after all?

When you analyzed your obsessions in Step 2, you identified what triggers obsessional fear and discomfort for you. Situational exposure involves practicing confronting these triggers and remaining in the feared situation long enough to see that anxiety decreases. The graph on the next page shows what typically happens: when you start exposure for the first time, it's normal for anxiety to increase; but if you remain in the situation, the anxiety begins to diminish on its own—even if you don't ritualize or leave the situation. This is called *habituation*. Your body simply has had enough of feeling anxious (the fight-or-flight response) and begins to calm itself down. You've probably never (or rarely) experienced habituation because you either avoid your fear triggers or use rituals to escape as soon as you feel your anxiety grow.

Using avoidance or rituals to quell anxiety is like giving up on exercise the minute you start to breathe hard: you never build fitness, and so every day you feel like you're exercising for the first time in years.

Notice that the graph also shows that anxiety decreases *between* exposure practices. The fourth time you practice an exposure, you don't feel nearly as anxious as you did when you practiced for the first time. Also, the more you practice, the quicker anxiety subsides. In other words, after repeated exposure practice, the anxiety associated with an obsessional trigger becomes weakened or *extinguished*. Again, since you probably haven't confronted your obsessional triggers

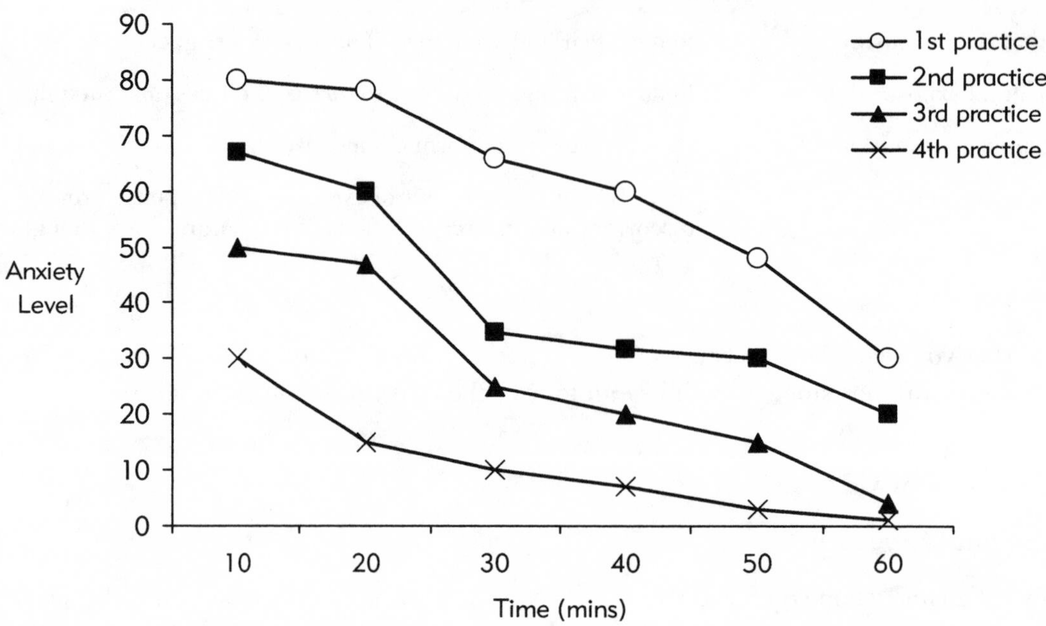

repeatedly, and remained exposed to them long enough, you have most likely never had the chance to see that this extinction occurs.

Many types of obsessions lend themselves well to situational exposure. If you have contamination fears and are afraid to touch certain objects (garbage cans, sweaty towels) or be in certain situations or places (public restrooms, homeless shelters), exposure should involve practice facing these situations. If you have obsessions about accidents that are triggered by driving near pedestrians, exposure to driving on roadways with pedestrians would be helpful. If you have violent or religious obsessions, exposure might entail watching horror movies or confronting unlucky numbers, knives, or religious icons that provoke anxiety and unwanted thoughts. If you confront your particular triggers repeatedly, and remain exposed to them for extended periods, they will soon no longer make you feel as anxious as they once did. Later in this step, I'll help you tailor a situational exposure plan for your specific needs.

The more you expose yourself to a feared situation, the weaker your anxiety becomes.

Imaginal Exposure

If your obsessions involve a fear that you'll transmit AIDS to your family and friends, there's no practical and ethical way to expose yourself to having or spreading this disease. If you have an obsession that you've hit a pedestrian with your car and the police are looking for you, you can't really confront this situation. Violent, sexual, and religious obsessions present similar dilemmas. I would never actually have someone stab a loved one, act in a sexually inappropriate way, or commit a religious sin simply to practice situational exposure! For these obsessional thoughts and doubts we use *imaginal* exposure.

Imaginal exposure involves creating mental pictures of the thoughts, images, and doubts about the catastrophes you fear might result if you don't perform rituals. As with situational exposure, imaginal exposure initially provokes anxiety, but with repeated and prolonged practice lowers anxiety and distress. *With imaginal exposure you weaken the connection between these obsessional thoughts and anxiety.* A bit later in this step we'll create an imaginal exposure plan tailored specifically for your needs.

Imaginal exposure gives you a way to confront your fears about violent or otherwise harmful situations that you can't expose yourself to in real life.

Response Prevention

Situational and imaginal exposure will probably provoke the urge to perform rituals. If you give in to those urges, exposure cannot lead to habituation because you're no longer truly exposing yourself to what you fear. So you need a tool to defeat those urges and disrupt the vicious cycle of OCD. That tool is response prevention. If you have contamination obsessions, you'll gradually refrain from washing and cleaning rituals. If your obsessions concern fears of being responsible for harm, you'll practice resisting urges to perform checking and reassurance-seeking rituals. If you have mental rituals, counting, repeating, or ordering compulsions, we'll work toward ending these as well when we develop a response prevention plan later in this step.

"Cold turkey" or a little at a time? Your CBT plan can be custom designed so you do response prevention at exactly the rate that will free you from OCD fastest.

Cognitive Therapy

If doing exposure and response prevention sounds very frightening or difficult, it's probably because—as you learned in Step 3—certain beliefs you hold are causing you to misinterpret your obsessional thoughts and triggers as realistic and dangerous. Garth, for example, believed strongly that intrusive thoughts are personally significant. He took his obsessional images of stabbing his wife and children to mean that he had a cruel underlying *desire* to harm those he loved. Cognitive therapy is a set of tools that teach you to recognize and correct such problematic thinking patterns. It helps you step back from the obsession and examine it more carefully and logically than you probably do when you're feeling anxious. Doing so provides such a strong foundation for exposure and response prevention that I'll teach you cognitive therapy techniques first in Part III.

Can you finish OCD off with cognitive therapy techniques alone?

In fact it's possible that cognitive therapy by itself will reduce your obsessions and rituals. But will it be enough? The available research says probably not. That's why I recommend using cognitive therapy to weaken the beliefs and interpretations that are the foundation of your obsessions to make your exposure and response prevention practices maximally effective.

Cognitive therapy is a way of gathering your forces and arming yourself to beat OCD—an important foundation but not the whole battle plan.

Designing Your Situational Exposure Plan

As you know, the situational exposure component of your self-help treatment program will involve confronting objects and situations that provoke obsessional anxiety and discomfort. Of course, this is going to be hard work; and while it's one thing to *say* you're going to face your fears, actually doing this in a therapeutic way requires careful preparation. To begin with, we need to generate a list of the specific situations you'll practice confronting.

The first step in creating a battle plan against OCD is deciding on your targets:

- **What situations and thoughts should you practice confronting?**
- **What rituals should you work on resisting?**

This list is called an *exposure hierarchy*. It's based on your own obsessions and personal experiences. The items listed on your hierarchy are ranked from the *least* fear-provoking to the *most* fear-provoking. Ideally, your hierarchy should consist of 10 to 20 items that provide a good sampling of the situations and objects that trigger obsessional fear. The sample hierarchy below was developed by Carlos, who had obsessions about bad luck, harm, or death befalling his school-age children.

As you can see, Carlos's hierarchy contains 10 items. Although Carlos probably avoids or feels frightened in more than 10 situations, the items he chose to put on his hierarchy provide a good representation of the situations that are most difficult for him. As you

Carlos's Situational Exposure Hierarchy

Item	Description	Discomfort level
1	*Pictures of black cats*	*35*
2	*Use a knife while alone*	*40*
3	*Use a knife while the children are nearby*	*55*
4	*The number 13*	*65*
5	*The number 666*	*65*
6	*The words death, dead, die, decapitate, accident*	*70*
7	*Wearing black clothes*	*80*
8	*Cemeteries*	*85*
9	*Funeral homes*	*90*
10	*Attending a funeral*	*100*

begin thinking about your own hierarchy, keep in mind that you don't need to include every single situation that presents a problem for you. Instead, select 10 to 20 items that best capture the types of situations that give you difficulty. Also, try to be as specific as possible. For example, if you're more afraid of *public* restrooms than restrooms in people's homes, you'll want to be sure to specify the location of the restroom you will practice with for exposure.

Subjective Units of Discomfort (SUDs)

Also notice that Carlos's hierarchy items are arranged by the level of discomfort they provoke. The first item is the *least* distressing, and the last item is the *most* anxiety-provoking. These discomfort ratings are based on an imaginary scale running from 0 (no discomfort) to 100 (extreme discomfort). If you are at a 0, then you're feeling as calm as you could possibly feel—like being in a very peaceful and contented state of mind. Now imagine the most intense fear or anxiety you've ever experienced—like you're tied down to the railroad tracks and the train is coming around the bend! This would be 100 on the scale. Usually, scores between 80 and 100 are associated with physical symptoms of anxiety (the fight-or-flight response) such as sweating, feeling tense, racing or pounding heart, trouble catching your breath, feelings of dizziness, or upset stomach. Once you have an idea of what 0 and 100 would be, you can figure out the various points in between. A score of 25 usually indicates mild distress or anxiety, 50 indicates a moderate level, and 75 means relatively high anxiety. These ratings are personalized—they're based only on how you experience your OCD symptoms. For this reason, we often refer to them as *subjective units of discomfort*—or *SUDs* for short (see the scale below). If at first you find it difficult to rate your fears using the SUDs scale, that's okay. It usually gets easier with practice.

The Subjective Units of Discomfort (SUDs) Rating Scale

0 10 20 30 40 50 60 70 80 90 100

No discomfort — Mild discomfort — Moderate discomfort — High discomfort — Extreme discomfort

Building Your Situational Exposure Hierarchy

To start building your own hierarchy, go back to Step 2 and look over your OCD Analysis Worksheet (page 39) and the lists you generated of your own obsessional triggers (page 41) and situations you avoid (page 50). Next, use the SUDs rating scale to give each trigger and avoided situation a rating from 0 to 100. When rating these items, try to ask yourself "If I had to face this situation *without ritualizing*, how anxious or distressed would I be?" Remember that the scale is personal. There's no right or wrong answer. All you're doing is making it easier to compare one situation with another so that you can put them in order according to how uncomfortable they might make you feel.

When you have given a SUDs rating to each trigger and situation you avoid, choose 10 to 20 items that best characterize the sorts of situations that are difficult for you. Then list these items on the Situational Exposure Hierarchy form on the facing page. These will be the items you practice confronting in situational exposure (Step 7). I recommend starting your list with items that have SUDs ratings in the moderate range: about 40 to 50. This will give you enough of a challenge, while helping to ensure that your first experiences with exposure are successful and not too overwhelming. Use the SUDs ratings to arrange the rest of your list so that, like Carlos, you are gradually working your way from moderately difficult situations to the most difficult ones (from the lowest to the highest SUDs ratings). If you have more than one type of obsessional theme, such as sexual *and* contamination obsessions, you can create separate hierarchies. I'll give you several examples a little later in this chapter.

Starting your hierarchy at a SUDs of 40–50 is like planning aerobic exercise to get you into the training heart rate. There's no point in doing exercise that doesn't get your heart pumping, and there's no point in targeting situations that cause you very little anxiety.

You might think of your hierarchy as a wish list and include the activities and events you'd like to be able to include in your normal routine without catering to OCD. I suggest looking at the sample hierarchies and consulting with someone who knows about your problems with OCD when you assemble your own hierarchy.

Include Your Worst Fears

When Carlos was constructing his hierarchy, he could never have imagined actually going to a cemetery, visiting a funeral home, or attending a funeral. These were his worst fears because they made him think about his own children's death. Still, Carlos wrote these situations on his hierarchy because he knew that if he *could* confront them, he would conquer his obsession. When you're creating your hierarchy, you too will need to "push the envelope." You'll probably be tempted to leave your worst fears off the list. Try, however, to include difficult items you may not be able to face *now* but that you will need to confront in order to defeat OCD. In other words, keep an open mind.

Try to "push the envelope" when creating your hierarchy. It's just a plan, and you'll work your way up to your worst fears once you're ready to face them.

Be Specific

One thing you might also notice in Carlos's hierarchy is that using a knife when he was alone was less anxiety-provoking than using a knife when his children were around. You too might find that some hierarchy items would receive higher or lower SUDs ratings depending on the circumstances, such as whether you're at home or away from the house and whether you're alone or with someone else. As Carlos did, you should clarify the specific factors that make some situations worse than others and incorporate them into your hierarchy. You can also use the factors that influence your fear to help you make your progression up the hier-

Situational Exposure Hierarchy		
Item	**Description** (type of obsession)	**SUDs rating**
1		
2		
3		
4		
5		
6		
7		
8		
9		
10		
11		
12		
13		
14		
15		
16		
17		
18		
19		
20		

archy more gradual. For example, if "touching doorknobs" is on your hierarchy, you might begin with easier doorknobs, such as those in your home; then move on to moderately difficult ones, such as in a doctor's office or professional building; and finally to the most difficult of all, perhaps those in a school or bus station. If you practice confronting less distressing items first, you'll be better off when it comes to facing your more intense fears.

Get Input from Others

Showing your completed hierarchy to someone who knows you well can be a big help in filling in the blanks. Perhaps this person can offer some advice on whether you've left any important situations off the hierarchy and whether the order of your items seems practical. You, of course, have the final say on your SUDs ratings and on what to include in your hierarchy. But keep in mind that family members or friends who spend a lot of time with you could be aware of avoidance strategies and other problems that you might not have noticed or that have become so ingrained that you've forgotten to include them. In Step 5, I'll help you choose someone in particular—a "treatment buddy"—to help you with doing exposure and response prevention exercises.

Is there someone you trust who could review your hierarchy to help you fill in any blanks?

Sample Situational Exposure Hierarchies

Here are some examples of situational exposure hierarchies for different types of obsessions. These samples are meant to give you ideas for how to build your own hierarchy (or hierarchies). Remember, most of the items for your own hierarchy will come from your lists of triggers and avoidances from Step 2.

Ronnie: Responsibility for Harm or Damage

Ronnie was a real estate agent who had obsessions that he might cause property damage and injure others by mistake. Seeing a fire truck, police car, or ambulance made Ronnie worry about whether he had started a fire, caused an accident, or even assaulted or killed someone without realizing it. He watched the news on TV, scoured the newspapers, and even checked with the police to ensure he wasn't responsible for any disasters. If Ronnie had taken home buyers to visit a house for sale, he worried that maybe he'd caused a fire by leaving a light or appliance on. He was also concerned about fires from electrical appliances in his own home.

Ronnie's Situational Exposure Hierarchy: Responsibility for Harm or Damage

Item	Description	Discomfort level
1	Leave light on in own home overnight	45
2	Leave a light on in a "for sale" home overnight	50

3	Keep toaster plugged in (own home) while at home	60
4	Plug in toaster and leave the house for the day	65
5	Be the last person to leave the house for the day	70
6	Read stories of assaults/murders	70
7	Drive past firehouse/police station	75
8	Use the iron and quickly leave the house	80
9	Read stories about house fires	85
10	Leave oven on while out of the house for 15 min., 30 min., etc.	85

Andrea: Contamination

Andrea was terrified of contracting illnesses. She avoided public bathrooms and contact with surfaces such as door handles and garbage cans. She also avoided contact with certain people she considered "dirty" and their belongings (pens, office telephones, and so on). Bodily fluids (urine, sweat), using the bathroom, touching her genitals, and contact with dirty laundry also evoked obsessive fear. Andrea washed her hands over 50 times daily and changed her clothes multiple times each day to reduce her fears of contamination.

Andrea's Situational Exposure Hierarchy: Contamination

Item	Description	SUDs rating
1	Touch door handles and railings in public places	40
2	Shake hands with a stranger	40
3	Shake hands with someone who looks "dirty"	45
4	Borrow and use someone else's pen	45
5	Contact with garbage cans at home	50
6	Contact with garbage cans at work	55
7	Contact with garbage cans at cafeteria or food court	60
8	Contact with dumpster at the apartment complex	65
9	Touch equipment at the gym without gloves	65
10	Use a public telephone (touch the mouthpiece)	70

11	Touch public bathroom door	80
12	Touch sink, faucet, toilet in public bathroom	85
13	Touch floor of a public bathroom	90
14	Touch my dirty laundry (pants)	90
15	Urinating	95
16	Touch my dirty underwear	95
17	Touch my own genitals	95
18	Defecating	100
19	Touch my own anus	100

Judy: Order and Balance

Judy engaged in ordering and balancing rituals triggered by obsessive thoughts of "imperfection" and "imbalance." Activities such as completing paperwork sometimes took hours because Judy had to painstakingly make sure letters were formed "perfectly." Household items had to be arranged in certain ways, and Judy had to check that order was maintained. Her most pervasive symptoms focused on left–right balance. If she used her right hand to open a door, touch, or grab something (such as from the refrigerator), she had to repeat the behavior using her left hand (and vice versa) to achieve "balance."

Judy's Situational Exposure Hierarchy: Order and Balance

Item	Description	SUDs rating
1	Write letters "imperfectly" on scrap paper	45
2	Write imperfectly in checkbook, notebook, forms	55
3	Write imperfectly in my own diary	60
4	Leave items in the family room "out of order"	65
5	Leave items in own room "out of order"	70
6	Say "left" without saying "right"	75
7	Say "right" without saying "left"	75
8	Hear someone say "left" without saying "right"	80
9	Hear someone say "right" without saying "left"	80

10	Write the word left without writing right	85
11	Write the word right without writing left	85
12	Take special note of left–right imbalance	90
13	Touch items with right (or left) hand (or side) only	95

Alan: Violent Obsessions

Alan was married and had a 6-month-old son, Kyle. His obsessions included senseless, intrusive thoughts of murdering his family. Alan was afraid of "losing his mind" and acting on these thoughts, which were invariably triggered by the sight of items that could be used as weapons (for example, knives, hammers). He avoided these items, as well as stories about people who had harmed or killed their loved ones. Alan was also avoiding being alone with his son.

Alan's Situational Exposure Hierarchy: Violent Obsessions

Item	Description	SUDs rating
1	Words kill, murder, stab, bludgeon	50
2	Read stories of fathers killing their own children	60
3	Knives	65
4	Baseball bats	70
5	Plastic bags	70
6	Cut meat or vegetables with a knife while Kyle is nearby	80
7	Give Kyle a bath	85
8	Stay at home alone with Kyle	90
9	Pick up and hold Kyle	93
10	Drive into rural area alone with Kyle	100

Marla: Sexual Obsessions

Marla, who was 42 years old, had been married for 17 years. Although she had never had any homosexual relationships, Marla had obsessional thoughts and doubts that perhaps she was a lesbian. These obsessions were triggered by seeing attractive women (including some of her friends), hearing sexually suggestive words (for example, sex, bed) or sounds (for example, kissing, moaning), and by the sight of anything that could be construed as sexual (for example, anything that vibrated, two women hugging). Marla feared that having so many lesbian thoughts meant she was "turning gay" and that she would have to give up the family life that she loved so much. When these thoughts came to mind, Marla tried to "think through" or "analyze" their meaning and "test" herself by looking at (or thinking of) her husband to reassure herself that she was still heterosexual. These mental rituals sometimes lasted for hours. Marla also prayed ritualistically that she was not gay. Her situational exposure hierarchy was as follows:

Marla's Situational Exposure Hierarchy: Homosexual Obsessions

Item	Description	SUDs rating
1	The words kiss, love, lover, bed, affair	40
2	The sound of a kiss	45
3	Moan, sex, vagina, wet, and other sexually charged words	50
4	Pictures of female models (for example, Victoria's Secret catalog)	55
5	Sound of a woman moaning or saying "Oh God!"	60
6	Visual diagram of the female sexual organs	65
7	Pictures of attractive friends	65
8	Visiting a lingerie store (for example, Victoria's Secret)	70
9	Going to the health club and watching women work out	75
10	Women's locker room at the health club	80
11	Watching a movie/reading a book about lesbians	80
12	Visiting a store that sells sexual products for lesbians (for example, vibrators)	90

Gene: Religious Obsessional Doubts

Gene was a devoutly religious Christian man with obsessional doubts that he was not faithful or devoted enough to God or his religion. In other words, he obsessed over whether he was really a "good Christian." For example, if he read or heard a sermon about the importance of living a life devoted to God, Gene wondered whether he was really living this sort of life. He avoided reading certain biblical passages and inspirational books that described the type of relationships Christians should have with God since this material provoked obsessions. Gene's hierarchy appears on the next page.

Gene's Situational Exposure Hierarchy: Religious Obsessions

Item	Description	SUDs rating
1	*Read from inspirational books*	40
2	*Read from the Bible*	50
3	*Watch a sermon on TV about living the Christian life*	55
4	*Read from books about how a Christian should have strong faith*	55
5	*Listen to Christian and inspirational music*	60
6	*Words grace, hope, faith*	61
7	*Words devil, hell, possessed*	62
8	*Read Bible verses pertaining to the importance of faith in God*	65
9	*Read transcripts of sermons about relationships with God*	70
10	*Sermon about the importance of being faithful and having a strong relationship with God*	80

Preparing Your Imaginal Exposure Plan

As you now know, you probably need not just situational exposure practice to win your battle against OCD, but also imaginal exposure. Imaginal exposure enables you to confront the mental components of your obsessions. The intrusions—the unwanted ideas, thoughts, doubts, or images that appear in your mind and evoke anxiety—are one mental component. Examples include images of germs spreading on your skin, thoughts of death and destruction, impulses to harm someone, images of people's genitals, blasphemous thoughts of the Virgin Mary having sex, and doubts about whether you're an atheist, child molester, or cold-blooded killer deep down inside. Sometimes intrusions are triggered by the situations or objects you'll be confronting in situational exposure (for example, knives, garbage cans, religious symbols), but sometimes these thoughts just come to mind spontaneously—without any identifiable triggers. Imaginal exposure, which you will learn to use in Step 8, involves confronting these distressing intrusions by purposely conjuring them up as if conducting situational exposure to a thought, image, or doubt. In some cases, the images will be like snapshots. In other cases, they may be more like scenes from a nightmare or horror movie.

The other mental component of your obsessions is the feared consequence. For example:

- The fear of being arrested for causing a hit-and-run accident
- The fear of getting cancer in 40 years because you might have inhaled carcinogens

- The fear that thoughts about violence imply you are becoming a serial killer
- The fear of getting ill if you don't wash
- The fear that you haven't done enough to prevent bad luck from befalling loved ones.

Imaginal exposures, which are similar to movies in which the upsetting scene unfolds, will help you confront these thoughts and doubts and weaken the feelings of anxiety and discomfort that have become associated with these ideas.

As with situational exposure, imaginal exposure is hierarchy-driven. Again, I recommend beginning with less distressing thoughts and images and gradually increasing the intensity until you're facing your most distressing obsessions. Another strategy is to link the imaginal exposures with situational exposures. For example, if you conduct a situational exposure to touching the floor, you might follow this with an imaginal exposure to images of floor germs and thoughts of causing loved ones to get sick. When you get to Step 8, I'll help you with the particulars of setting up imaginal exposures. For now, though, you need to plot your plan of attack. Remember Carlos? His obsessional thoughts concerned his own children being injured or killed. Carlos's imaginal exposure hierarchy appears below. He began by imagining bad luck, minor accidents, and injuries. Images of his children's death, which were his most distressing obsessional thoughts, came last.

Do your obsessions involve violent thoughts, unacceptable religious images or doubts, or offensive sexual ideas? I recognize that *purposely* imagining these things for exposure

Carlos's Imaginal Exposure Hierarchy

Item	Description	SUDs rating
1	*Images of the children dropping and breaking their favorite toys*	30
2	*Images of the children stubbing their toes*	40
3	*Images of the children getting bad grades in school*	50
4	*Images of the children accidentally cutting themselves with scissors*	55
5	*Images of the children getting the flu and being seriously ill*	60
6	*Images of the children falling and breaking an arm or leg*	70
7	*Images of the children in a minor car accident*	75
8	*Images of the children in a serious car accident*	80
9	*Images of the children dying in an accident*	95
10	*Images of the children's funeral*	100

therapy might be extremely distressing for you. Let me suggest you keep two things in mind. First, whether you realize it or not, you're *already* thinking these thoughts—they're your obsessions. So, in imaginal exposure, you won't have to think about anything you haven't already thought about. The only difference is that in imaginal exposure you'll confront these thoughts in a deliberate and therapeutic way. And this will help you practice new and healthier strategies for coping with these thoughts, images, and doubts, rather than trying to avoid them or do rituals—which don't work anyway.

The second thing to keep in mind is that obsessions come from normal and universal thoughts. In other words, everyone has strange, vulgar, violent, sexual, or otherwise negative thoughts, images, impulses, and doubts. So, as with situational exposure, I encourage you to push the envelope when developing your imaginal hierarchy. Try to include thoughts, images, and doubts you may feel very uncomfortable with, but that creep into your mind anyway. You know, the deep, dark, unacceptable thoughts or "dirty little secrets" that you try to fight, analyze, or understand; or perhaps that you wouldn't tell another soul about. In Step 8, I'll teach you how to face even these most distressing obsessions so that they no longer have to provoke anxiety.

Could you "push the envelope" in imaginal exposure if you remembered that these thoughts already come into your head anyway?

Building Your Imaginal Hierarchy

When you're ready to start building your imaginal hierarchy, go back to Step 2 and look over your OCD Analysis Worksheet (page 39) lists of obsessional intrusions (page 44) and feared consequences (page 47). Next, give each a SUDs rating: Ask yourself, "If I had to let this thought just stay in my mind—without using any rituals or strategies to control it or push it away—how distressed would I be?" Then choose between five to 10 intrusions and feared consequences and list these on the Imaginal Exposure Hierarchy form on page 104. You might have fewer images if you have only one main obsession. If you have multiple types of obsessions, like contamination fears and violent impulses, you might draw up separate hierarchies. List your hierarchy items according to their SUDs ratings from lowest to highest.

Sample Imaginal Hierarchies

Let's take a look at imaginal exposure hierarchies prepared by the six people with different types of OCD symptoms described earlier. You might use these examples as you think about your own hierarchy, although keep in mind that items for your own exposure plan should come from the lists of intrusions and feared consequences you generated in Step 2.

Ronnie: Responsibility for Harm or Damage

Ronnie's obsessional thoughts were about being responsible for property damage and injuries to others, such as "What if I started a fire by mistake?" and "What if I caused an accident, assaulted, or killed someone without realizing it?" Notice that in his imaginal exposure hierarchy he planned to practice purposely thinking about the feared consequences of his obsessions.

Imaginal Exposure Hierarchy

Item	**Description** (intrusive thought or feared consequences)	SUDs rating
1		
2		
3		
4		
5		
6		
7		
8		
9		
10		

Ronnie's Imaginal Exposure Hierarchy: Responsibility for Harm or Damage

Item	Description	SUDs rating
1	*Imagine someone broke into my home because I didn't lock the doors carefully enough*	40
2	*Imagine a home that I was selling burned down because I didn't turn the lights and appliances off and check them*	50
3	*Imagine my house burned down because I left appliances plugged in*	70
4	*I assaulted someone without realizing it and the police are after me*	80
5	*I killed someone without realizing it, and now the police are after me*	90

Andrea: Contamination

As is the case for most people with contamination obsessions, Andrea's triggers provoked upsetting images of germs and sickness, which she incorporated into her imaginal hierarchy.

Andrea's Imaginal Exposure Hierarchy: Contamination

Item	Description	SUDs rating
1	*Images of germs crawling all over my hands and skin*	45
2	*Images of germs on my things (pillows, cell phone, and the like)*	55
3	*Images of germs in my body*	75
4	*The thought that I will be contaminated forever and anxious about it forever*	80
5	*Images of my becoming sick*	90

Judy: Order and Balance

Order and balance obsessions can be tricky to address in imaginal exposure. Judy focused on the feeling of things being "not just right" and on the uncertainty of having to deal with this discomfort indefinitely. Some people with order obsessions have fears of other sorts of disastrous consequences that repeating, ordering, and arranging rituals serve to protect against. For example, "If I don't get dressed in just the 'just right' way, Mother will die." If you have these types of obsessions, you should incorporate these fears into your hierarchy.

Judy's Imaginal Exposure Hierarchy: Order and Balance

Item	Description	SUDs rating
1	Thoughts about how things are out of order	45
2	Images of my own diary having messy handwriting	55
3	Thinking of the word right (or left) without thinking the opposite	60
4	The thought that I will be anxious forever	75
5	The image of anxiety getting so intense that I go crazy or lose my mind	80

Alan: Violent Obsessions

Imaginal exposure for Alan was straightforward, although his hierarchy included very distressing doubts and violent images. First he practiced confronting his images of murdering his family, especially Kyle. Second, he confronted his doubts and uncertainty that he was a cold-blooded murderer. Notice the last item on Alan's hierarchy involved not knowing for sure whether he was a killer. This type of imaginal exposure to uncertainty is a useful tool for battling persistent obsessional doubts. We'll come back to this in Step 8.

Alan's Imaginal Exposure Hierarchy: Violent Obsessions

Item	Description	SUDs rating
1	Images of losing control and stabbing my wife	40
2	Images of stabbing Kyle	55
3	Images of killing my family with a baseball bat	60
4	Images of me suffocating Kyle with a plastic bag	70
5	Images of me drowning Kyle in the bathtub	80
6	I don't know for sure that I am not a cold-blooded killer who will one day act on these thoughts	85

Marla: Sexual Obsessions

Marla's imaginal exposure hierarchy was also clear-cut. She practiced purposely confronting her anxiety-provoking thoughts and fears that she was becoming a lesbian. Notice again, the first item is an "uncertainty exposure" (not knowing for sure).

Marla's Imaginal Exposure Hierarchy: Homosexual Obsessions

Item	Description	SUDs rating
1	*I don't know for sure whether I'm gay or straight*	*50*
2	*Thoughts that I am becoming a lesbian*	*60*
3	*Ideas of being in love with another woman*	*70*
4	*Images of hugging and kissing another woman*	*85*
5	*Images of being sexual with another woman*	*90*
6	*Images of having a lesbian relationship with my friend*	*95*
7	*Images of coming out of the closet to my friends and family*	*100*

Gene: Religious Obsessional Doubts

Gene's obsessions focused on doubts about whether he was a good Christian and whether he was being truly faithful to God. He was also concerned about what could happen in the afterlife if God didn't accept him (for example, "Will I go to heaven or hell?"). He confronted these doubts in imaginal exposure. Exposure to uncertainty also plays a role in several of Gene's hierarchy items.

Gene's Imaginal Exposure Hierarchy: Religious Obsessions

Item	Description	SUDs rating
1	*Doubt: I might not truly be living the Christian life*	*40*
2	*Doubt: I am not sure I have enough faith*	*50*
3	*The idea that other people might not think I am a good Christian*	*55*
4	*Doubt: I don't know whether I have a good relationship with God*	*55*

5	*The idea that God is upset with me*	*65*
6	*I don't know what will happen to me in the afterlife (heaven or hell?)*	*65*

Preparing Your Response Prevention Plan

Staying in the exposure situation until anxiety subsides (and doing so repeatedly) *without using rituals*—the *response prevention* part of your work—will teach you that you can weather the anxiety and that it will eventually diminish without your having to do anything to make it go away. It will also teach you that obsessional triggers and thoughts are less threatening than you had feared. Doing any rituals to reduce anxiety, on the other hand, will foil your exposure practices and prevent you from learning that you're safe even without rituals. Doing rituals also keeps you from learning more helpful strategies for coping with obsessional anxiety.

Deciding on Target Rituals

It's one thing to *know* that stopping rituals is an important part of overcoming OCD, but quite another to abstain successfully when you're in the midst of obsessional fear. After all, using rituals might seem like an automatic reaction. In this step, I'll help you develop a list of rituals to target once you begin exposure practice. Taking the time to carefully plan this list (as opposed to merely deciding to stop ritualizing) is an important part of defeating OCD since it will help you prepare for when you experience strong urges to ritualize. You might use one or more types of ritual to respond to your particular obsessions, which is another reason it's so important to develop a response prevention plan. In Step 9, I'll give you lots of tips and suggestions for how to implement your response prevention plan. At that point, we'll address common questions like:

- Do I need to stop rituals completely or just part of the way?
- How do I stop mental rituals?
- What do I do if my rituals are automatic and beyond my control?
- How do I manage my anxiety when I'm trying to stop ritualizing?

To begin preparing your list of target rituals, flip back and review your OCD Analysis Worksheet (page 39) and lists of compulsive rituals (page 54), mini-rituals (page 56), mental rituals (page 57), and reassurance-seeking strategies (page 58). Then, look back over the situational and imaginal exposure hierarchies you developed earlier in this chapter. When you do exposure practices that provoke obsessional anxiety, you'll probably also have urges to perform one or more of these rituals. It's also possible that your rituals have become so routine that you perform them even when you're not exposed to an obsessional trigger. For example, Ann Louise's ritual of making the sign of a cross with her fingers had become so automatic that she was doing this behavior throughout the day—even when she wasn't obsessing. It had simply developed into a habit. Leif's showering ritual was the same way. Whether or not he was having contamination obsessions, he took a 30-minute shower that involved very ritualized washing and cleaning of his body and the shower itself.

Carlos, whose situational and imaginal exposure hierarchies appear earlier in this chapter, used a variety of rituals in response to his obsessional thoughts and fears. The most prominent ones were mental rituals to "neutralize" or "cancel out" thoughts about death. For example, he would repeat the word *life* over and over to himself until any thoughts about death were no longer in his mind. When upsetting obsessional images of his children came to mind, Carlos had to imagine that his children were safe and repeat to himself "Everyone is safe and sound" until the upsetting thoughts were gone. Often he did these mental rituals along with repeating rituals: if an obsession occurred while he was doing an activity, Carlos repeated the action until it could be completed with a "good" thought, rather than with a "bad" one. Actions such as going through doorways, putting on clothes, turning on lights, and starting his car often had to be repeated many times while mentally neutralizing. Finally, Carlos engaged in counting rituals. To offset his fears of bad luck—and especially unlucky numbers (13 and 666)—Carlos would count to 4, which he considered a safe number. He would do things four times (turning on the light switch, chewing his food), and multiples of 4 (8, 12, 16, and so on), as a way of preventing bad luck from befalling his family. Carlos decided to target the following rituals in his response prevention plan:

> Have any of your rituals taken on a life of their own, becoming things you do all day long and not just when the associated obsession comes up?

- Repeating phrases ("life," "good luck," "everyone is safe and happy")
- Repeating actions (getting dressed, opening doors, turning on lights, starting the car, and so on)
- Counting to four and multiples of four
- Repeating something four (or multiples of four) times

You can use the Response Prevention Targets form on page 110 to list the rituals you wish to target. I understand if you're very worried about ending rituals that seem realistic, important, or necessary, such as checking the rearview mirror for accidents, praying to God, washing after using the bathroom, and checking that appliances are turned off. Don't worry about stopping these behaviors just yet—when you get to Step 9, I'll teach you what you need to know to help you cut down on these rituals more easily. All I'm asking you to do right now is make a list of the ritualistic behaviors you perform—and to keep an open mind about stopping them later in the program. Remember, these rituals are part of the vicious cycle of OCD.

Sample Response Prevention Plans

Let's take a look at how the six people with OCD described earlier in this step planned to implement response prevention. You can use their examples to help with your own planning, again keeping in mind that your own lists should be made up of the rituals associated with the situations and thoughts on your exposure hierarchies that you recorded in Step 2.

Response Prevention Targets

Item	Description of Ritual
1	
2	
3	
4	
5	
6	
7	
8	
9	
10	

Ronnie: Responsibility for Harm or Damage

Ronnie engaged in checking and reassurance-seeking rituals to reduce anxiety and uncertainty about possible disasters. He sometimes used excessive prayer to quell his fears. Ronnie's response prevention plan targeted the following rituals:

- *Checking appliances and locks in my own house*
- *Checking on houses I have shown to potential buyers*
- *Praying that my feared disasters don't come true*
- *Calling the police and hospitals to make sure no disasters were reported*
- *Calling neighbors to make sure my house is okay*
- *Asking my relatives for reassurance about how dangerous they think certain situations are*

Andrea: Contamination

Andrea's main rituals were excessive washing and cleaning herself and her possessions. Sometimes she even asked other people to wash or clean if they were going to come into contact with her things. Andrea's response prevention plan addressed the following rituals:

- *Hand washing*
- *Using disinfectant hand gels*
- *Using sleeve or other barrier to open doors or touch things*
- *Washing other parts of my body to excess (genitals, face)*
- *Showering more than once per day*
- *Changing my clothes in the middle of the day*
- *Doing extra loads of laundry*
- *Cleaning things around the house to excess (pillows, couch)*
- *Asking other people to wash especially for me*
- *Asking doctors about germs/illnesses or looking up information on the Internet*

Judy: Order and Balance

Items on Judy's exposure hierarchies evoked urges to rewrite things perfectly, organize them "just right," and try to achieve left–right "balance" by thinking these words, or by touching or doing things with her right or left hand. Thus, her target rituals were as follows:

- *"Balancing" out a room so that it has left–right "evenness"*
- *Saying "left" or "right" if I hear (or think) the opposite word*
- *Doing something with my left (or right) side to balance out if I did it with the other side*
- *Rewriting letters and words if they look messy*
- *Arranging items in the house "just right"*

Alan: Violent Obsessions

Alan had a number of subtle and mini-rituals he used to reduce his fears of acting on his violent obsessions. He also tried to analyze the meaning of his intrusive thoughts and sometimes asked others for reassurance about this ("Do you think I will kill the kids?"). Alan frequently searched the Internet for information about murderers and compared himself to the people he read about as a way of gauging whether he was the "kind of person" who might commit murder. The following rituals appeared on his response prevention list:

- *Asking other people (wife, mother) for reassurance about my thoughts*
- *Mentally trying to figure out what the thoughts mean and why I have them*
- *Praying for the thoughts to stop and for me not to kill anyone*
- *Locking up the knives and other potential weapons*

- *Purposely touching the children gently*
- *Searching the Internet for information about child/family murderers*

Marla: Sexual Obsessions

Marla engaged in mental rituals involving trying to push homosexual thoughts out of her mind. She also had reassurance-seeking and analyzing rituals in which she tried to figure out what her unwanted sexual thoughts "really" meant. In a similar vein, she mentally reviewed her sexual and dating history to reassure herself that she had never been attracted to (or sexually active with) other women. Finally, Marla had a "testing" ritual that involved looking at (or thinking about) attractive men (and women) and trying to determine whether or not she had any sort of sexual response that could be an indicator of how she "really felt." Marla's response prevention plan included working on stopping the following rituals:

- *Fighting, resisting, suppressing, or pushing away unwanted homosexual thoughts*
- *Trying to figure out why I am having these thoughts and what they really mean (mental analyzing)*
- *Reviewing my dating and sexual relationships to prove I am not a lesbian*
- *Asking my husband about the thoughts and whether he thinks I am gay*
- *"Testing" my sexual preference for men or women*

Gene: Religious Obsessional Doubts

Gene's obsessions provoked urges to seek reassurance about his faith and relationship with God. He repeatedly asked his pastor, counselor, wife, parents, and friends about whether they thought he was living a "good Christian life" and whether they thought he had been sinful. Gene also engaged in constant confessing and prayer rituals that involved apologizing to God for any possible moral missteps or lapses in faith. He chose to target the following rituals:

- *Asking for reassurances about my faith in God*
- *Asking people if they think I am a "good Christian" or living a "good Christian life"*
- *Asking people if they think I have committed a sin*
- *Excessive praying about my obsessional doubts*
- *Excessive confessing and apologizing to God*

Are You Ready to Move On to Step 5?

We've covered a lot of ground in Step 4, from how the components of CBT work to which obsessions and rituals you plan to target when you use these CBT techniques in your exposure and response prevention work in Part III. At this point it's normal to feel overwhelmed about embarking on a treatment program that will include facing your fears and resisting your rituals. You may even be thinking that the cure sounds worse than the disease—a belief that causes some people with OCD to refuse to try CBT. It's very unfortunate for them that they do, and this is the exact reason I've included Step 5 in this book. In the next step I'll help you carefully examine your own mixed feelings about moving forward from the planning phase into the action phase of your battle against OCD. I think you'll leave Step 5 armed with the conviction that facing your obsessional fears is well worth the effort. After all, it's *your* life you're taking back from OCD.

STEP 5

Strengthening Your Resolve to Move Forward

Tonya had intrusive obsessional doubts that she might have accidentally killed a childhood friend she hadn't heard from in over 30 years. Of course, she couldn't recall *actually* hurting anyone—Tonya thought of herself as a very gentle person and had no history of violent behavior. Still, the doubts seemed very real, and she couldn't bear the possibility that she might be a murderer. To reduce her obsessional distress, Tonya often tried to remember back through her childhood to see if she could recall committing murder. She also checked local newspaper archives for stories of mysterious deaths around the time the mythical murder would have happened. These rituals did little to provide the reassurance she was looking for.

Tonya often thought about getting help for her problem and had accumulated a large pile of referral information and self-help books about OCD. Occasionally (usually on days when her obsessions were especially intense), she would look through this information and start to read the material. However, instead of making her feel hopeful, her reading usually made her think about how immoral it would be to ignore the possibility that she had murdered someone. A few times she even thought of just turning herself in to the police. Reading about CBT (exposure and response prevention) also made Tonya anxious and depressed. Although on some level she understood the senselessness of her obsessions and the potential benefit of treatment, she was also uneasy about trying the therapy and thought all she needed was a guarantee that she was not a murderer. Tonya was stuck.

If you're like the majority of people I've worked with, you (like Tonya) probably have mixed feelings about obsessions and rituals and about moving forward with your program for change. You'd like to be rid of OCD, but there's also a faint (or maybe not so faint) voice in your head telling you that your fears and rituals might be realistic or that facing your fears by doing exposure and response prevention isn't such a good idea. These kinds of mixed feelings about change are normal. We call them *ambivalence*, the state of having opposing positive and negative feelings *at the same time*. Maybe you view checking rituals as senseless and excessive on the one hand, but on the other hand you worry that they're crucial to preventing disaster. You might be completely fed up with how your religious and scrupulous obsessions are ruining your life, yet also believe that treatment might turn you into an atheist. You might have had it with your compulsive washing but at the same time think that these rituals are necessary to avoid becoming sick.

Ambivalence is not an all-or-nothing thing—it's a matter of degree. Some people have only a small amount, whereas others experience a great deal. Furthermore, a person's degree of ambivalence can change over time. If you experience very little ambivalence, you might be able to work through it yourself. In fact, you might be reading this book because you've already done so. But if you're feeling very indecisive, like Tonya, you probably have high levels of ambivalence. And like Tonya, your ambivalence might result in your maintaining the status quo—which means not working on OCD and continuing to live with its negative effects.

Most self-help books assume that readers feel little or no ambivalence and expect them to eagerly follow any instructions that might mean improving their life. I can't make that assumption. I know there are many people just like Tonya who will read about the details of the treatment program in this workbook and decide it just isn't worth it. I don't want you to miss the opportunity to make significant improvements in your life, so this chapter is designed to help you examine your ambivalence toward the program and avoid getting stalled before you even begin.

Tonya did the important work in this step, and as a result her story had a happy ending. She happened to attend a forum about OCD that I led at her local library and decided to make an appointment at our clinic. At her consultation, and for several sessions thereafter, we explored her desire to get over OCD and her reluctance to do exposure therapy. I never pushed her to confront her fears or to stop ritualizing. We focused only on the pros and cons of having OCD and the pros and cons of working to overcome it. In the end, Tonya concluded that she had much to gain by trying CBT—even if it meant temporarily feeling anxious. Ultimately she was extremely successful and thankful she made the decision to do what she did.

Are You Ready to Work on OCD?

I'm reading this book, aren't I? Of course I want to change!

When you ask yourself whether you're ready for change, is your honest answer "yes and no"?

If your answer is that simple, you're not dealing with ambivalence and might consider skipping this step and moving on to Step 6. But if your answer is more like "yes and no," let's find out what's holding you back. What Tonya discovered during her examination of her own ambivalence was that she wasn't ready for change until she had more reasons for changing than for not changing.

One of the first things I asked Tonya to do when she came to see me was to make two lists: a list of reasons why she wanted to work on her OCD and a list of her reasons for not wanting to work on it. Tonya's lists appear at the bottom of the page.

Tonya's lists were very revealing. On the one hand, she felt she was managing pretty well, her symptoms weren't hurting anyone else, and participating in treatment could be scary. On the other hand, Tonya's symptoms caused her a great deal of anxiety, her self-concept was suffering, her OCD symptoms often interfered with her life, and she was concerned her kids would grow up and develop OCD themselves unless she got treatment. Tonya looked at me skeptically when I pointed out that she actually had a number of good reasons for *and* against working on OCD. She was sure I was only using this exercise to set up an argument for treatment and was quite surprised when I suggested that we talk about her reasons for *not* changing. Sure, I wanted to help Tonya change since OCD was causing her pain. But I knew from experience with many other people dealing with the same struggles that if her reasons for not changing overshadowed her reasons for changing, Tonya was not ready to work on the problem, and trying to do so would probably end in frustration for her. The same is true for you, and this is why it's so important to look thoroughly at both sides of the coin.

A pearl I can pass on to you from my extensive clinical experience is that *you will begin to work on your problems with OCD only when your reasons for changing outweigh your reasons for not changing.* It's that simple.

Tonya's reasons to work on OCD	Tonya's reasons not to work on OCD
1. I don't want this to rub off on my kids.	*1. Exposure and response prevention will make me too anxious. I couldn't stand it.*
2. I want to have control over my life.	*2. I can't imagine not knowing for sure whether I killed someone.*
3. Rituals take more and more time away from things I would rather be doing.	*3. It's not the best situation, but I can get by with the way things are now.*
4. I could be myself again.	*4. My problems aren't hurting anyone else.*
5. I spend too much time worried about things that are probably senseless.	*5. I don't want to give in to everyone who tells me I'm crazy or I need help.*
6. My relationships would be a lot richer if I didn't have OCD.	*6. I don't have the time to devote to treatment.*
7. OCD makes me feel bad about myself.	
8. My thoughts and rituals get in the way of too many things and keep me from enjoying myself.	

Determining Your Readiness for Change

The statements in the Readiness for Change Survey below describe how a person might feel when thinking about OCD. Circle the number that corresponds to how much you agree or disagree with each statement. Make your choices based on how you feel *right now*, not how you have felt in the past or how you would like to feel. You'll get the most benefit from this exercise if you use a pencil or pen and write your answers down rather than just thinking about them. There's something about writing that forces you to think more clearly and carefully about your answers.

Readiness for Change Survey

Circle the number that corresponds to how much you agree or disagree with each statement.

1 = Strongly Disagree (SD)
2 = Disagree (D)
3 = Undecided (U)
4 = Agree (A)
5 = Strongly Agree (SA)

	SD	D	U	A	SA
1. As far as I'm concerned, I don't have a problem with OCD that needs changing.	1	2	3	4	5
2. I'm not the problem. It doesn't make sense for me to be using the program in this book.	1	2	3	4	5
3. I have a problem with OCD, and I really think I should work on it.	1	2	3	4	5
4. I'm hoping the program in this workbook will help me better understand myself and my OCD.	1	2	3	4	5
5. I am already doing something about OCD.	1	2	3	4	5
6. Anyone can *talk* about changing. I am actually *doing* something more.	1	2	3	4	5
7. It worries me that I might slip back on the gains I have already made against OCD, so I am hoping this workbook can help.	1	2	3	4	5
8. I am doing much better with OCD than I had been doing, but sometimes I still find myself struggling.	1	2	3	4	5

Adapted from McConnaughy, E., Prochaska, J., & Velicer, W. (1983). Stages of change in psychotherapy: measurement and sample profiles. *Psychotherapy: Theory, Research, and Practice*, *20*, 368–375.

Now make a few easy calculations:

- Add up your responses to items 1 and 2: ____________. This is your *precontemplation* score.
- Add up your responses to items 3 and 4: ____________. This is your *contemplation* score.
- Add up your responses to items 5 and 6: ____________. This is your *action* score.
- Add up your responses to items 7 and 8: ____________. This is your *maintenance* score.

Which of these four scores is the highest? If your highest score is for *precontemplation*, it means that right now you don't consider OCD a big enough problem to invest the time and energy it takes for a successful battle. Perhaps working through the exercises in this chapter will help you see things a different way; perhaps not. If your highest score is for *contemplation*, you are bothered by OCD but have not yet committed to doing something about it. This chapter is definitely an important one for you. Work through it thoughtfully and carefully. If *action* is your highest score, you've probably started the change process but may need a helping hand. The exercises in this chapter are geared toward enhancing your motivation and your resolve to push onward. If your highest score is for *maintenance*, you've already made noticeable progress in your battle with OCD, but you could use some help with staying on track. If so, you might think about moving on to Step 6, as Step 5 might not apply to you.

What Are the Pros and Cons of Change?

If you're pretty certain you need to work through this chapter, the worksheet on the facing page will help you begin to explore your own personal feelings about using the CBT techniques in this workbook to battle against OCD. "My Feelings about Working on OCD" has two columns. On the left side, write down your reasons for working on OCD. Then, on the right side, list your reasons for *not* working on OCD. If you need help coming up with ideas, take a look at Tonya's lists on page 116.

Which list is longer? If it's the list of reasons *for* working on OCD, you're on the right track. On the other hand, if you have more reasons for *not* working, you might have a difficult time staying motivated and being successful with this program. In fact, unless you find more reasons to change, there probably isn't much point in even trying to use the strategies in this workbook. Chances are your reasons for not working on OCD will become excuses for not fully or properly doing the challenging work that lies ahead. Maybe the exercise in the next section can help.

When you list your reasons for changing and your reasons for **not** changing, which list is longer?

What Is OCD Costing You?

If your reasons for *not* working on OCD outweigh your reasons for working on it, maybe your obsessions and rituals aren't terribly bothersome for you. Aroon worked for a pharma-

My Feelings about Working on OCD	
Reasons to work on OCD	**Reasons not to work on OCD**

ceutical company and lived by himself. He traveled a lot for his job and could set his own schedule most of the time. This allowed him to adjust his life around his obsessive fears of certain "bad luck" numbers (666, 13, and multiples of 7) and his repeating and mental rituals. Consequently, these symptoms didn't interfere much with his work life, and Aroon didn't have much of a social life. When traveling, he didn't mind asking for a different hotel room if he was initially assigned a room on the seventh floor. He also adjusted his daily schedule to include time for other avoidance strategies and rituals. Having OCD cost Aroon very little, and therefore he avoided getting help.

How much does OCD interfere in your life?

Perhaps your problems with OCD are not very bothersome because significant others in your life bear the brunt of your obsessions and rituals. Do you have the people around you (for example, your family or close friends) avoid situations that trigger your obsessions? Do they help you complete your rituals, do them for you, allow you extra time to do them, or give you constant reassurance? If other people are helping you avoid and carry out rituals, it might make it easier for you to live with OCD, and you might not fully recognize all the true disadvantages of having this problem. Esther's story illustrates what happens when a person's family accommodates his or her OCD symptoms.

Esther was 35 and unemployed. She lived with her mother and father. She had contamination fears and demanded that her parents carry out elaborate washing and cleansing rituals every time they entered the house so they would not bring germs inside. Esther refused to touch mail, groceries, or dirty laundry unless it had been washed down. She also refused to enter the laundry room and insisted her mother do all of the family's laundry in a certain excessive and ritualized way. Among other things, parts of the house were "off limits" to any family member unless proper decontamination rituals had been performed. When Esther finally decided to see me for a consultation—only after strong urging and threats from her parents—she said that OCD was not really a big problem for her. And in a sense she was right. OCD had become her *parents'* problem. By giving in to Esther's demands, they were bearing the brunt of her OCD and dealing with its consequences. Esther never recognized all the negatives.

> If OCD is only a minor problem for you, could it be a major problem for those trying to help you deal with it?

Following is a list of emotional, social, financial, and practical consequences of having OCD. Consider each one carefully; they come from people with OCD that I have evaluated and treated. Check each one that applies to you.

Emotional consequences

- ☐ Anxiety
- ☐ Depression
- ☐ Guilt
- ☐ Shame and embarrassment
- ☐ Dissatisfaction
- ☐ Insecurity
- ☐ Loneliness
- ☐ Feelings of worthlessness
- ☐ Anger and irritability
- ☐ Concern that your children will develop OCD
- ☐ Other emotional consequences: ______________________________

Social consequences

- ☐ Stress on family relationships
- ☐ Arguments with family members
- ☐ Fear of being teased, embarrassed, ridiculed, laughed at, or rejected
- ☐ Problems with dating and intimate relationships
- ☐ Fear of losing someone in your life
- ☐ Unemployment or problems with working
- ☐ Problems with developing friendships
- ☐ Unable to enjoy social or leisure activities
- ☐ Having to make excuses or lying about the problem

- ☐ Problems with school
- ☐ Turning to alcohol or drugs to cope
- ☐ Other social consequences: ________________________________

Financial consequences

- ☐ Costs of treatment (psychological treatment and medication)
- ☐ Costs of products such as soaps, lotions, toilet paper, gasoline, water
- ☐ Missed days of work
- ☐ Other financial costs: ________________________________

Practical consequences

- ☐ Difficulty sleeping
- ☐ Problems with sexual functioning
- ☐ Difficulty with using the bathroom, taking a shower, and other self-care behaviors
- ☐ Difficulty driving
- ☐ Problems with traveling (specify): ________________________________
- ☐ Chronic lateness
- ☐ Medical problems (for example, dry, cracked hands from too much washing) _____ ________________________________
- ☐ Problems with practicing your religion
- ☐ Avoidance of activities you would like to do (going to parties, eating out)
- ☐ Avoidance of certain people or places
- ☐ Avoidance of certain rooms or items in your home
- ☐ Avoidance of routine activities such as driving, shaking hands, opening doors, reading certain books, watching certain TV programs or movies, and so on.
- ☐ Other practical consequences: ________________________________

With your answers to the checklist items in mind, answer the questions in the worksheet on the next two pages to help you see the negative consequences of having OCD. Again, this activity will be most beneficial if you actually write down your answers rather than just thinking about them.

Now that you've thought more carefully about the negative consequences of OCD, do you want to change? Would you like to be able to control your obsessive thoughts and fears and your urges to perform compulsive behaviors and other kinds of rituals? Wouldn't it be great if you didn't have to worry about negative consequences? Let's consider these questions in the next section.

How Would Fighting (and Winning) the Battle against OCD Make Your Life Better?

I know it's not easy to really stop and think about all the negatives associated with OCD. Now it's time to look at the flip side: the positives of working on OCD and making some

The Negative Consequences of Having OCD

What bothers you most about your problems with OCD?

To begin with, write down the five things that bother you most about your problems with OCD. These might be items from the checklist you just reviewed, or they might be new things you think of.

1. ________________________________
2. ________________________________
3. ________________________________
4. ________________________________
5. ________________________________

How have these most bothersome problems interfered in various areas of your life?

First, how have they disrupted your social life?

- How do they get in the way of friendships and intimate relationships?
- How do they restrict activities with other people?

Describe in your own words how OCD impacts this part of your life:

Next, how have they impacted your family life?

- How does OCD cause tension, bad feelings, or arguments with relatives?
- How does it keep you from reaching your full potential as a spouse or partner, parent, grandparent, son, daughter, sibling?
- How does it interfere with family activities such as celebrating holidays?
- How do your family members feel about it?

The Negative Consequences of Having OCD *(cont.)*

Third, what about your performance at work or school?

- Are you able to work?
- If not, how does OCD keep you from working?
- If you can work, how does having OCD hold you back from achieving at your peak level on the job?
- If you are a student, how has your academic work been stifled by OCD?

Last, but not least, how does OCD affect you financially?

- Have obsessional fears and rituals led to unemployment or being passed over for promotions?
- Do you use extra gas because you turn the car around to check or drive out of your way?
- Do you frequently have to buy soap, detergent, toilet paper, or other cleaning products?
- How has OCD been a financial burden?

changes. By working hard at this program, you have the opportunity to improve your relationships with other people, increase your productivity, and step up your personal accomplishments. You might also develop more self-confidence and self-esteem and become more satisfied with life.

How have you dealt with personal challenges in the past?

Maybe you don't believe you have the discipline or willpower to change. To enhance your motivation to work on OCD, think about some of the personal challenges you've faced in the past. How have you coped with or overcome them? You might find battling OCD to be easier, harder, or about the same as working through previous challenges. But, if you've ever overcome adversity before, you can surely muster the courage to do it again!

Below, describe important challenges you have had to deal with in the past:

____

____

____

____

____

What are the advantages of working on OCD?

- How would your life be different if you weren't bothered by obsessive thoughts, the need to avoid certain things, urges to do rituals, and other emotional difficulties associated with these problems?
- What would you do if fear and anxiety didn't hold you back?
- What would you accomplish with the time wasted on repeating compulsive rituals?

Think about these questions and then below write down several ways your life would be better without OCD in the picture:

____

____

____

____

____

Earlier, I asked you to think about how significant others in your life are affected by your problems with OCD.

- Do they act negatively toward you?
- Do they get angry or critical?

- What would they think if you, on your own, decided to put an end to your problems with OCD?
- Would accomplishing something like defeating OCD get them off your back?
- Wouldn't it be nice to show them that you're stronger than they think?

Many people I see in my clinical practice are highly motivated by the idea that if they worked on OCD, others would treat them differently—with greater respect. Describe below how people in *your* life might think of you and treat you better if you were to win your battle against OCD:

____

____

____

____

____

At this point, you've explored disadvantages of the status quo and advantages of making changes. Perhaps you see that you could be better off in lots of ways if you worked on OCD. But CBT itself—especially exposure and response prevention—seems very hard. Is coping with all that anxiety worthwhile? In the next section, you'll explore your feelings about these treatment strategies.

The Pros and Cons of Treatment

I've said all along that overcoming OCD is challenging. Unfortunately, there is no way around it. If you're going to learn to control obsessions and compulsions, you are going to have to face your fears and reduce (or stop) your ritualizing at some point. But as scary as this might sound, the truth is that the anxiety and fear provoked by exposure and response prevention are only temporary side effects. They don't persist, and they don't have any long-lasting harmful consequences. A good analogy is getting an injection. Vaccinations, for example, can be painful in the short term, but they have very important long-term benefits: they keep you from getting serious illnesses. What would happen if people focused only on the pain of getting an injection? No one would ever choose to be vaccinated! In a similar way, you will need to look beyond the short-term anxiety when you do exposure and response prevention and keep your focus on the long-term benefits. You'll need to *choose to be anxious*. I will give you more specific techniques in later steps to help you cope with this anxiety, but *you* still have to make the decision to face your fears rather than run and hide from them.

> **There are concrete techniques you can use to cope with anxiety during exposure and response prevention, but the decision to face your fears is yours to make.**

Robert had violent obsessions and repeating rituals. If a violent thought about a loved one came to mind, Robert had to repeat whatever he was doing until he could complete the

	Pros of Doing CBT	*Cons of Doing CBT*
Short term		• *I'll have lots of bad thoughts in my mind.* • *I'll feel very afraid.* • *It will take up lots of time.* • *I'll lose sleep because of the fear.* • *I'll be tense and irritable.*
Long term	• *I'll learn that I won't be anxious forever.* • *I'll eventually stop worrying so much about other people.* • *I'll learn to control the urges to repeat tasks.* • *My kids and coworkers won't see me acting so strangely.* • *My family will be happier.*	

task without the obsessional thought in his mind. Closing doors, putting on shoes, doing chores at work—all were affected by his problems with OCD. Robert weighed the pros and cons of working on his problems using CBT. He wanted badly to get better, but knew that facing his fears would be challenging. When Robert divided the pros and cons of doing CBT into *short-* and *long*-term groups, he found something very interesting. Can you see a pattern in the chart of Robert's pros and cons?

Hard CBT work up front pays off in disproportionate gains over the long term.

It's pretty obvious: Robert's cons are short-term, while his pros are long-term. This explains why *you* might have trouble following through with working on OCD; you probably become too focused on how anxious you are feeling in the moment and don't stop to think about the long-term consequences of facing your fears and resisting rituals. Psychologist Richard Heimberg coined the phrase "*Invest anxiety now in order to have a calmer future*," which I think makes the exact point you need to consider if you are to change your attitude toward doing CBT. When working through this workbook, you're probably going to have to make a substantial effort to face anxiety and resist doing rituals. But it's worth it. Doing this hard work up front is likely to pay off "big time" in the long run, and you'll eventually get to enjoy the long-term benefits of beating OCD.

Setting Goals for Yourself

"*If you aim at nothing, you will surely hit it.*" This simple yet inspirational adage captures the importance of setting goals for your battle against OCD. Imagine you're playing base-

> Could you win a baseball game if there were no bases on the field?

ball and you've just hit the ball. You're running to first base, but wait ... there are no bases! Are you safe or out? To win, you have to round the bases and score runs for your team. So when there are no bases, there's no way of knowing if you've won the game, right? It's the same thing with battling OCD. You need to have a target—a goal—that helps you measure your success. In this section, we'll set goals for your self-help program.

How to Set SMART Goals

Goal setting is the process of deciding on (1) what's important for you to achieve and (2) in what time frame you aim to achieve it. But not all goals people set for themselves are effective or motivating; in fact, sometimes we choose goals that actually make us *less* likely to change. I recommend using the acronym SMART to help you decide on your goals to keep you motivated through this program. Your goals should be:

S = Specific
M = Measurable
A = Achievable
R = Relevant
T = Time bound

Specific

Think of your goals as your road map to success. They need to be as detailed and specific as possible. State exactly what you want to achieve. This will help you focus your efforts and clearly define what you are striving to do. For example, if you were out of shape, the goal of "getting in shape" would be too vague. It would be more helpful to set a specific goal to "take a 1-mile walk three times this week" or "eat three servings of vegetables every day." Achieving these goals will help you get in shape. In OCD terms, simply saying "My goal is to get over OCD" or "I want to get more out of life" is not enough.

One thing you might have noticed about the goals listed in the box below is that they

Sample Specific Goals for People with OCD

- Cut down on time spent washing my hands by 50% (someone with washing rituals)
- Leave the house without checking the appliances or locks (person with checking rituals)
- Go to confession but do not confess any sins more than once (scrupulosity)
- Leave my room with the clothes and books out of order (ordering obsessions and rituals)
- Drive without turning the car around to check for injured persons (checking rituals)
- Stay at home alone with the baby (this person has violent obsessional thoughts)
- Use the locker room at the gym (someone with homosexual obsessions)
- Conduct two exposure practices every day for 1 week (anyone with OCD)

are all based on personal performance. Setting *performance goals* allows *you* to determine whether you meet your goals and get satisfaction from them. *Outcome goals*, on the other hand, are based on the rewards of achieving something, such as getting recognition for working on OCD. The problem with outcome goals is that you can't always depend on other people (or situations) to give you rewards. For example, what if you completely stop your hand-washing rituals but still have trouble with dating? If you had set an outcome goal of getting more dates (which requires someone else to say "yes"), then you would not meet your goal. But, if you set a performance goal of stopping your washing rituals, you would have achieved the goal and could draw satisfaction and self-confidence from this success.

Are your goals based on what you can do, or do they depend on what someone else does?

Measurable

Goals need to be measurable so that you know when you've succeeded. So choose concrete goals you can easily keep track of. The examples you just read all adhere to this rule. "I will spend 50% less time doing compulsive rituals" gives a specific target to be measured: time spent ritualizing. On the other hand, "I want to control my compulsive rituals" is not a measurable goal: How will you decide when you've got *control*? The symptom rating forms you completed back in Step 2 (page 62) provide tangible ways of measuring progress with obsessional fears, avoidance, and rituals. So, setting goals of reducing scores (for example, the number or timing of rituals) on these forms is an excellent idea.

Do your goals include a number, making them measurable?

Achievable

Your goals should also challenge you to stay focused and committed to your treatment plan, but at the same time they need to be realistic. If you set goals that stretch you slightly—that require *some* effort to achieve—you will feel like you can achieve them and stay motivated. On the other hand, you probably won't stay committed to goals you set that are too far out of reach. For example, "I will never do an OCD ritual again" is probably unattainable, especially if you're just beginning to work on OCD. When you eventually realize trying for such a goal is a lost cause, you'll feel demoralized and risk losing momentum. Instead, "I will reduce my counting rituals by 50% by the end of this week" is probably a more reasonable (and also a more *specific*) goal. Don't bite off more than you can chew!

Can you position your goals somewhere between effortless to achieve and impossible?

On the other hand, be careful not to set goals *too* low. Aim for goals that are *just out of reach*. When you accomplish one, you'll have the momentum to move on to another. Many people with OCD, for instance, aim to reduce their rituals by 50% the first week, another 50% the next week, and another 50% the week after that. The eventual result is a dramatic decrease in rituals, but they've broken it down into smaller, achievable goals (steps) rather than trying to do it all at once. Think about it: if it takes you 15 minutes to run 1 mile, but you want to be able to run it in 7 minutes, you wouldn't expect to cut your time down all at once (this would be next to impossible). Instead, you would first aim for 14 minutes, then for 13, 12, and so on until you could run the mile in 7 minutes. Try to apply the same strategy to working on OCD. When you pick achievable goals, you figure out new ways to reach them. This, along with being successful, helps you stay motivated. In time, your smaller achievements add up and you will be able to look back at how far you've come.

Relevant

Without some sort of emotional tie to your goals, you will have trouble keeping up the motivation to achieve them. In other words, your goals should mean something to you—they should be *relevant*. If you're working on OCD, they should obviously relate to success in battling this problem. Of course, this doesn't rule out striving for goals in related areas such as relationships (I will do three more activities with my family this week), finances (I will spend half as much money on cleaning supplies), or work/school (I will hand in assignments on time this semester). However, make sure you stick to *performance* goals rather than *outcome* goals. Tying goals to something that is important to you will build your commitment to achieving it. To ensure that a goal is relevant, ask yourself how achieving it will affect (1) your overall success in getting control of OCD, (2) those around you, and (3) your quality of life.

Will reaching your goals result in personally meaningful gains?

Time-Bound

Finally, your goals should have a time frame. That is, you need a start date and an end date. For example, "by the end of the day," "in 1 week," or "in 3 months." By putting an end point on your goal you make it a priority, which increases motivation. Goals without specific time frames are less likely to be met because you feel you can put them off. As with goals in general, the time frame you choose should be realistic. It should also be fairly short term. Setting short-term goals will keep you active in your battle against OCD. Long-term goals (more than a few weeks) don't provide the same sense of urgency and motivation to start taking action as short-term goals do. Here are some examples of short-term goals:

Could you win a baseball game that never ended?

- I will not call the rabbi for reassurance this week.
- I will go out to dinner tomorrow night and not call the babysitter to check on the kids.
- I will take out the trash this week without changing my clothes afterwards.
- I will conduct two exposure practices every day this week.
- I will review Step 5 of this workbook once every day.
- I will shake hands with everyone in the reception line after the wedding this weekend.

Choosing *Your* Goals

Keeping the SMART guidelines in mind, take some time to think about what you want to achieve for yourself:

- Why are you reading this book?
- What would you like to change?
- What do you want to be able to do more easily?
- What do you have to gain by battling your OCD?
- What negative consequences of OCD would you like to remove from your life?
- Where should you start?
- Where would you like to end up?

Actually writing down your goals greatly increases your chances of success. Simply thinking about them is not enough; you must write them down, using the worksheet on the facing page. This worksheet also contains questions to help you think carefully about your goals. I recommend making copies of the blank form so you can use it for additional sets of goals. There is also little point in setting goals unless you *review* them on a regular basis—*weekly* is good; *daily* is better!—to monitor and steer your progress. Post your written goals where you can easily see them: the refrigerator, your mirror, your desk. If significant others are helping you with your battle against OCD (see the section below), post your goals where they can view your progress and help cheer you on. Knowing that others are aware of your goals can be highly motivating. On page 132 is a sample Personal Goals form that was completed by Candice, who had problems with compulsive checking.

Rewarding Yourself

Don't fall into the trap of trying to keep yourself motivated by approaching this program from a position of guilt, doubt, or shame. Never beat yourself up about the problems you haven't overcome yet. Imagine if you tried to motivate someone else this way. Do you think they'd stick around? How successful would they be?

> How does it feel when someone tries to get you to do something by trying to make you feel guilty?

Instead of focusing on what you haven't yet accomplished, let me recommend rewarding yourself each time you achieve one of your goals. Giving yourself a pat on the back and a word of encouragement will not only make you feel good; it will motivate you to work even harder to achieve your next goal. Even the smallest of rewards can work wonders as you move from goal to goal. Think about how you will reward yourself for accomplishing each of your goals (there is space on the Personal Goals for Battling OCD worksheet for writing down your reward system). Make your rewards meaningful and pleasurable to you (see Candice's examples, as well as some more below). Use smaller rewards for meeting smaller goals and bigger ones after you've accomplished larger goals over the longer term. Involve other people if you like. Create a celebration that you can anticipate and then keep it within sight all the time. Finally, be honest with yourself. Fudging the numbers mentally, or "borrowing" against the next

Personal Goals for Battling OCD

My personal goals for this program are:

1. ______________________________
2. ______________________________
3. ______________________________
4. ______________________________
5. ______________________________

Next, think about what made you choose these goals? Why are they important to you? Fill in the blanks to complete the sentences below:

It's important for me to work on OCD because:

1. ______________________________
2. ______________________________
3. ______________________________
4. ______________________________
5. ______________________________

If I work hard on getting over OCD, my life is likely to change in the following ways:

1. ______________________________
2. ______________________________
3. ______________________________
4. ______________________________
5. ______________________________

If I do *not* work on my OCD problem, the following negative things will happen:

1. ______________________________
2. ______________________________
3. ______________________________
4. ______________________________
5. ______________________________

When I accomplish each goal, I will reward myself with:

1. ______________________________
2. ______________________________
3. ______________________________
4. ______________________________
5. ______________________________

Candice's Personal Goals for Battling OCD

My personal goals for this program are:

1. *Reduce the number of times I call Mom to once per day this week.*
2. *Stop visiting OCD chat rooms to check that other people have similar experiences as me.*
3. *Spend at least 1 hour per day this week working on my OCD.*
4. *Reduce the scores on the Symptom Rating Form by at least 50% in 3 months.*

Next, think about what made you choose these goals? Why are they important to you? Fill in the blanks to complete the sentences below:

It's important for me to work on OCD because:

1. *OCD is getting in the way of my relationship with Mom.*
2. *I want to show my family that I'm stronger than they think I am.*
3. *I don't want Mom to be so upset with me for calling her all the time.*
4. *Having OCD is like dragging a 500-pound weight everywhere I go.*

If I work hard on getting over OCD, my life is likely to change in the following ways:

1. *I will feel more confident dating.*
2. *I'll feel better about myself and seem more attractive to others.*
3. *Better relationships with family (Mom).*
4. *I won't have to rely on checking and reassurance seeking to feel better.*
5. *I won't have problems with lateness or getting stuck doing senseless things.*

If I do *not* work on my OCD problem, the following negative things will continue to happen:

1. *I'll continue to struggle with bad thoughts and checking.*
2. *I'll continue to be worried about disasters all the time, like Mom dying in an accident.*
3. *I'll never feel comfortable in my own skin.*
4. *How can I find true love if I don't even love myself?*

When I accomplish each goal, I will reward myself with:

1. *After each exposure practice I do, I will take a nice bubble bath.*
2. *After I finish a week of daily practices, I will get a massage.*
3. *When I reduce my scores, I will buy the new computer I've been saving up for.*

reward, will hurt you in the long run. Remember to keep your focus on the battle against OCD, not just figuring out how to get the reward.

If you need help thinking of rewards, some examples my patients have used appear in the box at the bottom of this page.

Understand that your drive to do CBT might waver as you work your way through the steps in this workbook. When the going gets rough, you can help sustain your motivation by reviewing your goals. Luckily, one advantage of the CBT techniques we will use in Steps 6 through 10 is that they get easier as you go along. Getting started is the hardest part—and there will be occasional bumps in the road ahead—but for the most part, your successes in helping yourself will provide ongoing motivation.

Don't Go It Alone: Getting a "Treatment Buddy"

Earl was seeing a professional for help with obsessions and compulsions concerning order and the need for symmetry and exactness. He was doing a nice job with CBT when his therapist was able to coach him through exposure sessions in the clinic office. Earl was having a hard time, though, when it came to conducting therapy practices on his own. In particular, he was not fully engaging in exposure practices because it provoked anxiety. He was also cutting corners with his response prevention plan. As a result, Earl was not improving as much as he had hoped.

To help, Earl recruited his father, Hank (who lived with Earl), as a "treatment buddy." Hank had been confident that Earl could beat his OCD problem if only he put forth enough effort. Hank was respectful of Earl and never criticized him or belittled him. On the other hand, Hank was honest and assertive with Earl. If Earl was having trouble with rituals, Hank offered words of encouragement, such as "I know this is difficult for you. But if you get some help, I bet you can overcome this." For these reasons, Hank was an excellent treatment buddy. He was around for Earl when Earl needed the help, but Hank wasn't intrusive. He didn't meddle in Earl's business or badger Earl about doing CBT exercises. With Hank's support, Earl soon got the treatment results he was looking for.

Real Rewards Chosen by Real People

- Take a vacation or weekend getaway.
- See a movie.
- Go for a spa treatment or massage.
- Take a limo ride.
- Watch your favorite TV show.
- Buy something for your hobby.
- Pay someone to do the yardwork or housecleaning this week.
- Put $1 in a jar every time you meet a goal. When it gets to $50, treat yourself.
- Buy a new CD or DVD.
- Buy yourself a gift certificate.
- Subscribe to a magazine you always wanted.
- Enjoy a nice meal at a fancy restaurant.
- Find some time to be by yourself.

A treatment buddy can help you plan your treatment and choose goals, aid and cheer you on if you run into trouble with treatment, and participate in your rewards for success.

Even if you're ready to use the treatment strategies in this workbook, an encouraging friend or relative—a *treatment buddy*—can be very helpful and motivating. The more team members you have in your battle against OCD, the better! A treatment buddy can help you develop your treatment plan and your goals, provide assistance and encouragement if you run into difficulties using the treatment techniques, and help with rewarding you when you succeed. A supportive and encouraging relationship will make exposure and response prevention practices easier to bear. In this section, I'll help you decide whom you might choose as a treatment buddy, and we'll review some dos and don'ts for your treatment buddy to keep in mind when he or she is helping with your program. If you decide to work with a treatment buddy, encourage him or her to read this workbook so that he or she understands OCD and its treatment.

Who Would Make a Good Treatment Buddy?

Your friends and relatives probably react to your problems with obsessions and rituals in different ways. Some might be considerate, supportive, and optimistic about getting help. Others might be critical or even hostile. You should choose a treatment buddy who is warm, thoughtful, and sensitive. Another thing your treatment buddy must be able to do is be willing to challenge or confront you about your symptoms, but in a firm, constructive, and nonjudgmental way. If your treatment buddy always seems pessimistic, argumentative, or critical of you, it will add to your stress and make matters worse. On the other hand, your treatment buddy should not be too lenient or overly involved in your symptoms. Someone who is too tolerant of your problems with OCD might not be firm enough and might let you get away with avoidance and rituals when it's not in your best interests. Someone overly involved in your symptoms might even do rituals for you, or help you avoid obsessional anxiety, rather than push you to use the treatment strategies in this workbook that involve provoking anxiety. The qualities to look for in your treatment buddy are summarized in the box below.

Can your prospective treatment buddy be objective and firm but also warm and supportive?

Qualities to look for in a treatment buddy	Qualities to avoid in a treatment buddy
• Considerate	• Pessimistic
• Supportive	• Argumentative
• Optimistic	• Critical
• Warm, thoughtful	• Pushy
• Sensitive	• Lenient and tolerant of your OCD symptoms
• Trustworthy and consistent	• Overly involved in your symptoms
• Firm and assertive	

Teaming Up with Your Treatment Buddy

Your treatment buddy is your teammate in your war on OCD. But as the captain, or head coach, of your team, it is *your* job to deploy your treatment buddy as you see fit. In other words, you're in charge. You ask your treatment buddy for assistance when you need it, and it's your buddy's job to provide this help. "Treatment Buddy Tips" are placed throughout the remaining steps in this workbook to help your buddy help you. Your treatment buddy should not do the treatment for you, nor should he or she be constantly on your back nagging you about how much you've worked on OCD—remember, this is ultimately *your* responsibility. Finally, your treatment buddy should commit to being able to spend time with you each day (up to 1 hour, if necessary) to help you with your treatment.

Another way to think about your treatment buddy's role is that of a consultant. A company hires a consultant when it needs advice from someone who can provide expert help. The consultant is not a full-time employee of the company. Rather, he or she is involved only when the company needs advice with specific tasks and decides to ask the consultant for guidance. Similarly, your treatment buddy should understand your problems, realize the demands of the treatment program, and be available to make suggestions, recommendations, and give you encouragement *when you feel you need this support*. No threats, ridicule, or physical force are ever to be used to change your behavior. Rather, your treatment buddy should remind you of your commitment to working on OCD if he or she notices you're having problems.

> Is the person you're considering as a treatment buddy willing to accept the role you define and to prepare for it by reading the Introduction and Part I of this book?

Are You Ready to Get to Work?

In some ways, it seems like there is never a good time to start on a new project. But the fact that you're reading this workbook means that when asked if you're ready to change, your answer would be at least half "yes." If you've fully explored your mixed feelings about working on OCD, you should now be ready to find out whether your answer is *more* than half "yes." Circle YES or NO in response to each of the following questions:

- Are you motivated to reduce your obsessions, anxiety, and ritualistic behavior? Is this something you really care about?

  Yes No

- Are you willing to live with more anxiety and uncertainty in the short term in order to reduce your obsessional anxiety and urges to perform rituals in the future?

  Yes No

- Can you put aside, at least to some extent, other problems and stresses in your life (family or work issues) so you can focus on learning to manage problems with OCD?

Yes No

- Can you set aside blocks of time each day to practice the techniques described in this workbook?

Yes No

Your chances of getting the most out of this workbook are greatest if you answered "yes" to most of these questions. It means you're willing to work on overcoming OCD even though it will require lots of time and energy and at times involve feeling anxious. On the other hand, you might decide that now is not the best time to start a program like this. If so, you might still find reading Steps 6 through 10 helpful since they provide detailed instructions for how to take advantage of the particular strategies for learning to control obsessions and rituals. You can certainly use these strategies from time to time as you need them. Once you see that they can make some improvement in your life, you might find yourself ready to commit to the program more fully so you can achieve substantial and long-lasting change. Ready to give it a try?

PART III

Your Treatment Program

Gathering Your Forces

You've got everything you need to start battling OCD in earnest: knowledge of how OCD works, a thorough understanding of your own symptoms, and a plan for using CBT strategies to break the vicious cycle of obsessions and compulsions. Before you start, I want to give you some tactical suggestions to help you get the best possible results from your efforts.

Your Weapons against OCD

You'll be using four essential strategies in the coming weeks:

Cognitive therapy: Identifying, analyzing, and challenging maladaptive beliefs, interpretations, and other thinking patterns that underlie your obsessional fears and urges to perform rituals.

Situational exposure: Gradually confronting the real-life situations and objects that trigger obsessional fear (for example, actual contact with contaminants).

Imaginal exposure: Mentally confronting the obsessional thoughts, ideas, and images that provoke fear, and visualizing the feared consequences of not doing rituals (for example, violent thoughts to kill family members that you fear might lead you to become a murderer).

Response prevention: Resisting urges to do rituals (for example, driving past pedestrians without checking that you haven't hit anyone).

How to Structure Your Treatment Program

Our OCD Program in the Anxiety and Stress Disorders Clinic at the University of North Carolina is highly effective and provides a good model for how you might structure your own self-help program.

What We Do in Our Clinic

In our clinic, treatment includes about 15 90-minute sessions with the therapist; these meetings occur either once or twice a week (or more frequently), depending on the severity of the OCD, the person's schedule, and practical considerations like driving distance. In addition, there is at least 2 hours of daily self-supervised ("homework") practice. So, regardless of the frequency of treatment sessions, CBT strategies are used every day for at least 2 hours. The first three sessions involve learning about OCD, developing a treatment plan, and enhancing motivation. You have already worked through these components of the program by completing Parts I and II of this workbook. Cognitive therapy, therapist-guided exposure, and response prevention begin in session four and are practiced in each session until treatment ends. Beginning with the first exposure practice, the response prevention component is in effect: the patient starts working on resisting urges to ritualize. The final treatment session is dedicated to wrapping up and discussing strategies for how to maintain improvement (which is included in Step 10).

Each therapist-guided exposure session starts with a discussion of that day's exposure practice. Beliefs and interpretations about the feared item are identified, and cognitive therapy strategies are used to help the patient challenge these maladaptive thinking patterns and prepare to face the feared item. Doing cognitive therapy prior to starting exposure gives the patient a more realistic perspective on the feared situation or obsessional thought he or she is about to confront. This jump-starts the exposure practice and helps the patient change his or her problematic thinking patterns. Alberto, for example, was afraid to conduct exposure to cemeteries—his worst fear—because it would make him think about death. Through cognitive therapy, he realized that everyone has upsetting death-related thoughts from time to time but that, although they might temporarily create some distress, such thoughts are normal and harmless. Looking at it this way helped Alberto take the plunge and visit a cemetery for exposure.

When exposure is ready to begin, the therapist coaches the patient to face the feared item or enter the exposure situation. This usually provokes the urge to ritualize, but the patient is practicing response prevention, so the therapist also coaches him or her to resist doing rituals. When patients are afraid of disastrous consequences from facing their fears without ritualizing, imaginal exposure is used simultaneously. For example, Ava was confronting a butcher knife for situational exposure. But knives triggered violent obsessional thoughts of stabbing her husband and children. So once Ava's distress subsided somewhat in the presence of the knife, the therapist had her practice confronting her violent obsessional thoughts and feared consequences. Specifically, Ava practiced visualizing a fearful scenario in which she is using a knife, begins to think about stabbing her family, loses control, and kills them all in a bloodbath. For many years, Nikolai had avoided Bibles because of blasphemous obsessional thoughts of urinating and defecating on them. For situational exposure, he practiced reading from the Bible. At the same time, he practiced imaginal exposure to thinking the unwanted urination and defecation thoughts until he could do this without intense anxiety (obviously, no Bibles were ever soiled!). With consistent exposure practice, Ava substantially reduced her violent obsessions and Nikolai his sacrilegious obsessions.

Exposure is hierarchy-driven, which means it is done gradually over the course of the treatment program. It starts with situations and thoughts that trigger a *moderate* degree of anxiety. Starting with exposures that provoke very little anxiety wouldn't teach you to be brave and face your fears. On the other hand, beginning with situations that are extremely anxiety-provoking would make it too difficult. At each therapy session, a new, more challenging exposure item is confronted with the therapist's help until the most feared item is confronted. Between sessions, the patient continues (on his or her own) with confronting the situations and thoughts that were practiced in the therapy session. Response prevention rules also apply between sessions.

In addition to the exposure practices that are planned together with the therapist, we encourage our patients to *confront*, rather than *avoid*, all feared situations that arise unintentionally through the course of the day. In other words, *do what OCD tells you not to do*. For example:

- If OCD tells you that a trash can is dangerous to touch, *purposely* touch it when depositing garbage.
- If OCD says that the number 13 will cause bad luck, *choose* 13 as your password or identification number.
- If OCD tells you to take a detour to avoid the cemetery on your way home, *decide* to drive by the cemetery.
- If OCD tells you you're dirty or immoral if you look at other people naked in the gym locker room, *deliberately* glance at them.

I call this type of practice "lifestyle exposure" because it basically means choosing to practice exposure (instead of avoidance) as a *way of life*. I usually suggest that patients begin lifestyle exposure once they've got a few planned exposures under their belt and are comfortable with how exposure works.

A Timeline for Your Own Self-Help Program

In this book, I present the four CBT strategies in different steps so that I can show you how to apply each strategy to your particular types of obsessions, rituals, and avoidance behavior. However, as in our clinic, you'll probably combine these strategies when you begin working on your problems with OCD. So, here are some suggestions for how you might use Steps 6–10 most effectively.

1. *Begin by learning how to use cognitive therapy techniques by working through Step 6.* This will help you weaken the unhelpful thinking patterns that form the foundation of your obsessional fears. It will also help prepare you for doing exposure practice. *I suggest that each day for 1 to 2 weeks you spend at least 45 minutes per day practicing cognitive therapy.* Some of these strategies will involve sitting down with pencil and paper. Others you will use "on the fly" when you begin to obsess or run into something that triggers an urge to ritualize.

2. *After spending a week or two on Step 6, get started with exposure and response prevention*—even if your obsessional thoughts are still causing you distress. Start by reading all the way through Steps 7, 8, and 9 to get familiar with these techniques and how they are used together. I've included many examples that show how to apply situational and imaginal exposure and response prevention for different types of common and less common OCD symptoms. These chapters also explain how to use cognitive therapy as part of your exposure practices.

The chapter "Putting It All Together," which appears after Step 9, includes all the forms you'll need when you plan your timeline for practicing CBT.

3. *Practice planned situational, imaginal, or combined exposure twice every day for at least 1 hour at a time* (lots of patients I work with prefer to practice once in the morning and once in the afternoon or evening). The first 10 minutes of this time should be spent using cognitive therapy strategies to get you ready to face your fear. Then spend the rest of the time facing the feared situation, obsessive thought, or both. Of course, feel free to do more work if you like. The more time you put into doing these exercises, the faster you will improve and the more benefit you will get out of this program. After Step 9 (in the chapter "Putting It All Together") you'll find a form for keeping track of your SUDs levels during exposure and response prevention practices.

As I mentioned above, it will be easiest to face your fears gradually, starting with moderately fearful triggers and slowly working up to those that provoke more anxiety. Use the hierarchies you created in Step 4 (pages 95 and 104) to guide your exposure program. Practice with each hierarchy item until it provokes only minimal anxiety before moving on to a more difficult item. *A good rule of thumb is to spend at least 1 week focusing on each item before moving on to the next (more difficult) one.* This will ensure that you feel more comfortable with each situation before you jump to the next level of difficulty. I'll give you suggestions for dealing with anxiety in Step 7.

4. *When you start your first exposure practice, also begin applying the response prevention plan you tailored in Step 4 (page 110).* In Step 9 I'll help you decide on a strategy for stopping your rituals and give you techniques for resisting even strong urges to perform rituals.

5. *After about 3 weeks of practicing planned exposure exercises, start "lifestyle exposure"* by choosing to take advantage of opportunities to stand up to fear triggers and intrusive thoughts that happen to come your way in your daily life.

That's right, I said "take advantage of" and "opportunities"—which means learning to view unplanned encounters with triggers and intrusive thoughts as fortuitous circumstances where you get to practice exposure techniques and work on alleviating OCD, not as situations that you have to worry about or run away from. It's like losing weight by getting more exercise. You can't *just* rely on going to the gym—you have to start using the stairs instead of the elevator or escalator, and parking far away from the building (so you can walk further) instead of driving around for 15 minutes just to get the closest spot.

6. *Once you've completed exposure to all the items on your fear hierarchies, move on to Step 10.* Here you'll measure your progress with the program and learn about strategies for maintaining your improvement and continuing to get better.

As you can tell, your program will take up a good deal of your time over the next weeks and months. You might consider cutting back on other activities that would compete for your time and energy so that you can dedicate the necessary resources to getting better. As you've probably guessed, there will also be times when the going gets tough and you feel anxious. Facing each new fearful situation and obsessional thought while giving up your rituals will require courage, hard work, and persistence. But working hard and taking risks is likely to pay off: the more often you take advantage of opportunities to practice cognitive therapy and exposure, and the stricter you are about stopping your rituals, the faster you'll win your battle against OCD. *You can do it*—as have so many people before you.

STEP 6

Attacking OCD at Its Foundation

Thinking Errors

- Spend at least 45 minutes every day for 1 to 2 weeks practicing the techniques in this step before moving on to Steps 7, 8, and 9.
- Begin each exposure practice with 10 minutes of cognitive therapy.

All the strategies described in Steps 6–9 are important to your treatment. In fact, they really need to be used together—rather than trying them one at a time—in order for you to win your battle with OCD. So, although I present them as steps in this workbook, you should read through all four of these chapters to learn how the techniques are used together before actually beginning to practice them. Then read "Putting It All Together" following Step 9 and get to work. While you read Part III (and for up to about 2 weeks), you can practice the techniques you'll learn about in this step.

As you learned in Step 3, every time you feel anxious or feel the need to ritualize, it's the result of how you're interpreting obsessional triggers or intrusive thoughts. These interpretations aren't always trustworthy—especially if they lead to excessive fear and rituals. Everyone makes mistakes sometimes, and—just like everyone else—you're not immune to making illogical, inaccurate, or simply *unhelpful* (mis)interpretations of situations and thoughts. Have you ever felt convinced that things would turn out badly, but in reality they didn't? Have you ever judged someone only to find out later that they're the opposite of who you thought they were? It's similar kinds of thinking errors that contribute to the vicious cycle of OCD. In the following pages, I'll help you see this for yourself so you can begin correcting any problematic thinking patterns that have you caught in OCD's vicious cycle.

Cognitive therapy is the part of CBT that aims to change the types of cognitions that lead to anxiety. The term *cognition* refers to ways in which we think, interpret, assume, believe, pay attention, and remember. If you have problems with OCD, the goal of cognitive therapy is to change your belief that your negative intrusive thoughts are important, threatening, and must be controlled, as well as your interpretations of obsessional triggers as dangerous and harmful. In this step, I'll teach you strategies to help you challenge these unhealthy cognitions and replace them with healthy (and more accurate) ones that don't lead to anxiety and rituals. Many of the strategies I present have been developed and expanded on elsewhere by my colleagues Sabine Wilhelm, Mark Freeston, Gail Steketee, Maureen Whitall, Martin Antony, Christine Purdon, and David A. Clark.

The Cognitive Principle: Negative Feelings Come from Your Interpretations

It's a fact that how you feel depends on how you interpret (or *what you tell yourself about*) your situation. Negative feelings such as anxiety, depression, and anger are not caused by situations or events themselves, but rather by how you *think about* these situations and events. Furthermore, certain types of interpretations lead to certain feelings and emotions. Overly negative beliefs about your self-worth ("I am useless and unlovable") lead to feeling depressed. If you view yourself as not living up to high enough standards ("I *should* have made 100% on the exam—95% isn't good enough"), you'll feel guilty. When you interpret a situation as very dangerous, threatening, or unpredictable ("Dogs are very unpredictable animals that often bite for no reason"), anxiety and fear arise.

Let's say you're in school and before class begins your teacher comes up to you and says, "I want to talk to you after class." What kinds of thoughts might come to mind as you're sitting there during the class? What would you be telling yourself? Pick one of the following interpretations:

- **a.** The teacher is happy with my work and wants to tell me in person.
- **b.** The teacher wants to ask me if I'll help with a special project.
- **c.** The teacher just wants to get to know me a little better.
- **d.** I did something wrong and the teacher is upset with me.

If you picked *a* or *b*, you'd probably feel pretty good as a result of your interpretation. You might smile or get more confident by raising your hand and asking questions. If you picked c, you'd probably feel neutral and not really change from your normal routine. If you picked *d*, however, you'd probably feel anxious and worried, and you may keep quiet and ruminate about what could be wrong and what the teacher was going to say (or *do*) to you after class. All of these interpretations are possible, and the one you picked created your reality and determined how you felt and behaved. This relationship applies to most situations in life.

Remember the *cognitive principle*: it's not really what's happening to you that determines whether you feel anxious, sad, angry, happy, or neutral. It's how you interpret what's happening.

The Cognitive Principle and OCD

Likewise, as you learned in Step 3, erroneous and self-defeating beliefs and interpretations are the foundation of OCD symptoms. Consider Shawn, who had obsessions about contamination and hand-washing rituals that were triggered by touching money and doorknobs and by shaking hands with people. Shawn believed that if he touched any of these things, he would get very sick from the germs people have on their hands. He interpreted these items as dangerous. From the cognitive perspective, Shawn's beliefs about germs and his interpretations (for example, "If I shake someone's hand, I'll have his germs and get very sick") lead him to feel anxious in situations where he might come into contact with such germs. In turn, this anxiety triggers washing rituals to make him feel safer.

But are people's hands really that dangerous? Do activities like handling money, opening doors, and shaking hands routinely make people sick? Of course, no one can *completely* guarantee Shawn that he wouldn't get sick from these activities—the truth is that it's *possible*. But most people take this risk for granted and view these situations as "reasonably safe." Most people don't avoid these things, and they don't feel the need to compulsively wash their hands. In Shawn's case, the evidence from everyday experience is that the risk of contamination is *acceptably low*. If Shawn could change how he thinks about his triggers and somehow come to see them as being "acceptable risks," he'd feel less anxious in these situations, and he wouldn't need to turn to rituals to make him feel safe.

As I explained in Step 3, just as we interpret events and situations in the external world, we also make judgments and interpretations of our intrusive thoughts. Let's say you have an intrusive thought or image of murdering someone you love very much. How might you judge or interpret this intrusion? Choose one of the following:

- **a.** I've got to be absolutely certain that this is *just* a thought, and not something more.
- **b.** Thinking this thought increases the chances I will act on it.
- **c.** Only cold-blooded killers have these kinds of thoughts. Therefore, I must be one.
- **d.** This thought doesn't make sense. I wouldn't do this kind of thing.

As you've probably figured out by now, if you chose *a*, *b*, or *c*, you would become anxious and probably try to analyze, scrutinize, or pore over the thought—or try to get it out of your mind—using some sort of ritualistic or reassurance-seeking strategy that (temporarily) might make you feel better. But are *a*, *b*, and *c* accurate interpretations? Based on what you've learned so far about intrusive thoughts and obsessions, *d* is the only logical interpretation. And in addition to being true, this interpretation doesn't lead to obsessional anxiety. If you believed *d*, you wouldn't need to analyze or fight the intrusion, and you wouldn't need reassurance or rituals to help you cope.

Cognitive Therapy for OCD

So the same event, trigger, or intrusive thought can lead to totally different (even *opposite*) feelings—delight, neutrality, or anxiety—based on your own interpretation. It turns out that obsessional anxiety and fear result from *exaggerated* and *mistaken* (erroneous) interpretations. But these cognitions are often so automatic that you don't even have a chance to decide whether they're logical. If you can learn to identify, challenge, and modify these kinds of thinking errors, you'll be able to slow the process down and better control your feelings and emotions in any situation. As I mentioned above, this is the aim of the *cognitive* therapy part of CBT.

Notice that the aim of CBT is not to help you avoid obsessional triggers or to get rid of obsessional thoughts altogether—that would be impossible. You probably can't help encountering some of your obsessional triggers in your daily life, and upsetting intrusive thoughts are normal experiences. Rather, CBT is designed to help you identify and change problematic ways of thinking about and responding to these triggers. Specifically, cognitive therapy will help you see that your erroneous beliefs and interpretations are only one of several possible ways of reacting to obsessional triggers and thoughts. You'll find that there are more helpful ways of thinking about these stimuli that do not lead to anxiety.

Anxiety and fear are not caused by obsessional trigger situations and intrusive thoughts themselves, but by how you misinterpret these triggers and intrusions as significant and threatening. If you correct the misinterpretations, you'll reduce your anxiety and fear.

Maria, for example, was afraid of the word *cancer* based on her belief that saying, writing, or thinking this word would cause her to develop the disease. Maria used some of the cognitive therapy techniques in this step to help her consider alternate ways of thinking about the dangerousness of the word *cancer*. For instance, she hadn't considered that many doctors—especially oncologists—use this word many times every day. Authors of books about cancer and people posting information and personal stories on supportive websites write this word all the time. Considering these facts helped weaken Maria's strongly held beliefs about the word *cancer* to the point that she was willing to try exposure therapy practices in which she confronted the word without doing mental rituals to erase it.

How to Use (and How *Not* to Use) Cognitive Therapy Strategies

Maria benefited from trying *specific* cognitive therapy strategies—particularly examining the evidence—that are designed to challenge particular cognitive errors, which in her case were mainly a form of thought–action fusion (believing that thoughts—or words—are the equivalent of actions). As you learned in Chapter 3, cognitive errors can be divided up into various categories. CBT researchers and clinicians have discovered that certain thinking errors are best addressed using particular cognitive therapy strategies, as shown in the table on the facing page. So the *correct* way to use cognitive therapy strategies is to identify the types of errors you're making so you can use the right tool to challenge it. You might want to refresh your memory about the different types of cognitive errors by reviewing the material on pages 74–78; then read about the strategies on the following pages. At the end of the chapter I'll ask you to look back at the exposure hierarchies you created in Chapter

Strategy	Cognitive errors
Examining the evidence	All cognitive errors
Continuum technique	Thought–action fusion
Pie-chart technique	Exaggerated sense of responsibility
Life-savings wager technique	Need for certainty
Double-standard technique	All cognitive errors
Cost–benefit analysis	All cognitive errors
Experiment techniques	Thought–action fusion and the need to control thoughts

in Chapter 4 and try to match the appropriate cognitive therapy strategy with the cognitive errors involved in your hierarchy items.

It's important to know, however, that there is also a *wrong* way to use cognitive therapy. Because some of these techniques involve analyzing your feared situations and thoughts, it may be tempting to use them as reassurance. Doing so, however, turns these strategies into rituals in which you are trying to pin down a guarantee about your fears—like trying to get reassurance about something you can never be absolutely certain of ("Will I get cancer or not?"). Consider Art, for example, who was afraid of curse words because he thought that he might mistakenly make obscene gestures or use profanity when it was inappropriate, such as when conversing with his boss or his pastor. But he used cognitive techniques to try to reassure himself beyond the shadow of a doubt that his fear of cursing was irrational: he scoured OCD-related Internet chat rooms for any discussion about people acting on their intrusive thoughts. Then he pored over what he read until he figured out the "best" rational interpretation of his intrusions: "My thoughts about curse words are completely irrational. People with OCD never act on their obsessional thoughts." Art then recited this statement to himself whenever curse words came to mind. It was a way of reassuring himself that he wouldn't do anything embarrassing. This strategy was no different from using a mental ritual for reassurance. Art was using this statement to reduce his fear, rather than to generate alternative (more realistic) ways of thinking about intrusive unwanted thoughts. But he found himself reciting this statement ritualistically. A more helpful approach would have been to practice saying to himself something like "Everyone sometimes has senseless thoughts; I'm probably misinterpreting an intrusive thought as more important than it really is."

Instead of trying to prove that your obsessions are false, can you try telling yourself there's actually a *small* probability that they're valid? Can you focus on what is *probable*, instead of what is *possible*?

Cognitive strategies help you open yourself up and see whether your interpretations of obsessional triggers and thoughts are correct. Usually, there are other, more accurate ways of thinking about your obsessions that don't lead to high anxiety and rituals. When Maria tried the "examining the evidence" strategy, she was able to consider the possibility that her obsessive belief about cancer might not be entirely accurate; she knew it didn't guarantee her that she wouldn't develop cancer. She also knew that this strategy might be a good place to start since it was a good one to challenge thought–action fusion. But she could have tried any other cognitive strategy that appealed to her. The cognitive strategies are tools in a metaphorical sense, not in a literal sense, the way a screwdriver is guaranteed to tighten a screw and is the only tool designed to do so. Here are some tips to help you avoid falling into the trap of using cognitive therapy techniques as rituals.

1. Don't use cognitive strategies to try to convince yourself that your feared consequences *definitely* won't come true. In other words, don't use them to simply dismiss your obsessional fears as *illogical*.
2. Don't use cognitive strategies to come up with reasons why you definitely shouldn't be worried about your obsessional fears.
3. Instead, make sure you're using these strategies to open your mind to *new* and *possible* interpretations.
4. Use cognitive techniques to encourage you to confront your fears and risk being uncertain about the consequences. In the examples above, Maria decided it was worth conducting an exposure to the word *cancer* to test out her new beliefs that confronting this word would not lead to becoming sick. When Art used the cognitive strategies correctly, they helped him purposely think curse words in different situations to test out whether his fears of acting and speaking inappropriately would come true (*which they didn't!*).

Examining the Evidence

Bruce had obsessional thoughts and fears about food poisoning. Believing that food-borne illnesses were highly prevalent and very severe, he had developed elaborate food cleansing and checking rituals, and he generally avoided eating in restaurants. Whenever someone tried to convince Bruce that his fear, avoidance, and rituals were senseless and unnecessary, Bruce would say, "Yeah, but I *could* get sick if I'm not careful. Remember last year when they found that dead roach in the hamburger and it was on the news? It *could* happen."

An important step toward winning your battle against OCD is recognizing that just because you *feel* anxious about certain events, situations, and obsessional thoughts doesn't necessarily mean your beliefs, interpretations, and feared consequences are realistic. Likewise, just because something is *possible* doesn't mean it's *probable*. So, rather than simply assuming the worst-case scenario, it's better to treat your interpretations and beliefs as *guesses* or *hypotheses* as a scientist might do. A scientist who comes up with a hypothesis collects data—factual evidence—to test whether or not it holds up. By using the technique of examining the evidence, you'll learn how to consider evidence to help you get a better sense (without needing to be absolutely *certain*) of whether your beliefs are realistic and whether there might be alternative (and more helpful) ways of thinking about the situations and thoughts that trigger your obsessions and rituals. In Bruce's case, he was right—he *could* get sick. But the evidence strongly suggested that it was extremely unlikely. In other words, he didn't need to obsess about or avoid restaurants, and his food-related rituals were clearly excessive and unnecessary.

Actually collecting this evidence is harder than you might think. That's because OCD can make you focus more strongly on evidence that *confirms* your obsessional fears and make you ignore or discount evidence that would disprove your fears. The more anxious you're feeling, the more this will be the case. Bruce ignored the fact that no one he knew had ever had food poisoning and focused instead on one random incident in which a dead bug was found in a fast-food hamburger. This single confirmatory event was overblown so that it overshadowed other, more persuasive evidence to the contrary. To avoid this trap and get a fair and balanced perspective on your obsessional fear, you've got to get into the habit of routinely asking yourself the key questions in the box below. You might even write them on an index card, which you can then carry around as a reminder in your pocket or wallet.

The process of examining the evidence actually involves four basic steps:

1. Identify the mistaken beliefs and interpretations that underlie your obsessional fear.
2. Ask yourself the key questions and generate alternative cognitions.
3. Weigh the evidence supporting and contradicting these cognitions.
4. Come up with a more realistic cognition that is based on the evidence and will encourage you to expose yourself to fear triggers and intrusive thoughts.

Janet had recurring violent obsessional images of stabbing her husband, Brad, and mutilating his face. This image occurred out of the blue but was also triggered by the sight of knives, which Janet avoided. She believed these images meant that deep down she actu-

Key Questions to Help You Examine the Evidence for Your Obsessional Fears

- What does my past experience tell me about the likelihood that my fear will come true?
- What do other people's experiences tell me about my fears?
- Have there been times when I expected the feared consequences to happen, but they didn't?
- How might someone else look at this situation or intrusive thought?
- What have I learned about intrusive thoughts?
- Are my obsessional fears based on how I *feel* or on actual circumstances?
- Am I confusing a *high*-probability event with a *low*-probability event?

Examining the Evidence Worksheet: Janet's Example

1. Identify the mistaken beliefs and misinterpretations that underlie obsessional fear (cognitive error):
   - *My images of Brad's mutilated face mean I am an awful person who really wants this to happen (Type of cognitive error: importance of thoughts, thought–action fusion).*
2. Ask yourself the key questions and generate alternative beliefs:
   - Key questions: *What have I learned about intrusive thoughts? How would someone else look at this situation/thought?*
   - Alternative beliefs: *Everyone has mental images that are neither significant nor personally meaningful. My images are probably normal and harmless. Other people, including Brad, tell me it's nothing to worry about and are not scared of me.*
3. Weigh the evidence supporting and contradicting these cognitions:
   a. Evidence supporting the mistaken belief/interpretation
      - *When I have the obsessional images, I feel like I could act on them.*
      - *I once read a news article about someone stabbing her husband while he was asleep.*

   b. Evidence supporting the new, alternative belief
      - *Most people have strange thoughts that are out of sync with their personality.*
      - *I have other thoughts that are out of sync with who I am, but they don't bother me.*
      - *Being scared of your own thoughts makes the thoughts more intense.*
      - *I have never done anything violent in my life. I don't want to hurt anyone.*
      - *Brad even tells me he thinks I'm not dangerous. He's not even afraid of me.*
4. Come up with a more realistic cognition that is based on the evidence and that will encourage you to confront your triggers and intrusive thoughts:
   - *It looks like I'm overreacting to senseless, normal intrusive thoughts. It would really help if I practiced using knives, confronting my senseless images, and stopped the mental rituals.*

ally wanted to mutilate her husband and she was really a terrible, violent person. To try to neutralize her obsessions, Janet repeated phrases to herself (mental rituals; for example, "*I love him, I love him*").

You can use the blank worksheet on the facing page to start examining the evidence supporting and contradicting your own cognitive errors, as Janet did. Janet's worksheet appears above.

BATTLE PLAN Make copies of the Examining the Evidence Worksheet and keep them handy for when you're ready to begin working with your cognitive errors.

Examining the Evidence Worksheet

1. Cognitive error

____

____

2. Alternative belief(s)

____

____

____

3a. Evidence supporting the cognitive error

____

____

____

3b. Evidence supporting the alternative belief (*and contradicting the cognitive error*)

____

____

____

4. Evidence-based realistic belief and suggestion for exposure/response prevention

____

____

The Continuum Technique

This technique can help you take a more realistic approach to interpreting your intrusive unwanted thoughts. It's especially useful if you have sexual, violent, or sacrilegious obsessions and are afraid that these thoughts mean you have a bad moral character (that is, thought–action fusion and beliefs about the importance of thoughts: "I'm a bad person because I have bad thoughts," "The thoughts mean that I want this to happen," "Thinking is as bad as doing"). Paulina had sexual obsessions about molesting children. She couldn't look at a small child without experiencing unwanted images of touching the child inappropriately. Paulina believed these images meant she was secretly a predator who was sexually aroused by children. She figured it was only a matter of time before she lost control and acted on her "urges."

It might seem easy to confuse *unwanted* and *intrusive* obsessional thoughts with the *intention* to act. You might even experience what seems like an *urge* or an *impulse* to do the action. But clearly, your *actual behavior* is a more valid measure of your character than your thoughts, urges, and impulses—especially if these thoughts are *unwanted*. Let's flip this around by considering the unfortunate circumstances in which people actually do sexually assault children. If someone merely *thinks* about assaulting a child, but doesn't act on these thoughts, is that the same as actually assaulting a child? If you believe that who you are (your personality or moral standing) is determined by what you think, then how many bad thoughts must you have before you're truly "immoral"? Where's the cutoff? Is having one very immoral thought as bad as having 100 slightly immoral thoughts? And what about the fact that *everyone* has these kinds of thoughts? Surely we're not all immoral! The continuum technique is designed to help you see this even more vividly.

The line below (the continuum) runs from the "most immoral/worst person ever" to the "most moral/best person ever." Think of someone who would fit into each of these categories and write their names above the line at the appropriate end of the continuum.

Most immoral/ worst person ever ———————————————— **Most moral/ best person ever**

Next, mark an X on the line (or put your initials) where you'd place yourself on the continuum between best and worst person ever. Then consider the people listed below. Place each of them on the continuum by writing the number next to their name somewhere on the line.

1. Someone who commits murder
2. Someone who thinks about committing murder but never does it
3. Someone who shoplifts
4. Someone who thinks about shoplifting but doesn't actually do it
5. A married person who cheats on his or her spouse
6. A married person who thinks about cheating but doesn't go through with it

Where did you place yourself on the continuum? Where did you put the six other people? Next, write your answers to the following questions:

1. How did you decide where to place yourself and the others on the continuum? ____

____

____

2. Are you more like the people who *committed* bad behaviors, or those who merely *thought* about bad behaviors? Why? ______________________________

____

____

3. Are your obsessional thoughts *intentional* or *unwanted*? Where would you put yourself on the continuum if you intentionally thought about the immoral behaviors? Why? ______________________________

____

____

Completing this exercise should help you become more open to the idea that morality is based on a deliberate choice of action, rather than involuntary intrusive thoughts that you have never acted on. In other words, *bad deeds* are more important than ***unwanted*** *bad thoughts*.

Pie-Chart Technique

When you obsess about a negative event (a car accident, illness, bad luck, or the like), do you worry that perhaps you're responsible for *causing* it? Do you fear that you didn't do enough to *prevent* it from happening? Should you have ritualized more? Been more careful? The *pie-chart technique* can help you get some perspective on your own role in causing, or failing to prevent, negative events and catastrophes. Basically, it involves four steps:

1. List the factors (other than yourself) that could contribute to the negative event.
2. Judge each factor's role in causing the event.
3. Draw a pie chart.
4. Reconsider your own role in causing the event.

In Step 3 I described Melissa, whose obsessional fear of harming others through her own carelessness provides a nice example of how to use the pie-chart technique. Melissa constantly checked that she hadn't done anything that could lead to any sort of negative consequences—for example, dropping glass on the floor, which could lead to injury, and leaving the refrigerator open, which could lead to spoilage and food poisoning. Her main obsession was that she could mistakenly drop her medication on the floor and a small child would think it was candy, ingest the pills, and become very sick or even die. Melissa believed she alone would be responsible if this happened, so she rarely left the house (just in case a loose pill was in her pants pocket). She also counted her pills twice a day to make sure all were accounted for. Of course, every negative event that happens has multiple factors that could directly or indirectly influence it. The pie-chart technique helped Melissa see that her negligence is not the only factor that could play a role if this unlikely event were ever to occur. Here's how Melissa worked through the four steps:

1. *Identify factors (other than yourself) that could contribute to the negative event,* and
2. *Judge how much responsibility each factor contributes (these should add up to 100%):*
   - The bottle manufacturer for producing a defective pill bottle (about 15%)
   - Bad luck (about 20%)
   - The young child who doesn't have good judgment (25%)
   - The child's parents for not keeping an eye on the child (40%)
3. *Draw a pie chart using the percent responsibility for each factor.*

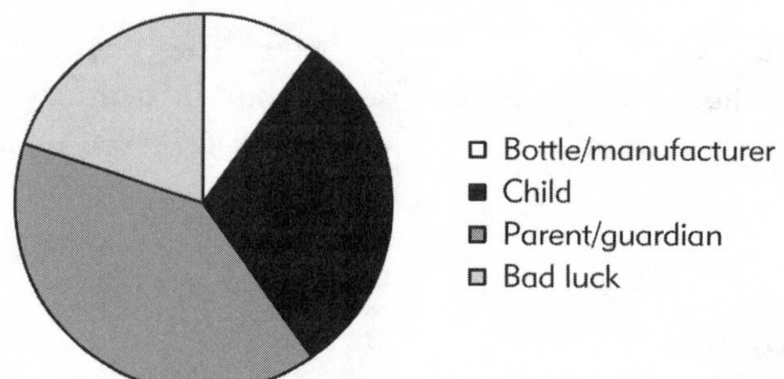

4. *Consider your own contribution to the cause of the event relative to the other factors.* After considering the pie chart and thinking more carefully about the different sources of potential responsibility, Melissa rated herself as being about 10–20% responsible for this event were it to actually happen. She decided that this was acceptable compared to living the way she had been. It encouraged her to do exposure therapy exercises in which she took her pills to public places (malls, playgrounds, the zoo) and even handled the pills *without checking and counting rituals that would reassure her that she'd put them away safely.*

BATTLE PLAN Make copies of this form so you can use it in different situations where exaggerated responsibility cognitions arise.

You can use the Pie-Chart Technique Worksheet (on the facing page) to help you with your own exaggerated responsibility beliefs so that you can gain a broader perspective on blame and accountability.

The Life-Savings Wager Technique

Patrick had obsessional doubts that he might have, without realizing it, struck a pedestrian while he was driving (so-called hit-and-run obsessions). He interpreted these senseless doubts as a sign that such an accident *could have happened* and was extremely distressed at not being able to *completely* convince himself that he hadn't injured anyone. As a result, he regularly retraced his route—sometimes driving many miles out of his way—to double-

Pie-Chart Technique Worksheet

Describe the situation or feared consequences about which you feel responsible:

____

____

List factors (*other than you*) that could contribute to the negative event or feared consequences:

	Contributing factors	Responsibility rating
1.		
2.		
3.		
4.		
5.		
6.		
7.		
8.		

Rate how much (what percent) of the overall responsibility can be attributed to each contributing factor (the percentages should add up to 100%)

Make a pie chart to depict the degree of responsibility for each contributing factor

Think about your own estimated degree of responsibility relative to the other factors:

____

____

check that there weren't any signs of a hit-and-run accident. When Patrick was in my office talking about his problem, he readily acknowledged the senselessness of these obsessions. But, when he was in the midst of an OCD episode, the anxiety took over and he became fixated on convincing himself that he hadn't hurt anyone.

Perhaps, when you're not feeling terribly anxious, you can intellectualize that your obsessional fears and rituals are illogical. But when anxiety strikes, this logic probably goes out the window and you end up reacting solely on your emotions. The life-savings wager technique is a strategy to help you distinguish what you logically *know* from what you *feel*. It can help you think rationally even when you're face to face with obsessional fear. The technique involves imagining yourself in the following scenario when you're having trouble with obsessional doubts:

THE LIFE-SAVINGS WAGER

Imagine that you have to place a bet in which you will wager your entire life savings on whether or not your feared consequence will come true (or has already occurred). If you bet wrong, you'll lose all the money you've saved up and be completely broke. You don't have to be 100% *confident* in your bet, but you do have to *place* the bet. Now, where would you put your money?

This imaginary bet is actually a fancy way of forcing you to make your best *guess* about the validity of your obsessions. I often use it in my own work with people who have OCD, and believe it or not, everyone always guesses "correctly"—meaning they make the same wager that people who *don't* have OCD would make! For instance, Patrick used this technique to bet on: (1) whether or not he had hit a pedestrian without realizing it and (2) whether or not he would realize if he did hit someone. Without hesitation, Patrick wagered that (1) he had *not* hit anyone with his car and that (2) he *would* know if he had.

So people with and without OCD arrive at the same intellectual conclusions. But while most people *without* OCD take for granted that even a best guess is not always the same thing as being certain of the answer, people with OCD sometimes have a hard time taking this for granted. You might become very anxious just knowing that your guess is just a *guess* (even if it's a well-informed one). That is, you probably feel as if you need a *guarantee* that you're absolutely safe—you cannot live with uncertainty. The life-savings wager won't make your guesses feel more correct, but it will teach you that you can overcome your problems with OCD without feeling like you know things for certain. If you made the same bet as someone without OCD, what kind of exposure exercises should you attempt? The answer is that you should try facing this fear trigger so you can learn to be more comfortable with your wager, or "guess."

The Double-Standard Technique

If you have OCD, you might apply faulty beliefs and interpretations to yourself, but not to other people. For example, if *you* have a violent thought about your infant, you might think of yourself as an awful person; but if you found out *your mother* had the same kinds of unwanted thoughts about you when you were a baby, it wouldn't change your feelings about her. Do you see the double standard? Here's another one: If *you* touch the floor, you worry about getting sick, but you don't see it as dangerous for *someone else* to touch the floor. It's a double standard when we use one set of rules and beliefs for ourselves and a different set for other people.

A powerful way to change strongly held beliefs is to look for your own double standards. And the best way to do this is to mentally "step out" of yourself and imagine that it's someone else (a friend or family member) who's experiencing the obsessional fear and coming to *you* for some advice. What would you tell this person? The double-standard technique involves thinking through what advice you'd give and then applying this advice to yourself.

Let's suppose a friend told you about obsessing over one of the following circumstances:

"I heard there was road construction near my child's school, and I'm worried about sending her today because she'll get poisoned by the fumes."

"I've been having strange thoughts about children lately, and I think they mean I am becoming a child molester."

"Sometimes curse words come to mind while I'm sitting in a religious service. I worry whether deep down I actually hate God."

"When I was driving earlier, I hit a bump in the road, but I think I might have hit a person by mistake."

"I parked in space #13 today, and now I think my family is going to have bad luck."

"When I picked up the money I dropped on the floor, I got germs on my hands that will make me sick. I had better shower and change my clothes."

"If I wake up in the middle of the night and my husband is asleep, I think of how vulnerable he is; and I get thoughts of hurting him. I think it means I have an evil heart."

Most likely you would comfort this person by saying something like "It's okay. That situation [or thought] probably isn't as bad as you think." Or maybe you would say something like "You know, I also feel anxious when I'm in that situation [or when I get that thought]. It feels awful for a little while, but eventually it passes." Do you see the double standard? Of course, it's much easier to challenge *someone else's* mistaken beliefs than it is to challenge your own. But why should you have a double standard? Can you think of any good reason that the advice you give someone else wouldn't also apply to you? Use the Double-Standard Technique Worksheet on the following page to use this strategy to help you with your own obsessional fear.

Another type of double standard involves applying faulty beliefs and interpretations inconsistently in your life. Do you have one set of cognitions when it comes to OCD-related situations, and a different set of beliefs that you apply to non-OCD situations? Crystal had

Double-Standard Technique Worksheet

Describe your obsessional fear: ____________________

____

____

What would you tell a friend who said he or she needed your help in dealing with this obsession?

____

____

____

Describe how you could use the advice you would give someone else to help with your own obsessional fear: ____________________

____

____

a problem with fears of bad luck and was afraid that thinking a *bad* thought (for example, about death) would cause a *negative* event (a loved one will die). Interestingly, she didn't believe that thinking a *good* thought (for example, winning the lottery) would cause a *positive* event. Do you see the inconsistency? If bad thoughts can cause bad events, why can't good thoughts cause positive events?

Can you live with uncertainty? You sure can! You probably take risks every day, like driving (accidents are *possible*), eating (you *could* choke on your food), climbing stairs (people *sometimes* fall), using a cell phone (*some* say it causes brain tumors), and so on. Think about the "risks" you take for granted in your daily life. If you'd react to your obsessional fears in the same way that you react to parallel situations that happen to fall outside of your OCD concerns, you'd be better able to control your obsessional anxiety and ritualistic behavior.

If you have contamination obsessions and washing rituals, you might exaggerate the dangerousness of germs but overlook the fact that too much washing can cause cracks in the skin that actually make you more susceptible to illness. If you have religious obsessions (scrupulosity), you might obsess over relatively minor aspects of your religion and overlook the more important observances or values. I've worked with people who have obsessional fears of fires and worry about making sure certain appliances such as irons and lights are turned off and unplugged; but they *don't* worry about other appliances that actually use much more electricity and could be just as dangerous—such as the furnace or the refrigerator. Finally, although you might have trouble with doubts and uncertainty where your obsessions are concerned, you probably have no problems accepting (even taking for granted) many other routine uncertainties of everyday life (for example, driving, crossing the street—to name a few).

In the space below, write down five "everyday risks" that you take without much hesitation:

1. ______________________________

2. ______________________________

3. ______________________________

4. ______________________________

5. ______________________________

Now, think about the negative consequences that these activities *could* have. If you can perform these activities with relatively little fear or anxiety, you're able to live with risk and uncertainty—the same kind of risk and uncertainty that your obsessional fears pose.

Maureen, whose obsessions centered around the fear of germs, and who engaged in constant avoidance and washing/cleaning rituals, identified the following everyday risks:

1. Driving short distances without a seatbelt
2. Running on the treadmill
3. Leaving the heat (furnace) running while out of the house
4. Rock climbing (not an everyday activity, but a few times per year)
5. Swimming

She hadn't ever considered that these behaviors, which she routinely takes for granted, actually pose a risk. The risk is small, but there *is* a risk. Maureen realized that each time she takes these "risks" she is making a guess that things will *probably* turn out okay. She realized that if she could apply this same logic to her obsessional fears of germs, she would be able to manage her obsessions and rituals much better. This encouraged her to practice exposure in which she confronted situations that provoked her obsessions.

BATTLE PLAN To use the double-standard technique correctly you need to try changing your own beliefs and behaviors based on how you would react to other people's obsessions and to situations that are outside the domain of your problems with OCD.

Cost–Benefit Analysis Technique

When Jed was growing up, he was taught, as most of us are, that it's important to stay clean—to bathe or shower, brush your teeth, change your clothes, wash your hands before eating and after using the bathroom, and so on. "Cleanliness," his parents told him, "protects you from looking and smelling bad and from getting sick." In other words, it's helpful for most of us to believe in the importance of keeping clean.

But when Jed developed OCD, his concern with cleanliness became excessive. He spent hours each day washing and cleaning because he was worried about germs, dirt, and other contaminants. Jed washed his hands so often, and with such intensity, that the skin of his hands had become dried out and cracked, which ironically increased his susceptibility to contamination and infection. Jed exaggerated the belief that "it is important to be clean." He took it way too far.

Consider the following beliefs:

"It's important to protect others from harm."
"I should have only good thoughts."
"I should be certain of things."
"It's important not to act sinfully."
"I should take responsibility for my actions."
"I should do things perfectly."

For most people, these ideas are generally realistic and healthy. But if you have problems with OCD, you might take one or more of them to the extreme—that is, to the point that they interfere with your life—like having too much of a good thing. So, in addition to examining the *accuracy* of your beliefs, it's useful to consider how *helpful* or *useful* these beliefs are for you. If they're helpful, they may be worth holding on to. But if not, perhaps it's time to let them go—or at least to tone them down.

Cost–benefit analysis is a tool to help you consider the pros and cons of holding certain beliefs. If the pros outweigh the cons, then the belief in question is probably helpful for you. If the cons outweigh the pros, it might be worth reconsidering.

Three easy steps are involved in cost–benefit analysis: (1) identifying a belief, (2) listing the *benefits* of holding this belief, and (3) listing the *costs* of this belief.

Preston had problems with religious OCD symptoms. He worried about upsetting God by accidentally committing sins. He avoided praying and taking part in religious ceremonies because he was concerned he might perform these activities incorrectly or with too little faith to satisfy God. He repeatedly asked his family, friends, and religious leaders whether they thought he was "faithful enough" and "a true believer." However, his incessant questioning started to anger members of his congregation, who began excluding Preston from religious activities. Ironically, Preston's scrupulosity was interfering with his religious observance. Talk about a self-fulfilling prophecy!

Preston conducted a cost–benefit analysis (shown in the form on the facing page) of his belief that "I must be perfectly faithful in everything that I do, or else God will be upset and punish me." He identified the various costs and benefits of holding this belief so rigidly.

This exercise helped Preston think about his problem with scrupulosity in new ways. Before, he had always thought of his obsessions as a sign that he needed to try harder to be perfectly faithful. But after taking a step back and considering the costs and benefits of his belief, he saw that he was actually trying *too* hard and that it was impossible to be *perfectly* faithful (or even to pin down exactly how faithful he was being). Preston also noticed that,

Cost–Benefit Analysis Worksheet: Preston's Example

Describe the belief, assumption, or prediction:
I must be perfectly faithful in everything that I do, or else God will be upset and punish me

Benefits of holding the belief	**Costs** of holding the belief
• *Makes me feel like I'm obeying the rules*	• *Very difficult (if not impossible) to achieve*
	• *Can't be certain that it's perfect—it always feels imperfect*
	• *I'm always worried about offending God*
	• *Leads to reassurance seeking*
	• *Reassurance seeking doesn't work*
	• *Gets in the way of social relationships*
	• *Other people don't really worry about this*
	• *Gets in the way of religious observance*

paradoxically, his beliefs were *interfering* with his religious observance. This new way of thinking led Preston to question whether it was worth trying so hard to be "perfectly faithful." He worked on learning to be no *more* or no *less* faithful than other members of his congregation whom he admired. As time passed, he found that he was able to practice his religion in a more meaningful way, patch up his social relationships, and even feel closer to God.

BATTLE PLAN As you use this technique, continue to review what you learned in Steps 1, 2, and 3. This review will help you identify the costs of your beliefs.

You can use the Cost–Benefit Analysis Worksheet on the following page for your own cost–benefit analyses. Go back to the beliefs you identified in Step 3 and try this exercise with each one (make copies of the form).

The costs of believing you can be *certain* are that it may be impossible to gain certainty and that it leads to endless reassurance rituals that cost you time and don't work in the long run. The costs of hyperresponsibility beliefs include excessive ruminating about the harm you might cause (or *might have* caused) and excessive checking behavior. The costs of believing that thoughts are the same as actions, and that you can and should control your unwanted obsessions are that this is an impossible way to win the battle with OCD—intrusive thoughts are normal and will always recur. Fighting them using avoidance and rituals only serves to make them stronger.

What's the cost of trying to be absolutely certain about your obsessional fears? Is such certainty even possible?

Cost–Benefit Analysis Worksheet

Describe the belief, assumption, or prediction: ______________________________

____

____

Benefits of holding the belief	**Costs** of holding the belief
______________________	______________________
______________________	______________________
______________________	______________________
______________________	______________________
______________________	______________________
______________________	______________________

Conducting Experiments

Rather than logically analyzing and writing about your cognitions, experimental strategies involve challenging and weakening these beliefs and interpretations by actually putting them to the test. This section describes three experiments that I find most helpful when working with people with OCD. The Cognitive Therapy Experiment Worksheet on the facing page is a tool for helping you set up these experiments and for keeping track of your results—just as a scientist would do. Read the descriptions of each experiment first, then use the worksheet to help you plan and work through the following steps:

1. Before conducting the experiment, specify the belief or interpretation you're going to test in the experiment.
2. Specify what the experiment will involve (where and when you'll conduct it).
3. Make predictions about what you expect the outcome of the experiment to be.
4. Then conduct the experiment.
5. Examine the outcome (the results).
6. Compare the outcome with your initial predictions and consider what you learned by conducting the experiment.

Power of Thoughts Experiment

If you worry that thinking bad thoughts will actually cause bad things to happen, this experiment can help you test your belief without taking too much of a risk. Specifically, you can try to make something "not too bad" happen. Follow these steps:

- Choose the "victim" of your thought (a friend, relative, or colleague—someone you can check in with to see if the experiment "worked"). *Don't let on that this person is the subject of your experiment since this could influence the results!*
- Decide what "not so bad" thing you will think about happening to this person. Make sure the mishap is something that would be somewhat out of the ordinary, but not com-

Cognitive Therapy Experiment Worksheet

1. The purpose of this experiment is to test the belief that: ____________________

____

2. On (date) ____________ at (time) ____________ I will (explain the experiment): ____________

____

____

____

3. My predictions about what will happen in the experiment are: ____________________

____

____

4. Conduct the experiment.

5. The results of the experiment were that (explain what happened and how you felt): ____________

____

____

6. How did the results compare to your predictions in #3? What did you learn by conducting the experiment? ____

____

____

pletely out of the question. Examples I often suggest are aggravating and annoying things like locking the keys in the car, getting a paper cut, getting a headache, losing power at home, having a flat tire, and the like. Also, make sure to specify a window of time so you can check on your results. For example, getting a flat tire *on the way to work tomorrow morning*.

- Then write down your "bad thought" on a piece of paper ("I hope Jasmine gets a headache sometime today").
- Keep the paper with you and remind yourself of this thought all day long. Think about it as much as you can. Wish for it. Go ahead—take the risk! If you're afraid, use the life-savings wager technique described on page 158. Where would you place your bet?
- At the end of the day (or the next day), check in and ask the person whether what you were thinking about actually happened ("I had a bad headache the other day; have you had any lately?").
- Repeat the experiment a few times with different victims and different situations to see if your first results were *luck* or the *real thing*.
- Then review the results of the experiment and what they mean for your prediction. Do your thoughts cause bad things to happen?

Vernon used the power-of-thoughts experiment to test his belief that thinking about misfortune would cause bad luck. Every day for a week he purposely thought about his wife getting a speeding ticket while driving to or from work (she commuted about 20 miles each way). When his wife didn't get any tickets, Vernon used this as evidence against his fear that he might cause mishaps simply by thinking about them. Vernon's completed Cognitive Therapy Experiment Worksheet appears on the facing page.

You might hold the belief that your thoughts could lead *you* to lose control and do inappropriate, immoral, or violent things that you wouldn't ordinarily do. If so, you can use a variation of the power-of-thoughts experiment in which you purposely think about doing something you don't wish to do. For example, try holding an object such as a cup or a pen in your hand and think about dropping it, but try not to drop it. Really focus intently on thinking of dropping the item. Does thinking about dropping this object make you drop it even though you are trying not to? Do your thoughts alone make you do things you don't want to do? Next, try something a little more challenging, such as thinking about dropping a fragile item (a glass, a lightbulb, an egg, your infant). Try to make yourself drop this item, or throw it against the nearest wall, *just by thinking about doing so*. Do your thoughts make you do things you don't want to do? The aim of this experiment is to demonstrate that you're capable of making decisions about whether to act on intrusive or unpleasant thoughts. Unwanted thoughts don't automatically lead to actions.

> Does this exercise seem too difficult? If so, try it with a **positive** event first: try to make someone win the lottery, get a promotion, find a dollar bill on the street, and so on, just by thinking about it.

Vernon's Cognitive Therapy Experiment Worksheet

1. The purpose of this experiment is to test the belief that:

   Thinking about something bad will cause something bad to really happen.

2. On (date) *Monday* at (time) *7:30 a. m.* I will (explain the experiment):

   Imagine that Joan is going above the speed limit on Interstate 40 (as she usually does) on her way to work, and that a police officer pulls her over and gives her a speeding ticket.

3. My predictions about what will happen in the experiment are:

   Joan will end up with a speeding ticket because I was thinking about it.

4. Conduct the experiment.

5. The results of the experiment were that (explain what happened and how you felt):

   Joan did not get any speeding tickets.

6. How did the results compare to your predictions in #3? What did you learn by conducting the experiment?

   The result was different than my prediction. Doing the experiment gave me evidence that I don't have to be so concerned that my obsessional thoughts will really cause bad things to happen. Maybe these thoughts are just senseless and meaningless.

Premonitions Experiment

A premonition is a situation in which you forecast a future event. A famous example is that of Abraham Lincoln, who apparently had a dream about his own funeral the night before he was assassinated (he supposedly told his wife about the dream the morning of the day he was shot). We all have premonitions from time to time. Have you ever turned on the radio and heard the very same song you were just humming to yourself? What about when the phone rings and it's the very person you were just thinking of? Perhaps it seems to you that there's more to these experiences than just coincidence—maybe our thoughts *can* influence external events. But what most people don't stop to think about are all the times we're humming a song and it *doesn't* come on the radio, or all the people we think about who *don't* call. When you look at it this way, it's easier to see that premonitions are just coincidental. The human mind, though, tends to remember the few coincidences (because they stand out) and forget about all the other times.

The premonitions experiment is another way to test beliefs about the importance of thoughts. It involves having premonitions and keeping track of whether they come true. For example, think about a good friend and see if she calls. Sing your favorite song and then turn on the radio. Can you predict these things? You can use the Premonitions Experiment Worksheet on page 168 to keep track of how often your premonitions turn out to be valid.

Premonitions Experiment Worksheet

Premonition	Valid? Yes	Valid? No
__________	☐	☐
__________	☐	☐
__________	☐	☐
__________	☐	☐
__________	☐	☐
__________	☐	☐
__________	☐	☐
__________	☐	☐
__________	☐	☐
__________	☐	☐
__________	☐	☐

Thought Suppression Experiment

Donna was a devout Christian whose main obsession was a recurring mental image of Jesus' penis. Naturally, she found the image extremely distressing and blasphemous. Thinking that she shouldn't be having such thoughts, Donna began trying to dismiss it by repeating to herself, "Don't think about Jesus' penis . . . Don't think about Jesus' penis. . . ." But this strategy didn't work. In fact, the image was getting more intense! Donna interpreted her failure to dismiss her unwanted image as catastrophic—a sign that her mind was possessed by the devil.

> Do you try to fight or suppress your obsessional thoughts even though this strategy doesn't work?

Whether your obsessions concern germs, illness, harm, bad luck, numbers, violence, sex, religion, order and symmetry, or other topics, you probably have unwanted thoughts that you try to dismiss. If you're bothered by these thoughts, it's only natural to want to get rid of them. But how well does this strategy work? Maybe you can *sometimes* control your obsessions, but most likely, they end up returning sooner or later. This is because of a well-known phenomenon called the *rebound effect*. Many studies show that when you deliberately try to dismiss a thought (a strategy called *thought suppression*), it paradoxically makes the thought more intense. It's not that your mind is spitefully working against you.

Instead, you should compare your mind to a radar scanner that picks up on thoughts that you've associated with high levels of negative emotion. By the way, this happens to people with and without OCD.

The thought suppression experiment can help you challenge the belief that you can and should control your upsetting obsessional thoughts. You'll learn that not only is it impossible to completely control a thought, but that trying to do so actually makes your obsessions worse. You'll need the Thought Suppression Experiment Worksheet (below) and a watch with a second hand to try out this experiment.

The rebound effect of thought suppression helps explain why obsessions develop a life of their own: the more you struggle against and try not to think a certain thought, the more you end up thinking about it.

How successful were you at stopping pink elephant thoughts? How many check marks did you have? Due to the rebound effect, most people can't control pink elephant thoughts when they try. Of course, this also applies to your obsessions. So, if you're trying hard *not* to think about sex, violence, germs, blasphemy, injuries, and so on, you'll probably end up failing. The implication here is that trying to stop these thoughts is not only a lost cause but likely to make you feel *worse*. Instead, as you will learn in Steps 7 and 8, the best strategy is to do the opposite—to *confront* these unwanted thoughts, images, and impulses and see that they're not worthy of your fruitless attempts at mental control. When you stop trying so hard to suppress or fight your obsessional thoughts, and befriend them instead, they'll actually start to leave you alone.

Using Cognitive Therapy to Help with Exposure Practice

Once you're familiar with the cognitive techniques, you'll find them very helpful to use right before an exposure practice. In a sense, cognitive therapy weakens the foundations of your obsessions so that exposure can completely take them out. Using cognitive therapy before an exposure practice may help alleviate some of your anticipation about facing your

Thought Suppression Experiment Worksheet

For the next 30 seconds, close your eyes and try *not* to think of a pink elephant. You can think about anything else in the world *except* for a pink elephant. Put a check mark in the space below for any pink elephant thoughts that *do* come to mind during the next 30 seconds.

fears. It will give you some perspective on the feared situation or thought you're about to confront so that the risks of exposure don't seem quite so high.

BATTLE PLAN After you've read about exposure and response prevention in the next three steps, I'll help you see how these techniques are used in combination, but you can use the Cognitive Therapy and Exposure Worksheet to help you prepare for using cognitive therapy when you begin exposure practice. Wait to fill out this form until after you've practiced cognitive therapy for a week or two and are ready to move on to exposure practice. That way, you'll know about which cognitive techniques might work best for you.

Completing the Cognitive Therapy and Exposure Worksheet is straightforward. In the left column, you'll see that I've listed all the cognitive therapy strategies described in this step. Your job is to think about which of these techniques you could use to weaken the cognitive errors associated with each of your exposure hierarchy items from Step 4. So fill in the right column with the situational and imaginal exposure hierarchy items that each cognitive strategy might be particularly helpful with.

Moving On to Step 7

Cognitive therapy techniques are powerful—they can help you challenge the mental gremlins that underlie obsessional fears and ritualistic urges. But they are not powerful enough to defeat OCD on their own. Practice them while you read about exposure and response prevention in the following steps. They'll only enhance the gains you get when you put Steps 7–9 into action.

BATTLE PLAN To help you match hierarchy items with cognitive therapy strategies, refer back to the table at the beginning of Step 6 (page 149) to identify which techniques work best with which cognitive errors. Then try to figure out which hierarchy items are associated with each cognitive error.

Cognitive Therapy and Exposure Worksheet

Cognitive technique	Exposure hierarchy item(s)
Examining the evidence	
Continuum technique	
Pie-chart technique	
Life-savings wager technique	
Double-standard technique	
Cost–benefit analysis	
Experiment techniques	

STEP 7

Defeating Avoidance Behavior

- Read Steps 7–9 before starting exposure practices.
- While you're learning about exposure and response prevention, you can practice the cognitive therapy techniques you learned in Step 6 for 45 minutes a day for 1–2 weeks.
- Need help? Troubleshooting tips for situational and imaginal exposure appear at the end of Step 8.

Like everyone else, you don't like feeling anxious, right? So it's only natural to try to avoid the situations, objects, and other stimuli that trigger your obsessions. When you avoid a fear trigger, it makes you feel safe and relieved—almost like you've narrowly escaped a terrible mishap or catastrophe (for example, "I must avoid bathrooms to stay germ-free and healthy"). But this sense of safety and relief is only temporary. You know from plenty of experience that it's just a matter of time before another obsessional thought or trigger sets you off again. What may not be so obvious from moment to moment is the huge cost of that temporary relief. When you avoid your obsessional triggers, you don't have a chance to see how things would have turned out had you not avoided them. If you *always* avoid, you'll never know. This is why avoidance keeps the OCD vicious cycle going. It literally keeps you from overcoming your obsessional fears.

What if the situation or object you avoided wasn't really as dangerous as you thought?

What if you could manage it better than you give yourself credit for?

Avoidance increases your fears by reducing your chances to learn that your obsessional fears aren't accurate. It also saps your confidence that you can handle the situation the next time it comes up.

Exposure therapy is the process of overcoming irrational fears and avoidance by facing whatever makes you anxious. I know this sounds very difficult. Maybe you're thinking, "You want me to do *what*!? Never happen! I'd be much too scared;

it's not worth the risk!" Don't worry; I'm not planning on overwhelming you. We'll do this step by step, at your own pace. You'll be in the driver's seat the whole time. In this step, I'll give you some tips for how to conduct successful exposure practices. Then I'll walk you through your first exposure exercise and give you suggestions for how to prepare for experiencing anxiety. Finally, I'll give you lots of ideas and examples of how to create exposure practices for your particular types of obsessions.

Let me tell you about the very first patient I treated with exposure therapy. Amelia was scared of elevators—she had avoided them her whole life and always used the stairs instead. Now she wanted to overcome her fear since she was getting older and couldn't climb stairs as easily. First Amelia practiced just walking on and off an elevator while it stayed on the ground floor. At first she felt afraid to do this, but after a little while her fear subsided and she found that nothing bad happened to her. So we moved on to the next step: Amelia rode up to the second floor of the building. At first she worried the elevator might get stuck and she'd be trapped for a long time without food, water, or a bathroom. She even worried that she'd run out of air! Amelia was visibly anxious—sweating, trembling, heart pounding. But she didn't give up. She stayed on that elevator, and after about half an hour of riding her anxiety subsided and she felt a lot more comfortable.

In total, Amelia completed four exposure therapy sessions with me. We charted her anxiety level (from 0—no anxiety—to 100, total panic) every 5 minutes during each session, and this is shown in the chart below. As you can see, when she first entered the elevator on the first day of practice, her anxiety level was quite high. But as she continued to ride, she felt less and less anxious. Also, with repeated practice, her peak anxiety level got lower and her anxiety subsided more quickly—the elevator no longer frightened Amelia. Exposure therapy helped her learn from her own experience that although she initially *felt* unsafe, it was unlikely that anything bad would actually happen (*even though there was no*

Amelia's Fear Level While Riding Elevators during Four Exposure Therapy Sessions

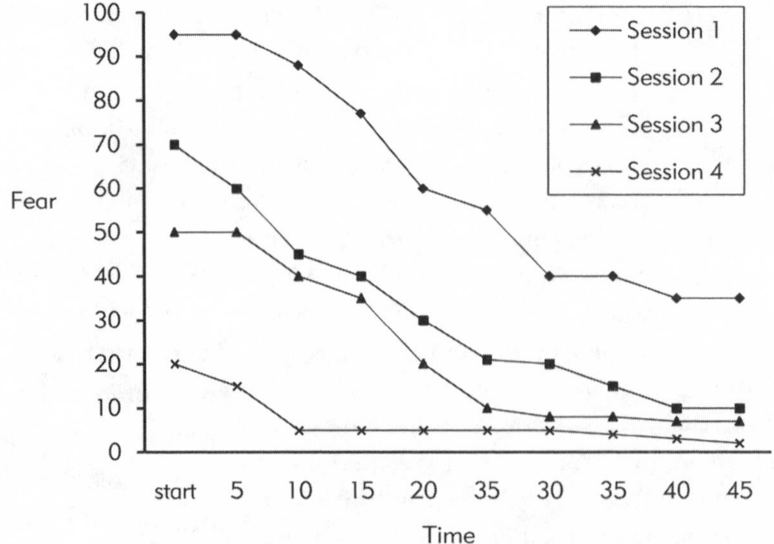

guarantee). "I feel so good about what I've done," Amelia said. "I never thought I'd be able to do that."

So exposure therapy means confronting situations that provoke feelings of anxiety, uncertainty, and risk and moving forward as if you're *reasonably* sure that your feared outcome won't materialize. Practicing exposure will teach you three things you must know to conquer your obsessional fears. First, as Amelia's chart clearly shows, the feelings of anxiety you have when you confront your obsessional triggers will not last forever. Instead, they'll dissipate by themselves if you give them a chance—even when you remain exposed to the trigger. Second, exposure will teach you the difference between the way feared situations *feel* and how they actually *are*. That is, just because you feel anxious doesn't mean that danger is lurking around the corner. You'll see that your trigger situations are not as dangerous as you had thought. Third, doing exposure therapy will help you feel more comfortable with a normal degree of risk and uncertainty. It's not always possible to get an *absolute* guarantee about something you fear. Through exposure, you'll practice managing with a *reasonable* degree of certainty.

The goal of exposure therapy is to tolerate your anxious thoughts and feelings long enough to see that anxiety subsides on its own, that your trigger situations are actually safe, and that you don't need an absolute guarantee of safety to feel comfortable.

Exposure is one of the main techniques used in the treatment of anxiety problems. Studies show that it is a very potent tool. I use it with my patients almost every day. These people are often amazed at how, after only a few sessions, they're going into situations they never thought they'd be able to handle and doing things they thought they were too frightened to do. They're allowing themselves to face risks and uncertainties in order to learn that these situations are nowhere near as dangerous as they had thought. As I said, we'll make sure that your exposure practices aren't overwhelming by starting with easier ones and working our way up to the harder ones. Also, you'll use cognitive therapy skills from Step 6 to help you get though the periods of high anxiety. Over time, you too will be able to handle more challenging situations than you probably can imagine right now.

How Can I Face My Obsessional Triggers If I'm Not *Absolutely* Sure It's Safe?

If you have problems with OCD, you might avoid taking chances and instead insist on an absolute guarantee of safety before you act. But unfortunately, there really are no absolute guarantees, and trying to get them before acting only leads to feeling trapped and overwhelmed. So an important goal of situational exposure is to help you learn to live with taking risks, even if you don't have an absolute guarantee.

Olga has contamination obsessions that are triggered by lawn fertilizers and pesticides because they can contain toxic chemicals. To protect herself, she washes her hands after using such products. But she doesn't feel completely safe, so she simply avoids using them. She still doesn't feel absolutely safe, so she avoids stores and shopping centers where these products are sold. *Still* not feeling completely safe, and realizing that many people she might encounter might have had contact with her feared contaminants (for example, from walking across a lawn treated with fertilizer), she decides to avoid interacting with anyone except two friends who know about her fears. Now, because of her fear of chemicals and her unwillingness to take risks, Olga has become socially isolated and can't work or enjoy leisure activities. Although she has good evidence that her fears are excessive (lots of people she knows use the products she's afraid of and remain healthy), she pays attention only to her obsessional fears: "I *could* get very sick." Olga would probably overcome her fear if she'd allow herself to have contact with a broader range of people and even use the feared substances. But she never puts her fears and assumptions to the test.

Do you waste too much time and energy trying to keep yourself safe by avoiding?

The moral of this story is that you pay a price for protecting yourself like this. As Olga's story illustrates, the costs of doing everything under the sun to eliminate all possible risk and uncertainty are very high: you lose your freedom and become a prisoner of your obsessions. As you learned in Step 6, however, most people without OCD choose to accept *some* risk and uncertainty because it's simply more practical than demanding an absolute guarantee of safety. For example, most people drive knowing they *could* be in a deadly accident. Most people leave appliances such as computers, furnaces, and refrigerators on when they're sleeping or away from home, even though there is a risk of fire. These situations (and many others like them) may not seem like risks because the chances of disaster are very small. But they're not 100% risk free either: there is no absolute guarantee of safety.

Your obsessional triggers fall into the same small-risk category. Yes, they may pose *some* risk, but it's minimal. In fact, other people have probably told you that they think the situations you fear are actually quite safe. Again, that doesn't mean they're *absolutely 100%* safe—just that the risks are minimal.

To overcome your obsessional fears you must decide to accept the small risks of facing your fears by doing exposure practices so you can learn how to treat your obsessions just as you would any other situation involving minimal everyday risk.

When you practice situational exposure, you'll work on facing the fearful situations you listed on your situational exposure hierarchy in Step 4 (page 95). You'll deliberately touch or use the objects you fear, visit places and confront numbers or words you've been staying away from, and put yourself in situations you might usually try to avoid. If you're ready to jump right in and do the really hard exposures, good for you. But most likely you'll want to take it slow and move through your hierarchy gradually from the least fearful to the most fearful items.

"I've Tried Exposure Before—It Doesn't Work for Me"

If your obsession involves cemeteries, will happening to drive past a cemetery once in a while eliminate that obsession? If you're afraid of germs from trash cans, does accidentally touching a garbage can in a fast-food restaurant mean your obsession about trash should be over? Some people mistakenly believe that because they continue to have obsessional anxiety after a few chance encounters with feared situations, it means that exposure therapy isn't going to work

At some point it's inevitable—you'll probably have unplanned run-ins with your feared situations as part of your daily life. Once you're experienced with doing the carefully planned exposure practices, you'll work on adding in more and more of these "lifestyle exposures" to your routine.

for them. It's important to understand, however, that inadvertently exposing yourself to your fears is not the same thing as therapeutic exposure. For it to have the effect of extinguishing your obsessions, exposure must be *intentional*, *prolonged*, and *repeated*. It also must be true exposure—you have to truly face the feared situation, rather than fighting or resisting the anxious feelings you get when you come face to face with a trigger.

Therapeutic exposure must be:

- **Planned**
- **Prolonged**
- **Repeated**

Exposure won't be therapeutic if it's accidental. The reason for planning is that it allows you to choose to face the easier, more manageable situations first. These early successes breed confidence and make it possible to gradually work your way up to the more frightening items at a pace that feels comfortable to you. If you had contamination obsessions about urine, for example, you might begin with touching the door of a bathroom, then the bathroom floor, then the toilet, then dirty underwear, then touching spots of urine on a piece of toilet paper.

Exposure that's too quick won't give you a chance to get used to normal levels of anxiety. Think of a time when you jumped into a swimming pool and the water felt cold. If you stay in the water long enough, it seems to warm up. Of course, the water temperature hasn't really changed; you've just gotten used to it—what we call "habituating" to it. The anxiety you feel when you do exposure therapy will also habituate if you give it enough time.

One-time confrontation with a feared situation is not enough to get you over your obsessions. Why? When you first confront a situation you've been avoiding, your fear of the unknown and the pattern of expecting the worst automatically kick in. Wearing down this pattern and learning not to be so fearful takes time and practice. You need to see, *over and over again*, that nothing awful happens when you confront the situation—and that your anxiety level decreases. This is similar to what occurs if you watch a horror movie 100 times. The first time you see it, you don't know what to expect and may find it very frightening. But if you watched the movie again and again, it would lose its ability to scare you. You'd get used to it. You'd know what's going to happen, and you'd become comfortable (or even bored) seeing it. You'll probably be anxious the first several times you try each exposure practice, but eventually your anxiety will decrease if you stick with it.

Therapeutic exposure must also:

- **Cause *some* anxiety**

For exposure to be helpful, you must "go with" the anxious feelings when they occur. Don't worry—exposure doesn't require *maximum* fear, only *some* degree of anxiety. If you were teaching your teenager to drive a car, you wouldn't have to throw him onto a busy highway the first time he got behind the wheel to help him get used to the pressure of driving in traffic. Rather, practicing on side streets, where driving techniques can be learned safely, is a good way to get started—even though the driver will experience *some* anxiety there. It's the same when you do exposure therapy. If you fight or resist anxious feelings using rituals, avoidance, reassurance seeking, distraction, or any other means, you won't overcome your fear. In fact, fighting your fear this way will only cause you to feel *worse*.

How to Make Sure Your Exposure Practices Are Effective

The way you conduct your exposure practices will determine how much improvement you get from this program. Here are 10 tips to help you optimize your exposures.

1. **Practice with situations that closely match those that trigger your obsessional fears.** For situational (and imaginal) exposure to be helpful, your exposure practices have to trigger the same kind of obsessional distress that you experience when obsessions occur in your daily life. The best way to make sure this happens is to pick situations that duplicate or closely match the real-life triggers of your obsessions and urges to ritualize. If you're mainly distressed by contamination from certain pesticides that have particular toxic ingredients, make sure you visit a home improvement store that carries these particular pesticides.

2. **Use your hierarchy for a gradual approach.** The whole point of creating your hierarchies in Step 4 (pages 95 and 104) was to give you a ladder by which to work your way through exposure gradually. Don't jump around and don't move on to a more difficult hierarchy item until practice with an easier one provokes only minimal anxiety.

BATTLE PLAN To be sure that you feel more comfortable with each situation before moving to the next level of difficulty, I recommend focusing on each hierarchy item for at least 1 week.

3. **Practice exposure every day.** It's a fact: the more often you practice exposure, the happier you'll be with your results. For example, if you're afraid of cemeteries, going to a cemetery once a week will decrease your obsessional fear more effectively than going once a month. But going every day, or several times a week, will be even more effective than going once a week, even if the number of times you visit the cemetery is the same. In other words, going to a cemetery 5 days in a row will likely lead to a greater decrease in your obsessional fear than will going once a week for 5 weeks. This is why I suggest daily exposure practice.

BATTLE PLAN Practice exposure twice every day (perhaps once in the morning and once in the afternoon or evening). Of course, feel free to do more work if you like. The more time you put into doing these exercises, the faster you'll improve and the more benefit you will get out of this program.

4. **Stay in the exposure situation until your anxiety decreases.** Stick it out! Each time you practice, force yourself to remain in the feared situation until your level of anxiety decreases by at least half. If for some reason you can't stay with an exposure until anxiety comes down, try to

practice the same situation again as soon as possible. You may also find that some of your exposures are naturally brief. An example is leaving the house (without checking) after you use an electrical appliance (if you're afraid of causing a fire). If you were to repeat this activity (returning home and leaving *again*), you'd see each time whether everything was turned off, and this would be like a checking ritual! In these cases, you'll use imaginal exposure techniques (see Step 8) to help you stay exposed to the uncertainty and doubt that triggers anxiety.

BATTLE PLAN Stay in your exposure situations for at least 1 hour. This is usually enough time for your anxiety to subside. If you're doing an exposure to driving, try to stay in your car for at least an hour. If you're confronting a fear of "floor germs," sit on the floor for the same amount of time. Timing, though, is not as important as your anxiety level. Later in this step you'll learn how to keep track of your anxiety level when you do exposure practices.

5. **Don't fight the anxiety.** It's hard to believe until you see it for yourself, but when you embrace your anxious feelings, they actually fizzle out more quickly than if you try to fight them. Just allow the anxious feelings to come, reminding yourself that it's okay to be anxious and that what's happening in your body is completely normal, harmless, and temporary. Tell yourself the worst thing that can happen is that you'll feel uncomfortable for a little while.

Some types of anti-anxiety medications (such as Xanax, Ativan, Valium, and Klonopin) and mood-altering substances (such as alcohol, marijuana, and cocaine) have the same effect as trying to fight anxiety. Using these drugs to help you cope with the anxiety that comes with confronting your fear might seem like a good idea, but these drugs will keep exposure from being effective. They'll prevent you from learning that anxiety isn't dangerous and that it will fizzle out on its own even if you don't take the drugs to help you.

Although quick-acting benzodiazepine medications such as Xanax and Klonopin defeat the purpose of doing exposure, other medications such as the SSRIs are okay to use along with CBT.

6. **Don't fight your obsessions.** Go ahead: let yourself worry about the disastrous things you're afraid will happen. When you practice letting your obsessional doubts "hang out" in your brain, you're taking the wind out of their sails, and they'll bother you less and less. OCD wants you to be afraid of your obsessions; when you try to resist them, you only reinforce OCD's hold over you. Instead, show OCD who's the boss! Doing imaginal exposure (Step 8) will also help you confront your upsetting obsessional thoughts.

Trying not to be anxious or worried is a little like trying not to think of a pink elephant. When you try to force yourself *not* to think of something, your mind gets stuck on the very thing you're trying not to think about. It's the same with anxiety and obsessions. Fighting and resisting these thoughts and feelings makes them more intense. As soon as you allow yourself to become anxious and welcome these unpleasant feelings, you'll start to feel more comfortable around your obsessional triggers. I realize this sounds contradictory, but that's how it works.

BATTLE PLAN Use the imaginal exposure techniques that you'll learn in Step 8 to help you confront upsetting obsessional thoughts, images, and doubts that come up during situational exposure. This will show you that they're just senseless thoughts and ideas.

Dede had contamination obsessions and was afraid of contact with her brother, Jeremiah, because he had diabetes. Dede was afraid she'd catch this disease if she touched anything that belonged to Jeremiah. For exposure, Dede practiced wearing Jeremiah's clothes and sleeping in his pajamas. While doing this, she allowed herself to feel anxious and even let herself imagine catching diabetes. Dede found that her discomfort subsided quicker than she had expected. She noticed herself thinking that her fear was senseless, and she became less and less obsessed about Jeremiah's diabetes.

7. **Use response prevention—don't ritualize!** Put everything you've got into resisting performing rituals. The whole point of situational exposure practice is to provoke urges to ritualize and then substitute new ways to respond. That means working on stopping compulsive behavior, mental rituals, mini-rituals, and even attempts to get reassurance in other ways such as asking questions or looking up information about your fear triggers. In Step 9 I'll give you more response prevention strategies, but for now understand that if you perform these rituals during and after exposure, you'll sap exposure of its ability to help you since you won't learn that anxiety subsides on its own and that you can manage uncertainty.

BATTLE PLAN Start applying your response prevention plan when you begin your first exposure practice. Read Step 9 for details on how to use response prevention along with exposure practice.

Response prevention also means not engaging in subtle safety behaviors. For example, Annette had obsessional thoughts of drowning her infant son in the bathtub. Fearing she might act on her obsessions, she avoided bathing her son. Finally, she worked up the courage to confront her fear, and she bathed her son every day for a week. However, she made sure her husband was there with her when she did these exposures *just in case anything bad happened.* Annette didn't realize it, but involving her husband in this way spoiled the exposure. It was like stringing up an extra safety net—one that she didn't really need. Knowing her husband would intervene if she began acting violently was like having a guarantee that she wouldn't commit any harm. It prevented Annette from really putting her fears to the test. How could she possibly learn to live with uncertainty if she conducted exposure this way?

"Safety behaviors" are subtle things you might do to make exposure practices easier and less frightening. Examples include having other people around (as in Annette's example) and saying prayers before exposure. Because they're usually brief, safety behaviors might seem insignificant. But as with rituals, they'll sabotage your exposures. So it's important to perform exposure exercises without them.

They might be quicker and more subtle than repetitive compulsive rituals, but brief safety behaviors, mental rituals, and mini-rituals are just as important to stop when you do CBT. These brief and covert behaviors can ruin your exposures just as much as blatant compulsive rituals can.

8. **Don't distract yourself.** When you practice exposure, don't try to ignore the upsetting parts of the situation you're confronting. Rather, pay attention to these aspects and stay emotionally involved in the experience. For example, if you're confronting a toilet for exposure, you should focus on what is disturbing to you about the toilet—perhaps the possibility of germs and getting a disease. Don't try to overlook these parts of the situation or pretend they're not there by trying to convince yourself that the toilet was just cleaned.

9. **Try something easier if anxiety doesn't decrease.** If your discomfort level hasn't started to go down after an hour of exposure, you might have jumped the gun and chosen something too difficult for where you are right now. Stop your practice and try to find a situation that's a little easier for you to confront. Then go back to the more difficult situation. For example, if you were trying to touch the floor, stop and try touching something a little less frightening, such as your shoes (or perhaps even your socks). This easier exposure is not a way to avoid facing the original, more fearful situation—you'll need to come back to it at some point. Instead, think of the intermediate exposure as a way of helping you gradually work up to the more difficult one.

BATTLE PLAN Give your anxiety 1 hour to go down. If it doesn't, switch your exposure practice to something a little easier.

10. **Face your fears in different settings.** Your improvement will be most complete if you conduct exposure in different situations and settings. For example, if it's restrooms that provoke fear, don't just practice exposure to one or two—confront many different restrooms. This will ensure that you learn to manage obsessional triggers wherever they might pop up—not just in your most comfortable environments.

If there's a big difference in how much distress is provoked by facing your fears in different situations, make these separate hierarchy items. For example, Bernie had a difficult time with exposure to curse words. Confronting them at home was hard enough, but doing so in a place of worship was a whole different ball game. So he split his original hierarchy item—curse words—into three separate items: (a) curse words at home (b) curse words at school, and (c) curse words at church (he wrote the words on a piece of paper, which he took to the church in his pocket). This helped him gradually confront his fear in different situations.

BATTLE PLAN Practicing exposure in the settings that match your obsessional fears doesn't mean limiting yourself to one "perfect" match. To ensure that your mind gets used to not just *that* bathroom but all bathrooms, the number 4 not just in restaurants filled with tables for four but the number 4 anywhere, and so forth, you have to practice in many situations that are close matches.

Isn't It Dangerous to Get So Anxious?

Harper was terrified. She knew she'd get very anxious when she tried exposure, and she thought it would make her "go crazy," lose control, and have a "nervous breakdown." She also worried it would lead to a heart attack or some other medical emergency.

If you have OCD, you're no stranger to feeling anxious. But actually, *everyone* knows what it's like to feel this way. In fact, there isn't a person alive who hasn't experienced the unpleasant feelings of fear and anxiety, whether it's the butterflies in the pit of your stomach before an important exam, interview, or date or the sense of anticipation when you feel something awful is about to happen. But what you might *not* know—and what Harper didn't know—is that anxiety is as harmless as it is unpleasant. In fact, *the very purpose of anxiety is to keep you safe and help you deal with danger.* Without it, you (and everyone else) simply wouldn't survive. Think of how anxiety makes you look both ways when crossing a busy street and how fear makes you jump out of the way of an oncoming car. Anxiety also helps us perform at our best. If you've ever had to prepare for an important presentation or test, you know that a little anxiety keeps you motivated and focused on what you're doing.

Anxiety feels so uncomfortable because it's intended to put you on "high alert" and push you to act. It's like an annoying alarm that won't stop until you do what it says—typically, to do whatever it takes to avoid danger and protect yourself. We call this the fight-or-flight (or adrenaline) response because it prepares you to defend yourself by making your heart beat faster, your breathing get deeper, and your muscles tense, and by providing more oxygen to your brain and muscles so that you are alert and have more energy to fight off danger or flee from it.

How has anxiety—the fight-or-flight response—been helpful for you?

Anxiety *won't* make you lose control or act destructively. Think about it; it would make no sense at all for humans to have a system like anxiety that protects us from harm but then double-crosses us and harms us. Once Harper learned to think of anxiety as a "friend," she was able to practice exposure, become anxious, and see for herself that she eventually calmed down.

Anxiety might feel uncomfortable, but it can't hurt you! Rather, it is there to *protect* you from danger and help you stay out of harm's way. The uncomfortable feelings that happen when you get anxious are part of the body's automatic way of preparing you to fight or flee from danger.

Don't worry that "too much" of the fight-or-flight feelings will harm your body or give you a heart attack or stroke. There is no such thing as being "too anxious." First, anxiety won't last forever. It has a limit—a ceiling—and then you begin to calm down. Second, although constant long-lasting stress over many years might increase your risk of certain diseases (for example, heart disease, stroke), this type of *chronic* stress is very different from the fight-or-flight response. In fact, the fight-or-flight response involves short bursts of adrenaline, which is very similar to what happens when you exercise—and we all know that exercise-related exertion is very healthy for your body. So, although high levels of stress can pose a *long-term* risk, this risk is minimal compared to the dangers associated with other unhealthy lifestyle factors, such as a poor diet, lack of exercise, smoking, and substance abuse.

Starting Your Exposure Practices

Planning the First Exposure

When you're ready to get started, choose the first item on your fear hierarchy (page 95). Think about when and how you will confront this situation or object. In some cases the exposure will be relatively straightforward, such as touching dirty laundry, hanging a picture off center, or holding a knife. In other instances exposure will require you to plan ahead, be creative, or arrange a specific situation, such as going to a gay bar, driving alone at night, or visiting a funeral home. You'll find suggestions on exposure practices for different types of obsessional fears later in this chapter. After Step 9, in the chapter "Putting It All Together," I show you how to keep track of your exposure practices using the Planned Exposure Practice Worksheet.

Dealing with Multiple Exposure Hierarchies

If you have obsessions with more than one theme and ended up creating more than one situational exposure hierarchy (for example, one for your contamination obsessions, another for your religious obsessions), I suggest you work through these one at a time. The questions below can help you choose which obsession (and hierarchy) to begin with:

List the themes of your hierarchies (for example, contamination fears and homosexuality obsessions):

____

____

____

1. Now list the hierarchy themes *in order* from the easiest to confront (the least distressing items) to the most difficult to confront (the most distressing items): ____________________

____

2. Which hierarchy contains the most feared items that interfere with your daily life? __________

____

3. Which hierarchy would close friends or family members suggest that you begin with? ________

____

4. Which hierarchy contains items that will be the most straightforward to practice exposure with? (Contamination exposures are often straightforward, as are symmetry/order exposures. Exposures for sexual, religious, violent, and responsibility obsessions tend to be more challenging to arrange—see the descriptions later in this step): ____________________

____

Once you've considered the answers to these questions, list your hierarchies in the order that you'll practice: ____

____

____

June had religious obsessions and was afraid of committing sins. For example, she worried that if she noticed a good-looking man (June was happily married), she would be "committing adultery in her heart." So the first item on June's hierarchy was "looking at attractive men." For her two daily exposures, June planned to look at pictures of good-looking male models in fitness magazines—something that many women do every day, and it hardly means they're cheating on their partners!

Treatment Buddy Tip

If you're having trouble getting up the nerve to begin an exposure practice, ask your treatment buddy to talk about the exercise with you. Let him or her know what you think will be stressful. Talk about how you will deal with the situation and the anxiety if it becomes very difficult. Plan with your treatment buddy what you want him or her to do if you run into trouble or want to stop the exposure practice.

For treatment buddies: If your friend or loved one requests it, try to be there when he or she attempts the first exposure practices; but it's important to gradually phase out your involvement in exposures over the course of the program so that your friend or loved one can learn to manage anxiety on his or her own.

Setting the Table with Cognitive Therapy

BATTLE PLAN Spend about 10 minutes at the beginning of each exposure using cognitive therapy techniques to prepare you for facing your fears.

Analyzing your beliefs and interpretations before and after each exposure will help you fix problematic cognitions and reduce anxiety about facing your fears. The Planned Exposure Practice Worksheet includes space for recording your cognitive therapy work so you'll have it in written form.

Before you enter the feared situation, consider what you're afraid might happen if you do this exposure without ritualizing or using any avoidance behaviors. For example, "I [or someone else] will get sick and die," "I'll become a child molester," "I'll go to hell," "I'll never know whether I injured someone," or "I'll be responsible for causing an injury." Try to make your negative prediction as specific as possible by identifying what will happen to whom. June's feared outcome was "I'll become a sinner and God will hate me."

Next, use one or more cognitive therapy strategies from Step 6 to help you challenge this negative cognition and come up with a more helpful and balanced way of thinking about the exposure situation. What's a more likely outcome than the overly negative prediction? Remember, the goal is not to try to reassure yourself that the exposure is totally safe—always keep in mind that the task carries *some* risk. Instead, acknowledge this risk without resorting to avoidance and rituals. Your new prediction should help you feel better (although not 100% reassured) about confronting the feared situation. If your fears have to do with very long-term negative consequences ("I'll get sick *50 years from now*"), use cognitive therapy strategies like the Life Savings Wager to help you better manage uncertainty.

June: Cognitive Challenges

June used the double-standard technique and examining the evidence to arrive at more helpful, realistic beliefs such as, "Everyone sometimes finds other people attractive—this is a fact of life, but it's not the same as lusting over someone with intent to commit adultery," and "I don't think God would *hate **other people** if they had similar thoughts—why am I any different?" Thinking about looking at pictures of male models in light of this new, more balanced perspective helped June see that facing her fear wouldn't be as bad as she had thought. She was ready to begin her exposures.*

Preparing to Experience Anxiety

Sometimes you know when an anxiety-provoking situation is coming up, but at other times obsessional triggers take you by surprise. You see an advertisement for a television show about pedophiles, you hear someone say a curse word you've been avoiding, or you see an "unlucky" number on a nearby license plate. When you conduct planned exposure exercises, you'll know the stressor is coming up, and this will help you prepare to experience the anxiety.

> Do you use coping statements haphazardly or intermittently? Try using them much more consistently.

When you know in advance that you'll be feeling anxious, you might automatically start telling yourself how awful it will be. But as you learned in Step 6, such thoughts only lead to more anxiety. Instead, I suggest you try making statements to yourself that will help you deal with your anxiety, such as those listed at the bottom of the page. These coping statements are not designed to magically reduce anxiety, but if you can change the things you say to yourself during exposure practice, it will help you stay in the feared situation until anxiety subsides on its own. You might have already tried using similar coping statements, but I find that most people don't try consistently or long enough for it to really help.

Using these types of coping statements might be very different from the way you've dealt with obsessional anxiety before, and may seem awkward at first. To learn to use these statements effectively, you're going to have to practice, as you do with any other skill. At first, it might be hard for you to think of these kinds of thoughts when you're very anxious, so you need to rehearse them. I suggest reading the list of coping statements at least once each day during a time when you are *not* doing an exposure. This will help you become

Coping Statements for Confronting Anxiety

- Anxiety is normal and temporary. Think how good you will feel when it subsides.
- Anxious sensations feel *uncomfortable*, but they're not *dangerous*.
- Anxiety won't hurt me. It's just my fight-or-flight/adrenaline system at work.
- I have to make myself anxious to get better.
- If I stop now, I'll only be making OCD worse.
- It's worth deciding to be anxious in the short run to get over this problem in the long run.
- When I've faced my fears before, I've always eventually felt better.
- Trying to control anxiety with rituals doesn't work. I need to "go with the anxiety" to get better.
- The trigger only bothers me because I give it so much negative meaning.
- I can handle this. I can let the anxiety decrease by itself—no matter how long it takes.

familiar with them. It will take some time and effort to learn how to use the statements the right way, but you'll get there.

Confronting Your Fear and Keeping Track of Your Anxiety Levels

With helpful beliefs and coping statements in mind, the next step is to confront the feared situation or object as planned. In Step 4 you learned to use the Subjective Units of Discomfort (SUDs) Rating Scale, rating frightening situations from 0 (no discomfort) to 100 (extreme discomfort). Now, you'll use this scale to keep track of how uncomfortable you feel as you go through the exposure practice.

The Subjective Units of Discomfort (SUDs) Rating Scale

0	10	20	30	40	50	60	70	80	90	100
No discomfort		Mild discomfort			Moderate discomfort		High discomfort			Extreme discomfort

The Exposure Graph on the facing page is part of the Planned Exposure Practice Worksheet that I'll introduce in its complete form after Step 9. You'll use this graph to keep track of your anxiety levels during planned exposure practices by charting your SUDs ratings every 5 minutes. Keeping track of your SUDs allows you to notice how you're responding to the fear trigger. You'll be able to see more objectively how your own anxiety habituates over time when you remain in the exposure. To assess anxiety levels, many people find it useful to simply ask themselves, "What's my SUDs level now?"

Note that you can use this graph to keep track of two exposures—the two you'll practice each day. As the legend at the top of the graph shows, during the first exposure you can chart your SUDs using dots and a solid connector line. During the second exposure of the day, use an X and a dashed line (to illustrate, I'll show June's exposure graph a little further on).

BATTLE PLAN While it's best to fill in your exposure graph in real time as you're practicing, this is sometimes impractical, such as when you're in a social situation. If this happens, keep a mental note of your SUDs and complete your graph when you have some privacy.

Always begin each practice by noting your SUDs level as you start the exposure and place a dot on the graph to indicate your SUDs level at the "start" time point. You'll feel pretty uncomfortable at this point, but your goal is to hang in there and remain focused on your task. If you need to, use the coping statements on the previous page to help you ride out the anxiety. Whatever you do, don't fight the anxiety or use rituals and other subtle avoidance strategies to reduce it artificially—it needs to go down on its own. Also, don't overanalyze whether your obsessional fear is true. Instead, just allow yourself to worry and feel uncertain about your fears. Your distress will subside as you practice letting yourself embrace the feelings. In other words, accept the anxiety and doubt. Allow these feelings to just "happen." Welcome them.

Does the discomfort you feel at the beginning of the exposure call for using coping statements?

Exposure Graph

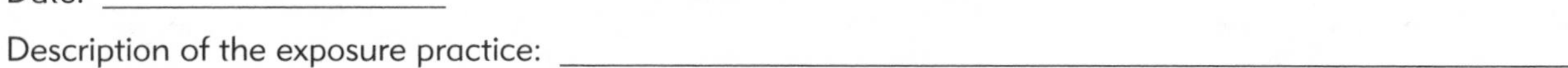

Date: ____________________

Description of the exposure practice: ____

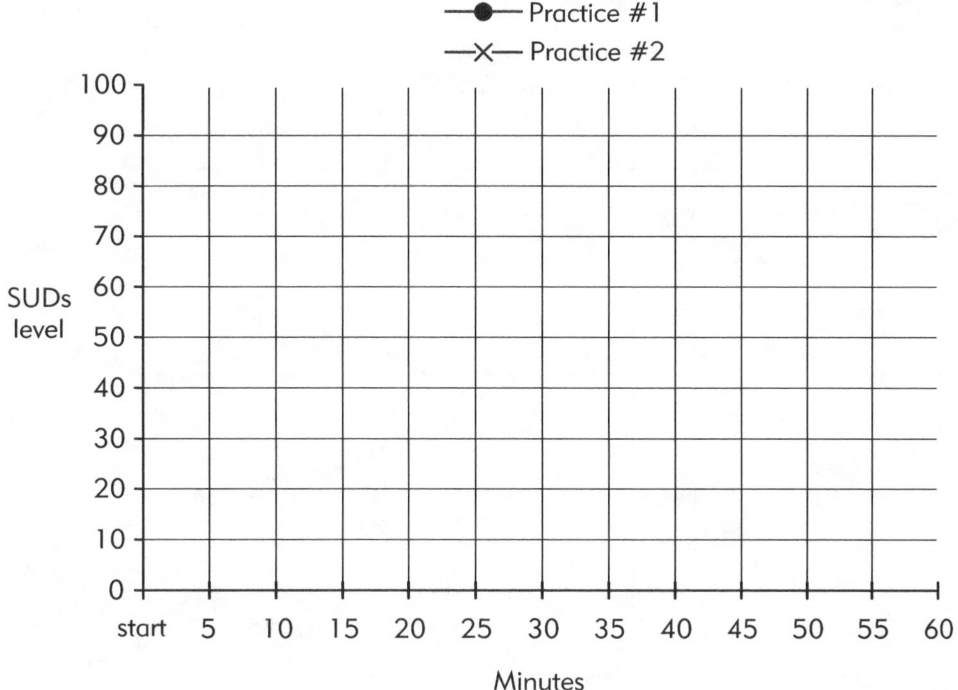

Do you feel no anxiety at all? Try moving on to the next item on your hierarchy.

Is your SUDs level soaring? Try backing off a bit or finding some way to expose yourself only partially to the feared situation without backing down entirely.

Take a look at June's exposure graph on the next page. When she began her first exposure to looking at pictures of male models in fashion and fitness magazines (indicated on the graph by the dots and solid lines), her SUDs level was about 80—after all, she had been avoiding this activity for a long time. She flipped through the magazines and just allowed herself to feel anxious—without fighting it or trying to make it go away. After about 20 minutes, she noticed that her SUDs had dropped to 70. Ten minutes later, she was at 65. After a half hour of looking at magazine models, she was still feeling moderately anxious, but then her distress began to decrease more rapidly so that she was only minimally anxious after 1 hour, when she ended the exposure.

Later that day, June conducted her second exposure practice to male magazine models. Notice that her SUDs dropped more quickly this time. After 20 minutes, she was at about 20 SUDs. As I mentioned before, you'll probably find that your anxiety decreases more and more rapidly each time you repeat an exposure. After an hour of practice (2 hours for the entire day), June could look at attractive men in magazines without feeling anxious. She repeated these exercises twice daily for the rest of the week.

June's Exposure Graph

Date: *example*

Description of the exposure practice: *look at attractive male models in magazines*

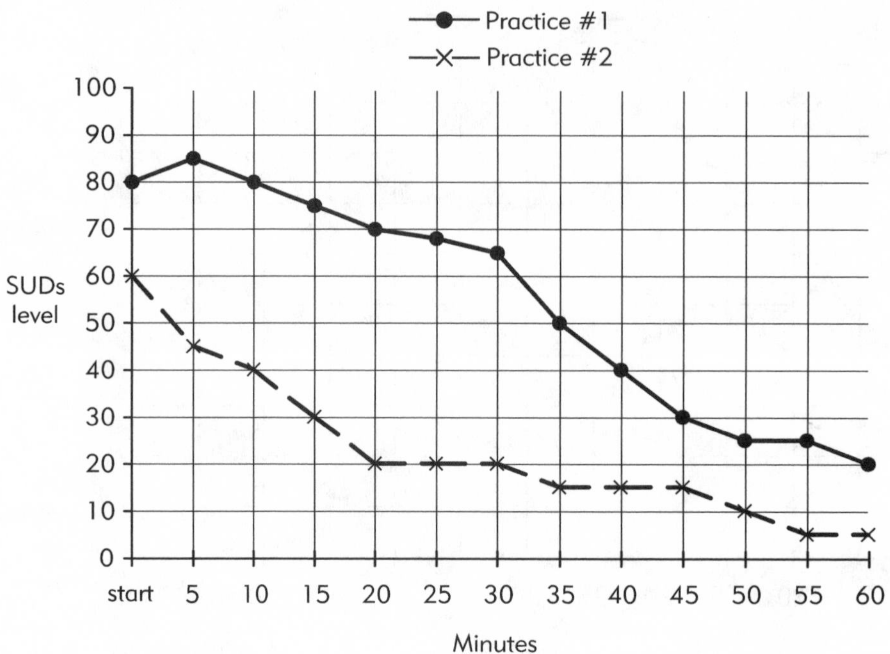

What Did You Learn?

After you complete the exposure exercise, give yourself a pat on the back. Look back over the experience to see what you can learn from it. Evaluate your attempt to cope with the situation and the anxiety, but don't expect perfection and success all of the time. Recognize even small gains. Praise yourself and don't belittle gradual progress. Keep in mind that overcoming OCD is very hard work and sometimes painful. At times you might wonder whether it is all worth it. That's why it's important to keep all of your gains in mind and reward yourself for each step. You must also keep your expectations realistic. Don't expect miracles, but if you work hard to confront the situations on the exposure list consistently, you are likely to see real progress.

After her exposure was over, June was still not 100% certain that God was not angry with her. But she realized that lightning wasn't going to strike her down if she looked at a cute guy. She also saw firsthand that she could control her excessive worries about sin by facing her fear and not ritualizing. Most of all, she learned that she could live with uncertainty and doubt just like everyone takes for granted. June realized that doing this exposure brought her closer to having faith—not fear—in God. After

> What did you find out in the exposure practice?
>
> Did anxiety go down?
>
> Can you manage uncertainty?
>
> Did anything awful happen?

each exposure practice, I encourage you to note what you've learned (there's actually space for writing this in the worksheet I'll introduce later). June noted the following : *After about 45 minutes I was not anxious anymore. Anxiety doesn't last forever. I can notice attractive men without being lustful, just like everyone else. I don't have to be afraid of this. Even though I don't know what God is thinking about me, I have no good reason to believe he's upset with me.* We'll talk more about doing exposure for religious obsessions later in this step.

Taking It to the Next Level: Moving Up the Hierarchy

Build on Your Early Successes

When you've had success with confronting your initial hierarchy items, it's time to gradually increase the difficulty of your exposures. If you're frightened by the idea of working your way up the hierarchy, think about what happened during your earlier exposure practices. Review your exposure graphs:

- ☐ Did you feel very uncomfortable at first?
- ☐ Did your SUDs eventually decrease?
- ☐ Did the negative consequences you were afraid of actually occur?
- ☐ Did you manage the uncertainty?
- ☐ You probably felt tired or exasperated afterward, but did you have a sense of accomplishment when you completed the exposure?

There is no reason to believe that higher level exposure practices will go differently from the earlier ones. Yes, they might provoke more anxiety at first, but you are also better prepared since you've got some practice under your belt.

Lifestyle Exposure

If you had a chronic disease like diabetes, but paid attention to your diet and your blood sugar levels only *part-time*, you'd suffer serious medical complications, possibly even death. Although anxiety won't kill you, OCD is also a *chronic* problem. And chronic problems require constant attention. This means you need to make exposure part of your *lifestyle*, rather than something you do only twice a day for a few hours.

As you move up your exposure hierarchy, don't stop confronting the triggers that you've already practiced with. That is, once you've faced a feared situation in planned exposure, you shouldn't go back to avoiding it if it comes up in your daily life. In fact, try seeking out opportunities to keep confronting these situations and objects wherever and whenever you can. This will help you bulldoze your obsessions over and keep them from creeping back into your life.

I've worked with some people who diligently complete the exposure practices they plan in advance, but then avoid other situations in which they could be facing their fear. This is like taking one step forward and two steps backward. Lucas had fears of contamination from gay people. For exposure, he ate at a restaurant in a part of town where lots of gay people lived, but then avoided the bookstore next door because he feared it would be contaminated with "gay germs." He also avoided wearing his favorite shirt during this exposure because he didn't want it to become contaminated. Further, after his exposure, Lucas slept on the couch because he didn't want to spread the contamination from the restaurant to his bed. But all of this avoidance negated a perfectly good exposure, and Lucas's contamination fear remained strong.

BATTLE PLAN Don't miss opportunities to face your fears in your daily life. Think of it as a game: every time you face a fear trigger without ritualizing, it's a point for you. But every time you avoid a trigger or perform a ritual, that's a point for OCD. Try to win with as big a margin as possible!

On the other hand, don't feel like you have to confront hierarchy items that you haven't yet practiced using planned exposure. If you happen to encounter one of these triggers and become so fearful that you absolutely must avoid or ritualize, do so, but make sure that later you go back and do a planned exposure practice so that you're back up on your horse. We'll deal with resisting rituals in detail in Step 9.

BATTLE PLAN As an *adjunct* to scheduled exposure practice, incidental "lifestyle exposure" can enhance your success. (Incidental exposure will still not be sufficient on its own, however.) So try to take advantage of any occasions that might arise in your daily life to practice confronting, rather than avoiding, your obsessional triggers. *Seek out* your feared situations and *choose* to be anxious.

Confronting Your Worst Fears and Managing High Anxiety

Do I really have to face my worst fears? I understand your trepidation, but the answer is *yes*. Avoiding exposure to your most frightening obsessional triggers only strengthens your belief that these situations really are dangerous or unmanageable. This will undermine your battle against OCD and could even undo all the hard work you've put in to this point. Your success with early and midlevel exposure exercises should boost your confidence level and prepare you for taking this challenging step. Use coping statements and cognitive therapy strategies to help put you in the right frame of mind for embracing anxiety and obsessional thoughts. Take it slow if you have to. What's important is that you get through these exposures without avoiding or ritualizing, not that you get through them quickly.

Did you include your most frightening obsessional trigger on your hierarchy?

As with less difficult exposure items, once you have mastered confronting your worst fears in a specific setting (your home, for example), try conducting similar exposures in different situations (work, school, other public places). Suppose you have violent obsessions and have been confronting knives and scissors that you used to avoid. Once you're relatively comfortable facing these objects when you're alone, try using them when you're around other people. If you have obsessions about responsibility for car accidents, try driving with more and more distractions, such as loud music or talking to a passenger. After practicing look-

BATTLE PLAN If you become extremely frightened when facing your worst fears, back off and try the cognitive techniques or coping statements, then try to reenter the situation.

Treatment Buddy Tip

Agree on a plan in which your treatment buddy will be available to help you if you run into trouble when facing your worst fears—or anytime you become very anxious during an exposure and feel you need to stop the exercise prematurely. Your treatment buddy can help you stay in the situation and learn something important from the exercise.

For treatment buddies: If the person you're helping is experiencing intense anxiety, it may be tempting to say something reassuring like "Don't worry about it, it will be okay. We'll do this another day." Instead, try to help your friend or loved one by being supportive and encouraging him or her to *confront* the anxiety and *remain* in the situation until anxiety subsides. No escaping or avoiding anymore. You can say things like "I know it's hard, but keep going; you're going to get through this." This acknowledges that doing exposure is difficult, but also encourages your friend or loved one to stay in the anxiety-provoking situation.

Here are some more things you can say for support if anxiety gets intense:

- "Try to remain in the situation. Look at it as an opportunity to practice, to change how you think and behave in the face of OCD. OCD is like a bully who bothers you only if you run away from him. Stand your ground and use your coping self-statements."
- "Stay focused on the present. Your anxiety will come down as time passes. Remember the graph of an exposure session? It might seem anxiety will last forever, but it won't. You can get through it."
- "Don't fight the anxiety or demand that you feel relaxed. That's like trying not to think of pink elephants. It will make things seem worse. Instead, accept the anxiety and wait for it to decrease. Let yourself feel anxious."

Don't distract. When someone you care about is very anxious, it's tempting to try to take his or her mind off of it by distracting with conversation or focusing on something else. This might have helped the person get through the immediate situation, but it doesn't help in the long term because it is an avoidance strategy. So a little *temporary* distraction is okay, but keep the discussion focused on the obsessional fear and exposure practice. This is because the person needs to stay in touch with the fear-evoking situation and thoughts during exposure. He or she needs to be mentally as well physically present and "in the moment." Maybe it *seems* cruel at the time, but you're actually doing your relative or friend a favor if you help him or her stay engaged; like "tough love." Instead of using *distraction* during exposures, remind the person you are helping to use *coping* statements.

What if the person I'm helping becomes so anxious that he or she threatens to stop the exposure? If this happens, respect and accept that doing exposure is very difficult. But don't let your friend or loved one off the hook too easily. Try saying something like, "I think we need to finish this exercise. It's the wrong decision to quit now. But this has to be your choice. You know what I think you need to do." Ultimately, you can't control what the person decides to do. It's up to the other person to decide whether to engage in exposure and work on improving, or continue to avoid and stay stuck with OCD. As the treatment buddy, all you can do is provide support and encouragement to make the right decisions.

ing at pictures of attractive men, June conducted exposure at a local swimming pool she had been avoiding because she knew she'd see men without their shirts. Research shows that facing your fears in different settings helps you get the best long-term results.

Situational Exposure for Different Types of Obsessions

Here are some tips for how to design and conduct situational exposure exercises for the different types of obsessional fears. Obviously, I can't cover every possible obsession, but I've included examples for most of the "classic" and less common types. Your job is to adapt what you read to your feared situations listed in your fear hierarchy. Have your treatment buddy give you suggestions if necessary.

BATTLE PLAN While you're planning and working on your exposure practices, turn to the following pages to read about the types of obsessions that apply to you:

As you read these examples and suggestions, keep in mind that *exposure is not just about doing what "most people" or what "normal people" would do*. Rather, it is about helping you overcome obsessional fear by teaching you to take acceptable risks and live with everyday levels of uncertainty. Sometimes you'll need to push the envelope of what seems sensible or "normal" to demonstrate that the situations you fear are not very risky and that you can manage them. This might mean doing things that most people don't do in their day-to-day lives, but that still pose minimal risk.

BATTLE PLAN Remember the guiding principle for designing each exposure: the situations and items you confront must closely match your particular fears.

As you read the descriptions below, also keep in mind that you'll be practicing imaginal exposure and response prevention along with situational exposure. I'll describe these techniques in Steps 8 and 9, but it's not too early to begin thinking about how you can use all three techniques together for each type of obsession.

Contamination Obsessions

If you worry about germs, illness, or causing others to get sick, you must practice direct contact with items you fear are sources of contamination. For example, floors, shoes, railings, dirty laundry, doorknobs, bathrooms, toilets, garbage cans, shoes, hospitals, people (and their belongings), and the like. You might conduct an exposure practice while sitting on a toilet, stretched out on the floor, or with a sweaty towel in your lap. I've accompanied people with fears of pesticides to gardening stores where they learned about and practiced the proper use of these chemicals. If you can't maintain contact with the feared item, try to "contaminate" a piece of cloth or paper towel that you can take with you for later exposures. If you're fearful of urine, feces, saliva, or other bodily fluids, try putting a few drops on your hand. If this seems difficult, try first contaminating a paper towel with a small amount of the feared substance (for example, a few drops of urine, blood, or semen), and then touch the part of the paper towel that is most contaminated.

It's important that you not just touch the feared contaminants with your fingertips, but rather that you make yourself feel "completely contaminated." This means getting the "germs" on your whole hand, your clothes, hair, arms, face, and even other belongings (for example, pillow, purse, cell phone, or car). Don't hold back—immerse yourself. The more you spread the contamination around in your surroundings, the more effective the exposure will be. If you're afraid of making others ill by spreading germs, do things like shaking hands, touching their belongings, or preparing food for them while you're feeling contaminated. The aim of repeatedly practicing exposure to feared contaminants is not to permanently alter your hygiene practices. Rather, it's to help you learn to live with everyday levels of risk and uncertainty. After you practice exposure over and over, you'll begin to worry less and less about germs.

Pearl was afraid of contracting the herpes virus. She avoided public bathrooms, door handles, and garbage cans. She also avoided contact with other people and their belongings (pens, telephones, and the like). Bodily waste and secretions such as urine, feces, and sweat also evoked obsessive fear. Pearl's situational exposure hierarchy was as follows:

Hierarchy Item	SUDs
Doorknobs and railings	45
Shaking hands with others	65
Public telephones	70
Garbage cans	75
Sweat	80
Public bathrooms	85
Urine	90
Feces	95

Here is what Pearl did each week for situational exposure:

- *Week 1:* Walked through her office building every day, touching doorknobs and railings, maintaining contact for several minutes at a time. She got "door germs" on a paper towel, which she used for a planned exposure by placing it on her lap for 1 hour. Similar exposures occurred at the local mall. During her exposures, Pearl focused on thinking about the possibility of getting a virus such as herpes.
- *Week 2:* Stopped avoiding shaking hands with strangers. Practiced touching and using phones that others had been using at work, concentrating on the receiver since she was concerned about getting cold sores from germs in other people's mouths. Let herself worry about herpes and other illnesses.

• *Week 3:* Practiced touching garbage cans (inside and out), first at home and then in public areas such as malls and restaurants.

• *Week 4:* Confronted sweat every day by running in place and then touching her armpits and the inside of her shoes. Also kept a soiled sock in her pocket and handled it every few hours.

• *Week 5:* Focused on bathrooms, starting with exposure to bathroom doorknobs, sink faucets, and soap dispensers, maintaining contact for several minutes. Sat next to the toilet and touched the flusher and seat. Practiced sitting on public toilets, such as the ones at a local mall she had been avoiding.

• *Week 6:* Did daily urine exposures, placing a few drops of her own urine on a paper towel and carrying it in her pocket, touching it frequently throughout the day. Also touched the contaminated paper towel to items such as her cell phone, lipstick, bed, and couch.

• *Week 7:* Added exposure to feces, lightly soiling a piece of toilet paper with her own excrement.

I haven't included Pearl's response prevention plans here, but we'll get to that in Step 9.

Obsessions about Responsibility for Harm or Mistakes

Exposure for these types of obsessions almost always involves both situational and imaginal practices. For situational exposure, you'll need to put yourself in circumstances where you feel at risk of causing the harm, damage, injury, mistakes, or other negative events (to yourself *or* someone else) that you're frightened of. But don't just enter these situations passively; you should actively take the risk that what you're afraid of will come true.

BATTLE PLAN To decide whether you're going too far, psychologist Dr. Jonathan Grayson suggests asking yourself whether people who do *not* have problems with OCD now and then engage in the same situations or do the same behaviors either accidentally or on purpose. If so, include the exercise in your exposure program.

• *If you're worried about starting fires*, you can keep appliances (for example, the iron and the toaster) plugged in, lights turned on, and so forth, when you leave the house.

• *If you worry about leaving appliances on*, you can also conduct exposures in which you actually use the appliance, then quickly turn it off *without looking at what you're doing* (for example, turn your back, close your eyes). Be sure not to try to feel that the switch is in the off position—just leave the room, the house, or go to bed without checking. Then allow yourself to worry about whether the appliance is *really* off or safe. You can use a similar strategy if you're afraid of leaving doors, windows, or other things unlocked. Of course (as we'll cover in Step 9), you mustn't go back and check that switches are off or locked once you've conducted the exposure. The aim of these exercises is to teach you to manage the distress provoked by uncertainty about danger.

• *If you have obsessions about hitting pedestrians or causing accidents with your car*, you can practice driving in busy areas (business districts, parking lots, neighborhoods) without checking the roadside or the mirrors. Begin with easier routes and gradually work up to more anxiety-provoking ones. Perhaps driving at night and in poorly lit areas would be a more difficult step up the hierarchy. Do you worry that having the radio on or talking to a passenger will increase your chances of hitting someone? If so, incorporate this into your exposure. Make sure you don't return to where you have already driven—you don't want to reassure yourself that you haven't hit anyone. Your job is to learn to manage your anxiety and obsessional doubts without using checking rituals.

- *If you're afraid that writing out a bad wish will cause the wish to come true*, try writing it out (for example, "I hope my son Howard dies in a car crash today").
- *If you're afraid of certain words or numbers because they're associated with bad luck*, you can purposely confront these numbers or write them on a piece of paper that you carry with you (I once had a patient who tattooed her feared numbers on her skin).
- *If you're worried about poisoning others by mistake*, you can put poisonous materials (detergent, pesticides) near where you're cooking.
- *If you're worried about causing harm by being irresponsible or negligent*, plan to do whatever you're afraid will cause harm—for example, spilling water in an aisle of the supermarket or the floor of the food court, walking on stairs where small children are also walking.

When possible, you can use exposure to test out what happens when you purposely make a mistake or carry out a behavior you're afraid will lead to harm. For example, write the number 13 on a picture of a relative and then see if this person has a string of bad luck. If you're afraid of causing a fire, leave an appliance (such as the stove) on and unattended for an acceptable period of time (for example, go into another room for a while or take a walk around the block). If you're afraid of miswriting an address on an envelope, purposely misspell something and see if your letter gets to the intended destination. If you're fearful of performing imperfectly, you could commit minor "imperfections" on purpose as exposure tasks.

Keep in mind that some situational exposures for responsibility obsessions will be spoiled if you repeat them right away. For example, plugging in the iron or turning on the stove can only be done once during an exposure practice session because repeating these exercises will allow you to check and see that no fire has started. Therefore, you need to plan how you'll conduct your exposures without getting reassurance. A good solution is to perform the situational exposure once and then quickly leave the premises (without checking). Then allow yourself to worry about the feared consequences. In Step 8 I'll show you how to use imaginal exposure to help with these kinds of practices.

BATTLE PLAN The guiding principle for conducting exposure for responsibility obsessions is that the exercises you practice should make you feel as if you'd be responsible for causing (or not doing enough to prevent) the very harm or mistakes that you fear.

You'll probably also need to practice these types of exposures on your own. That's because having a treatment buddy or anyone else with you in these situations could make you feel less responsible for a potential disaster and lessen your anxiety. For example, if someone else is in the car when you do a driving exposure, you might feel confident that he or she will warn you if you hit someone by mistake. This wouldn't really be facing your true fear of possibly being *responsible* for harm and therefore wouldn't be a helpful practice.

Angelo's checking rituals were provoked by obsessions that he'd be responsible for injuring someone else or their property. Seeing a fire truck triggered obsessions that maybe he'd started a fire without realizing it. He watched the TV news, scoured the newspapers, and checked with police to reassure himself that he didn't cause any disasters. After his wife and children went to sleep each night, Angelo checked the electrical appliances, locks, windows, and water faucets in his home, and the parking brake of his car. Angelo's fear hierarchy was as follows:

Hierarchy item	SUDs
Turn light switches on/off	45
Fire station/fire truck	50
Open and close windows	55
Open/close car doors	60
Disable/enable parking brake	70
Turn appliances (iron) on/off	75
Turn water faucets on/off	80

Here's what Angelo did for situational exposure:

- *Week 1:* Conducted light switch exposures by first turning *on* all the lights in his apartment. Then he went around (no one else was home) and turned them all off as quickly as he could. Next, he left the building, drove to work, and purposely passed a local fire station. He also forced himself to worry that perhaps he had missed a light or two, and now he would be responsible for a fire that would burn down the entire apartment complex.
- *Week 2:* Opened and closed windows on the ground floor of his apartment, later forcing himself to think about burglaries for imaginal exposure (we'll work on this in Step 8).
- *Week 3:* Whenever he parked his car, he rolled down the windows and unlocked all the doors. Then he quickly rolled up the windows, locked the doors, turned off the engine, and applied the parking brake. Then he quickly walked into a building without checking the car. Angelo forced himself to think about what might happen if he had neglected to properly engage the parking break, close the windows, or lock the doors.
- *Weeks 5 and 6:* He conducted exposures in his apartment: he turned appliances (iron, stove, toaster oven) and water faucets on and off and then left the room without checking. Again, he purposely worried about responsibility for starting fires and causing floods, and drove past the fire station to intensify these thoughts and images.

After he could leave his apartment without a great deal of anxiety, Angelo worked on conducting exposures in different settings, such as at work and at his daughter's home. He also conducted appliance, window, water faucet, car, and light switch exposures before going to bed at night.

Symmetry and Order Obsessions

Exposure for these types of obsessions should make you feel as if things are "not just right" and that you want to go back and "put them right"—in the correct place, order, or arranged "perfectly." You can practice facing *asymmetry, inexactness*, and *disorder* by putting things in the wrong order, messing up items that you usually try to keep orderly, putting clothes away sloppily, tying your right shoe tighter than your left, or intentionally using sloppy handwriting. Then allow the discomfort about these situations to gradually habituate without going back and "fixing" them. You will learn that your discomfort will decrease (habituate) with time.

If you have obsessions that inexactness, disorder, imperfection, or asymmetry will cause bad luck or something awful to happen (for example, "Mother will be injured if I don't put on my clothes in the 'correct' way"), you should do what you think will cause the awful consequences and then let yourself worry that these consequences might happen *because of what you did* (almost like an exposure for responsibility obsessions). Here again, imaginal exposure will help you with getting used to visualizing the feared consequences, as I'll show you in the next step.

Evelyn had obsessional thoughts of "imperfection" and "imbalance." Activities such as completing paperwork often took hours because she had to make sure letters were formed correctly and "perfectly." Items in the house had to be arranged in certain ways, and Evelyn had to ensure that such order was maintained. Her most pervasive symptoms focused on left–right balance. For example, if she used her *right* hand to open a door or to grab something (for example, from the refrigerator), she felt an urge to repeat the behavior using her *left* hand (and vice versa) to achieve balance.

Evelyn's fear hierarchy was as follows:

Hierarchy item	SUDs
Write letters imperfectly	40
Write imperfectly in checkbook	55
Leave items at home out of order (for example, pictures)	67
Confront "right" without "left"	75
Notice left–right imbalance wherever possible	75
Touch something on the left (or right) side only	85

Here's how Evelyn's situational exposure practice proceeded:

- *Week 1:* Practiced writing letters imperfectly (that is, sloppily), first on blank pieces of paper, then on notes she was sending to others, and finally on paperwork such as financial statements.
- *Week 2:* Purposely made mistakes when filling out her checkbook.

• *Weeks 3 and 4:* Practiced rearranging different items in her home so that they were not orderly or "balanced," such as slightly tilting picture frames and cluttering the books on her shelves. This began with items in her living room and eventually spread to her bedroom. For imaginal exposure, Evelyn constantly reminded herself that these items were "out of order." For response prevention, she refrained from rearranging them the "correct" way.

• *Week 4:* Confronting the word *left* without the word *right* by saying "left" and even writing it on the back of both of her hands. She also kept a piece of paper with this word in her pocket at all times.

• *Week 5:* Practiced noticing left–right imbalance in her environment—kept track and noticed that she made six left turns and only two right turns while driving one day. Also noted this kind of unevenness in other ways, such as how elevator buttons were on the *right* side of the elevator door in her office building and the fact that more people were sitting on the *right* side of the waiting room at the doctor's office.

• *Week 6:* Exposed herself to purposely brushing against objects such as walls and desks on her left *or* her right side without "balancing" this out. She even allowed her belt buckle to be slightly off center (facing left) and to tie her left shoe noticeably more tightly than her right shoe.

Violent Obsessions

Although imaginal exposure will be your main strategy for conquering violent obsessions, situational exposure is helpful for reducing your problems with avoidance of situations and objects that trigger these obsessions. For example, if you have obsessional thoughts and images about death, you might watch a violent movie (for example, *Schindler's List*), read a website or book describing violence (for example, *American Psycho*), or confront guns, knives, baseball bats, scissors, ropes, lawn mowers, axes, or pictures of these potential weapons. If being around potential victims triggers violent obsessions, you might plan to spend time (alone) with such people (for example, a child or an elderly person). You can also practice confronting words associated with violence such as *murder, kill, stab, victim, death, decapitate, bullet*, and the like.

Keep in mind that the goal of exposure for violent obsessions is not to desensitize you to violence or make you into someone who enjoys horror movies or novels about serial killers (not that these are necessarily bad things). Rather exposure is designed to help you change the way you respond to otherwise normally occurring thoughts about violence. You will learn that such thoughts are not *evil* or *appalling* (although they might be *uncomfortable*) and that you don't need to work so hard to control them. You'll also see that you're not an awful person for having such thoughts. Finally, you'll learn that just *thinking* violent thoughts—even if they're extremely intense, vivid, and sadistic—doesn't mean you'll act on them.

Paxton's wife had just given birth to their first baby (a son), but within a few days of bringing the baby home Paxton began having unwanted violent thoughts that he couldn't get out of his head. The thoughts focused on awful things Paxton could do to his innocent and completely dependent infant son. For example, whenever he mowed the lawn, he had an image of shredding his son with a lawn mower. When he saw a knife he had stabbing images. Paxton had no history of violence and was appalled that he was having these thoughts. He began avoiding the baby—especially being alone with him and taking him for walks in the stroller. He even quit his softball team because handling the bat triggered images of bashing the baby's skull. Paxton's situational exposure hierarchy was as follows:

Hierarchy item	SUDs
Hold and burp the baby	45
Hold baby near a flight of stairs	50
Take the baby for a walk near traffic	60
Hold the baby on a busy street corner	75
Give the baby a bath	75
Use a knife while the baby is nearby on the floor	80
Hold a baseball bat while the baby is nearby	80
Use lawn mower while the baby is outside	85
Hold blunt end of the knife to the baby's skin	90

Here's what Paxton did for situational exposure:

- *Week 1:* Practiced holding and burping the baby, which involved gently patting the baby on the back to elicit a burp. This helped him confront images of beating the baby.
- *Week 2:* Practiced holding the baby while standing at the top of the staircase.
- *Week 3:* Practiced taking the baby out in the stroller—first with his wife accompanying him, but later on his own—near busy streets. This helped him confront his fear of losing control and pushing the stroller out into traffic.
- *Week 4:* Practiced taking his son out of the stroller and holding him while standing on a busy street corner and thinking about throwing the baby into the road. This helped Paxton realize that thinking about doing terrible things would probably not make him do anything he didn't want to.
- *Week 5:* Practiced bathing the baby in the bathtub, which triggered thoughts of drowning his son. At first, his wife accompanied him during these exposures, but later Paxton practiced alone.
- *Weeks 6–9:* Practiced with the baby in various potentially dangerous situations that triggered upsetting obsessional thoughts. Held (and swung) a baseball bat while the baby was nearby (although safely out of range of being hit). Also, he mowed the lawn (which was something Paxton had been avoiding altogether) while his son was outside in a playpen. Finally, he practiced using a knife while being near the baby and even touched the blunt end of the knife to the baby's skin to demonstrate the difference between simply thinking violent thoughts and acting violently.

Sexual Obsessions

As you can probably figure out by now, situational exposure for these obsessions involves confronting the stimuli that you avoid or that trigger intrusive, upsetting sexual thoughts, images, or doubts. If your obsessions concern unwanted or "forbidden" sexual behaviors or thoughts (for example, incest, sex with animals, other upsetting themes), you might practice exposure to looking at pictures of people in the nude (or in revealing clothing if you prefer not to look at nude photos) and to provocative words such as *sex, erection, lubrication, orgasm*, and sexual parts of the body or their functions. You can look at men's crotches or women's chests and read or write your own sexual stories about incest, bestiality (sex with animals), or whatever your unacceptable sexual obsessions concern. You could even tell people who are the focus of your sexual obsessions (for example, a member of the same sex) that you think they look nice.

If your obsessions focus on doubts about your sexual preference ("Am I gay?"), ideas for exposure include viewing pictures of members of the same sex in the nude (or wearing very little clothing); looking at members of the same sex in a gym or a swimming pool, locker room, or shower; and visiting restaurants, bars, or bookstores frequented by homosexuals. You might look at pictures of cover models, watch homoerotic pornography, or read gay literature, and confront words such as *homosexual, anal sex*, and *lesbian*. If you're opposed to using pornography, that's okay—a human sexuality textbook or educational website with anatomical drawings will do just fine.

If your obsessions focus on sexual matters dealing with children or incest, you might go to playgrounds or schools, look at pictures of children (or relatives), or confront words such as *molest, pedophile*, or *rape*, and the like. You might compliment children or relatives by telling them how good they look.

If you have obsessions involving your own children, you can look at them naked and give them a bath if appropriate. *Please do not use child pornography in your exposure practice as this sort of material is illegal.* Also, make sure to keep any explicit sexual material you might use for exposure practice safely away from where children might find it.

As with exposure for violent obsessions, exposure to sexual obsessions doesn't change who you are. It doesn't turn you into a pervert, change your sexual preference, or make you more liberal than you'd prefer to be when it comes to matters of sex. Nevertheless, I can understand if you're afraid of such consequences. The goal of this kind of exposure, however, is to help you learn that even the most vulgar and depraved sexual thoughts are simply "mental noise" that most everyone experiences from time to time. These unwanted thoughts are not worth the effort of avoidance, suppression, or ritualistic behaviors which only make matters worse anyway.

Matt, a devoutly religious, heterosexual married man had problems with homosexual obsessions. These were triggered by hearing certain words (for example, *penis*) and by the sight of certain men—especially his friend Todd. Matt was avoiding spending time with his male friends and had stopped going to the gym, where he might see men undressed in the locker room. He was also avoiding sexual intercourse with his wife because, once, a homosexual thought crept into his mind during sex. Matt feared that the presence of his obsessions meant he was "turning gay," something that was strictly forbidden from his religious viewpoint.

Matt's fear hierarchy was as follows:

Hierarchy item	SUDs
Words (*gay, penis, homosexual*)	55
Pictures of handsome men (models)	65
Pictures of Todd	70
Make flattering comments to another man	75
Gym and locker room	75
View pictures of men in the nude	80
Stories of homosexuality	83
Have sexual intercourse with wife	85

Here's a description of what Matt did for situational exposure:

- *Week 1:* Practiced saying the words *penis, gay, homosexual, anal sex*, and *blow job*. He also wrote these words on sheets of paper that he kept in his pocket.
- *Week 2:* Viewed pictures of attractive men by looking through fitness and fashion magazines. He allowed himself to think about how good-looking these men were and confronted thoughts about sexual relations using imaginal exposure.
- *Week 3:* Looked at pictures of his friend Todd (fully dressed) for exposure. He allowed himself to visualize what Todd looked like nude, including images of his penis.
- *Week 4:* Visited the gym during the busiest time of day and purposely noticed men's physiques. He practiced complimenting some of the men on how "ripped" (muscular) they looked and on how he liked their clothes. He also went into the locker room and struck up a conversation with a man who was undressed and preparing to take a shower.
- *Week 5:* Matt reflected on his religious and moral values and even consulted with a member of the clergy when planning his exposure to viewing pictures of nude men. In the end, he decided that rather than using real-life pictures (that is, pornography), he would view textbook illustrations of the male body and genitalia. So Matt went to the library and checked out a few books on male sexuality that contained detailed anatomical drawings.
- *Week 6:* Wrote stories describing himself having sex with other men, including his friend Todd. The initial stories were somewhat tame, but as the week progressed and he felt more comfortable, Matt included more graphic descriptions of sexual acts.
- *Week 7:* Resumed having intercourse with his wife and, during the sexual activity, allowed himself to have intrusive images and doubts about whether he was gay.

Religious Obsessions (Scrupulosity)

Doing exposure for religious obsessions can be a very delicate matter. For one thing, religion involves faith and beliefs about supernatural things that can't be seen, touched, or tested out in the way that other problems with obsessions can. This means that uncertainty plays a large role: Is God upset with you? Are you going to heaven or hell when you die? Did you repent *enough*? We do not (and *cannot*) have guaranteed answers to these questions—they require you to have *faith*. Some of your feared consequences might not occur until after you've died. Exposure to your religious fears aims to make you more comfortable about this level of uncertainty. In other words, exposure is designed to make you comfortable with your *faith* rather than demanding to know what humans can't know for certain.

To overcome your religious fears, you'll also need to take some risks. Do you have to blatantly commit sins or violate religious commandments to do exposure successfully? Absolutely not! In all of my work, I have never asked a patient to deliberately do this. It would be terribly disrespectful. Rather, your exposure situations should be those you *perceive* as sacrilegious, but that really aren't severe violations, such as:

- Not paying attention (or thinking "impure" thoughts) during a religious service
- Reading literature that you disagree with
- Saying or doing things you've been avoiding
- Praying "imperfectly" or with distractions
- Saying things you don't really believe
- Reading or learning about beliefs that are contrary to your religious views

I realize that doing these things might *seem like* moral or religious violations to you. But let's face it: your obsessions are less about true religion and more about uncertainty and fear. Whereas people without OCD take for granted that normal religious faith comes with a certain degree of uncertainty and doubt, you might have trouble doing so. But in contrast to the fear that typifies OCD, religion is about faith, peace, and love. So I recommend that you keep the following in mind when conducting exposure for religious obsessions:

About scrupulosity and religious obsessions and compulsions

- Scrupulosity is unhealthy religious behavior. It's outside the norm.
- Religion is meant to be practiced out of love and faith, not fear.

About exposure therapy

- Confronting your religious fears will help you become a more faithful person who observes his or her religion in the way it was intended.
- Although it might seem as if you're jeopardizing your immortal soul, to win the battle over OCD you'll need to take a leap of faith.
- Exposure practices don't change your religious beliefs or turn you against your religion. To the contrary, they are actually designed to help you practice your religion in a more healthy and faithful way—to become closer to God.

About God

- Sometimes you need to put things in God's hands and trust that you'll be guided down the right path. That's what faith is all about.
- If God sees and knows everything, then He also understands what's in your heart

and understands that your obsessions are *unwanted* thoughts—not what you really believe.

- Since God already understands, you don't need to confess, pray, ritualize, or ask for forgiveness for having unacceptable obsessional thoughts.
- Doing exposure therapy and response prevention will help you gain stronger faith that God is understanding.
- You can have faith that God understands the point of exposure therapy—and that *you* don't need permission and *He* doesn't need reminders.
- If you view God as angry, vengeful, and waiting for you to slip up so you can be punished, doing CBT will give you renewed faith that God is loving and forgiving.

Hattie was a devout Christian for whom listening to religious music, reading religious material, and attending church or Bible studies triggered unwanted and highly distressing obsessional thoughts about sex and the devil. As a result, Hattie avoided these activities. She also avoided placing anything having to do with Christianity in her lap because it triggered distressing thoughts about having sex with God. Hattie worried that God was very upset because of her immoral thoughts (that is, that she wasn't a "good Christian"). Although she continued to pray before eating, at bedtime, and at various other points through the day, she ended up having to repeat her prayers until she could say them without being interrupted by intrusive sexual thoughts. Hattie devised the following situational exposure hierarchy:

Do you view God as angry and vengeful—just looking for a reason to punish you?

Hierarchy item	SUDs
Listen to religious songs	50
Read religious/inspirational magazine articles	65
Think about the devil	70
Read spiritual literature (devotionals)	75
Read from the Bible	80
Attend Bible study	80
Attend church	90
Place religious items in my lap	95

Hattie's situational exposure work proceeded as follows:

- *Week 1:* Listened to Christian music. This provoked unwanted obsessions, which she practiced not trying to fight (and even confronted using imaginal exposure; see Step 8).
- *Week 2:* Read articles in religious magazines and continued imaginal exposure.
- *Week 3:* Confronted items that reminded her of the devil, including books from the library, and devil worship websites.

- *Week 4:* Read spiritual and devotional literature and allowed herself to think blasphemous thoughts while doing so.
- *Week 5:* Read from the Bible and allowed unwanted thoughts and doubts to "hang out" in her mind.
- *Week 6:* Attended Bible study groups.
- *Week 7:* Started attending church and allowing herself to have unwanted obsessional thoughts there.
- *Week 8:* Placed religious items in her lap and allowed herself to experience the upsetting sexual thoughts that came to mind (for example, having sex with Jesus). She began with Christian CDs and religious magazines, which were less distressing. Then she practiced with her cross, a picture of her pastor, and finally her Bible, which was most distressing.

Each time she confronted a new hierarchy item, Hattie initially felt sinful. But she persisted with her treatment and didn't ask for forgiveness or permission from God or her pastor. Instead, when she faced these situations, she went forward assuming that God probably understood what exposure is all about—in other words, she practiced having *faith*. In time, she was able to confront each of the situations on her exposure hierarchy and to think unwanted thoughts about sex and the devil without too much distress. She also strengthened her faith that she and God shared a mutual respect, love, and understanding for one another.

Moving On to Step 8

In this step you learned about the nuts and bolts of preparing for and conducting situational exposure practices. Hopefully, you've got some good ideas for how you'll implement this part of your treatment program when it comes time for doing so. But now that you're familiar with situational exposure, it's time to turn to imaginal exposure—which you'll use to tackle obsessional thoughts, doubts, images, and fears that can't be confronted except in your imagination. As is hopefully clear by now, OCD is a complex problem that requires a multifaceted treatment. Following Step 9—when you've prepared for situational and imaginal exposure, and response prevention—I'll show you how to combine these strategies so that you can defeat OCD.

STEP 8

Defeating Obsessional Thoughts, Doubts, and Images

- Read Step 7 before starting Step 8.
- Read Steps 7–9 before starting exposure practices
- While you're learning about exposure and response prevention, you can practice the cognitive therapy techniques you learned in Step 6 for 45 minutes a day for 1–2 weeks.
- Troubleshooting tips for exposure appear on page 222.

As you probably know, OCD can turn your imagination into your worst enemy. Unlikely disasters begin to seem like foregone conclusions. Your mind takes *unrealistic* thoughts and makes them seem very real. Your brain gets stuck on seemingly unacceptable, gruesome, immoral, embarrassing, and otherwise troubling unwanted thoughts and images. Sometimes these obsessional thoughts seem even more difficult to deal with than the real-life situations you fear and avoid. But, believe it or not, you can turn your imagination into a powerful weapon *against* OCD. I'll help you do this in Step 8 by showing you how to use *imaginal* exposure along with the situational exposure techniques you learned in Step 7. In imaginal exposure, you'll reclaim your imagination and beat OCD at its own game.

How Do Situational and Imaginal Exposure Work Together?

As potent a weapon as situational exposure is in your battle against OCD, there are some fears you just can't confront in real life—for example, illnesses, fires, car accidents, violence, unacceptable sexual behavior, punishment from God, as well as disasters you're worried won't happen for a long time in the future (such as getting cancer or going to hell). These fears occur in the form of distressing obsessional thoughts, images, and doubts—that is, they occur in your imagination. So the best way to confront them is also in imagination.

Imaginal and situational exposure work very well together in helping you overcome your obsessional thoughts, images, and feared disasters. If you fear that you'll hit pedestrians when you drive, you wouldn't actually hit anyone with your car as an exposure exercise. However, you can practice driving at night on a dark country road (situational exposure) and then *imagine* that, without realizing it, you hit a pedestrian you didn't see (imaginal exposure). Similarly, if you have problems with scrupulosity, you would not actually do anything sinful or sacrilegious for situational exposure. However, you could practice behaviors that you are afraid *might* be sinful or sacrilegious (situational exposure) and then *imagine* that God is upset with you (imaginal exposure). In this step, I'll help you arrange a combination of situational and imaginal exposures that will work best for your particular obsessive fears.

You'll also use imaginal exposure to confront recurring obsessional thoughts that pop up "out of the blue" or are triggered by many different situations. For example, you might have unacceptable sexual images involving incest or child molestation that occur whenever you're reminded of a certain person. You might have horrific images of harm or violence when you spot something that could potentially be used as a weapon. You may experience upsetting sacrilegious thoughts that come up at various times. If these obsessions are triggered by cues in the environment, you can practice situational exposure to the triggers and imaginal exposure to the obsessional images. If your unacceptable obsessions have no identifiable triggers and just "pop" into your mind at any time, you'll use imaginal exposure by itself.

Do your obsessional thoughts just pop into your head?

How Does Imaginal Exposure Reduce Obsessions?

Remember that your obsessions are just harmless intrusive thoughts that have developed a life of their own because they've been misinterpreted as very important, dangerous, or otherwise threatening. As I explained, interpreting thoughts in this way creates obsessional anxiety and makes you want to use rituals, reassurance seeking, and thought suppression to try to fight or counteract the obsession. But these strategies backfire because they lead to more unwanted thoughts. Over time the obsessional thoughts become more intense. They seem more and more frightening. And you never have the opportunity to see that they're really just harmless "mental noise." So fighting your obsessions actually gets you caught in a vicious cycle, as shown in the diagram on the facing page.

Trying to avoid and fight your obsessional thoughts is futile. These strategies intensify the obsessions and keep you convinced that these thoughts are more harmful, dangerous, and important than they really are. You need a new plan for dealing with obsessions, a plan that won't get you stuck in a vicious cycle.

The Vicious Cycle of Obsessions

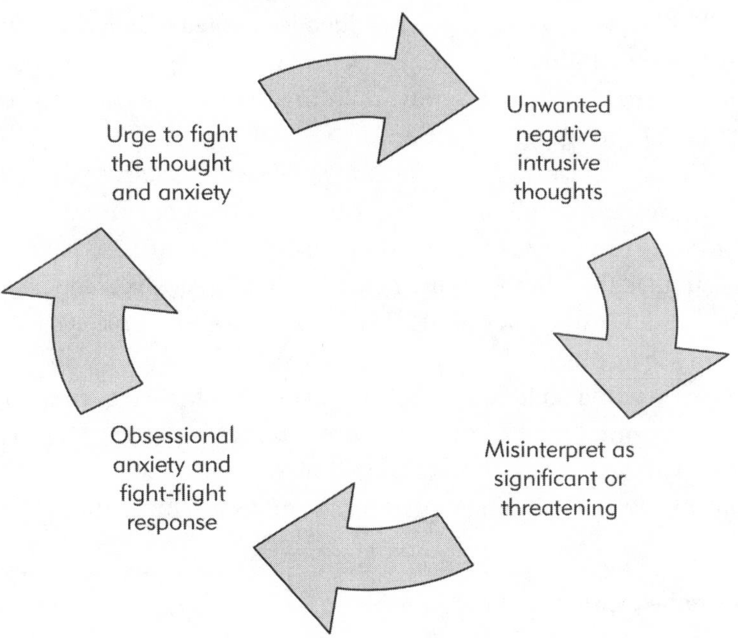

But when you reclaim your imagination and use it against OCD, you'll put an end to the vicious cycle of obsessions. I realize it sounds strange, but if over and over you make yourself confront the very thoughts, doubts, and images that frighten you the most—and you hold on to these thoughts instead of trying to distract, resist, or push them away—you'll take the wind out of their sails and win the upper hand. You'll stop obsessing. To put it another way, when you start treating your distressing obsessional thoughts like the harmless "mental driftwood" that they actually are, you'll gain the advantage.

Vladimir believed that his unwanted thoughts of attacking his elderly mother meant he was a dangerous and out-of-control man. He'd always tried to push these thoughts out of his mind. But when he forced himself to repeatedly imagine attacking his mother, he changed his tune and realized that the thoughts were meaningless. The idea that he'd act on them began to seem less and less realistic. So one way imaginal exposure reduces obsessions is by correcting mistaken perceptions of your intrusive thoughts (just like cognitive therapy). Repeatedly confronting your distressing thoughts helps you realize that they're *not* important and you *don't* need to control or suppress them using mental or compulsive rituals. By allowing yourself to imagine catastrophes and other awful ideas, you'll see that just thinking about awful things doesn't make them come true. My patients often tell me that when they practice imaginal exposure, the obsessional thoughts, ideas, and images that were extremely frightening seem to lose their punch, and the negative consequences they once feared begin to seem ridiculous.

Why do you have to purposely think your unwanted distressing thoughts to make them less frightening? Imaginal exposure works by the same principle of habituation that you read about in Step 7: when you repeatedly confront something frightening that's not really dangerous—in this case, an obsessional thought—you weaken your body's anxiety response. Again, think of this as similar to what happens if you were to watch a horror movie 100 times. At first, the movie might produce lots of fear. But as you watch it over and over, it eventually loses its ability to scare you. Why? Because you know that it's just images on a screen—not real life. In the same way, imaginal exposure will help you get over your fear of your obsessional thoughts.

Just like situational exposure, imaginal exposure also increases your tolerance for anxiety. By thinking distressing thoughts and holding them in your mind without ritualizing, you'll learn that anxiety won't last forever. You'll also see that anxiety, although uncomfortable, is safe and manageable. Remember: defeating OCD involves accepting anxiety as a helpful emotion that's a normal part of life. To do this, you must practice confronting your anxiety, not avoiding it or pushing it away.

Imaginal exposure will also help you defeat obsessions by increasing your tolerance for uncertainty. When you practice imaginal exposure, you'll resist the urge to check or seek reassurance, which will help you habituate to feeling uncertain about your feared disasters. This will be a major blow to OCD since OCD feeds off your fear of the unknown.

Imaginal exposure helps reduce obsessions by:

- **Correcting mistaken beliefs about your intrusive thoughts**
- **Weakening your body's anxiety response through repetition**
- **Strengthening your ability to tolerate anxiety, like building muscle**
- **Increasing your tolerance for uncertainty**

Imaginal Exposure in Action

If you haven't already, now is a good time to start thinking about how you can use imaginal exposure in your treatment program. To help you, here are three examples of how I use this technique when I work with people who have obsessional problems.

Gary's Parking Brake Obsessions

Gary was plagued by obsessional doubts that he'd forgotten to use the parking brake in his car. Maybe his car would roll down a hill and get damaged or, worse, cause damage to someone else's property for which Gary would be responsible. This fear led to constant "car checking" rituals that interrupted Gary's family and work life. As part of his treatment program, Gary placed a paper bag over the parking brake in his car to prevent him from checking and practiced parking in places he usually avoided, such as on a hill. When parking, he quickly reached under the bag to engage the parking brake and then left the car without any checking (note that Gary didn't purposely forget to use the brake since that could potentially be dangerous). But this exposure was too brief to allow Gary to habituate.

I explained to Gary that for his exposure to last long enough to produce habituation, he'd have to expose himself to his thoughts and doubts about the exact disasters he was afraid might transpire when he quickly left the car without checking the parking brake. So I asked him to write a few frightening stories in which his failure to engage the parking brake caused an accident. I reminded him to include every detail and make the scenes as lifelike as possible. At our next session, Gary showed me three stories that he'd written; each one took up about one sheet of lined paper. I've copied one of them here to show you what an imaginal exposure script is supposed to look like.

> *I am not sure whether I put the parking brake on in my car. What if I forgot? What if I didn't pull the lever enough and the brake isn't engaged? What if it comes undone? What if my car rolls away? I really want to go and check the car, but I know it's not a good idea. As I'm worrying about my car, I see two police officers coming toward me. My heart starts pounding. I can't concentrate on anything. Then one of the officers asks me if I drive a green Honda Civic. "Yes, that's my car," I say with my stomach all in knots. I'm having a panic attack as the officer tells me that my car rolled from its parking space and ran into another car. He suggests I take a look at the damage because it's very bad. He asks me if I forgot to use my parking brake. I go outside and see what happened. It's worse than I'd imagined. The front end of the other car is badly damaged. The repairs will be astronomical. My insurance premiums will go up. What am I going to do? I don't have a lot of money to pay for this. If only I'd been more careful about the parking brake.*

When I first read Gary's rough draft of this script, I noticed that he'd included several reassurances and rituals: phrases such as "I reassure myself that I've never actually forgotten to use the brake" and "God forbid this ever really happens." I explained to Gary that including these phrases prevented him from really facing his fears, and I asked him to cross them out.

Next I had Gary read his script aloud into a digital voice recorder (our clinic keeps several of these on hand to lend out to patients for this very purpose). The recorder has a "loop mode" that allowed him to listen to his obsessional thought repeatedly (like a loop tape) without the interruption of having to rewind it. This helped him stay focused on the distressing scene. I suggested that Gary use a serious tone when he recorded the script so that it would sound the way he thought about it. I then explained that listening to the thought would initially provoke anxiety but that, as with situational exposure, he'd gradually calm down as long as he allowed the thought to just "hang out" in his mind without any distraction or rituals. With repeated practice, I told him, he'd be able to end his obsessing about parking brakes, accidents, and checking. Then I gave him instructions to practice the following exposure once each day over the coming week:

1. Park the car on a hilly street.
2. Reach under the bag and engage the parking brake *once* without checking.
3. Quickly exit the car and walk to where you can't see it (inside, around the corner).
4. Listen to the recording over and over for at least 45 minutes or until your distress subsides.
5. DO NOT distract yourself, try to reassure yourself, or check the car.
6. Monitor your SUDs.

Although Gary was extremely anxious the first time he tried this exposure, he stuck with it and found that his SUDs decreased within about 15 minutes. When I saw him a week later, he said that each time he practiced, the exposure seemed easier and easier, until his fear and urges to check his car were virtually gone. When Gary monitored his SUDs, he found that (similar to Amelia's experience with elevators from Step 7) his anxiety subsided more quickly each time he listened to the recording. When I asked him how he felt, he said that thinking about leaving the brake off was still a little unsettling, but nowhere near as frightening as it *had* been.

Doing imaginal exposure helped Gary to separate his obsessions from reality. It made him realize just how farfetched and unrealistic his fears really were. He learned that just because he was *thinking about* negative events didn't mean they were really going to happen. He also learned how to tolerate uncertainty: during his exposure practices, Gary never received an *absolute guarantee* that his car was parked safely, but he learned to assume that it *probably* was okay. "I can just let go of the obsession now," he said. "I never thought exposure would help as much as it did."

Kiyana's Future-Oriented Obsessions

Do your obsessions involve fears and doubts about disasters that won't happen for a long time—perhaps many years in the future or even after you die? Maybe you're wondering how exposure could ever help you overcome fears of things like getting cancer when you're much older, turning into a child molester several years from now, or going to hell when you die (eternal damnation). After all, these things *could* happen, right?

Kiyana was afraid of glue—not because she would *immediately* become ill, but because she feared that the harmful vapors from glue would gradually lead to neuropathy (loss of control over her muscles) *many years from now*. She had read about exposure therapy but thought that it wouldn't work for her because she could never completely disprove her fears of what might happen in the distant future. There would always be some uncertainty.

If your obsessions involve fears of events in the distant future, your doubt about whether these feared consequences *could* happen someday might be as distressing (if not more so) as the knowledge that they actually *will* happen. In this case, imaginal exposure must focus on your uncertainty.

I explained to Kiyana that the purpose of exposure therapy would *not* be to disprove her fears—she was correct that it would be impossible to do so. Instead, it was to help her better manage the *uncertainty* of not knowing for sure whether this unlikely catastrophe would befall her someday. So for situational exposure Kiyana faced her real-life fear triggers by putting a small amount of glue on her skin and by keeping an open glue container in her office at work all day (situations that occur routinely; although at no point did she ever directly sniff any glue for exposure). Then she confronted her fears and images of getting neuropathy via the imaginal exposure script on the facing page. I helped her focus her script on her uncertainty, so that she could habituate to the thought of not knowing for sure if she would one day become ill. Indeed, everyone, with or without the burden of OCD, faces the same uncertainty.

I have been in contact with glue and even smelled the vapors. I've always avoided glue because they say that too much can lead to neurotoxicity and neuropathy. Now I'm afraid I might have these problems when I get older because of my exposure to glue. I want to find out for sure whether I've inhaled too much, but I can never know. Maybe I have, and maybe I haven't. I have to go on not knowing for sure. I can picture myself growing older and gradually losing control of my muscles. First I'll lose control of my fingers and toes. Then I won't be able to move my arms or legs. I'll have to be in a wheelchair. Other people will have to feed me. Soon I won't be able to move my mouth. Then my chest and lungs will stop working and I will die of lack of oxygen. I'll be a burden on my family. I'll miss out on all of what life has to offer. No one will want to be around me. Maybe this will happen to me. I don't know for sure.

Kiyana recorded her script and listened to it repeatedly during her situational exposure practice and whenever her obsessional doubts came to mind. At first she was extremely distressed to intentionally make herself face her doubts about not knowing for sure whether confronting glue would make her very ill someday. But she decided to work hard at using her imagination against OCD, and she challenged herself to vividly confront her worst fears. After a week of twice-daily extended imaginal exposure practice, without seeking reassurance from doctors (that is, to figure out how much glue was *too much*), she was obsessing less and less. Imaginal exposure helped her realize that although she didn't have a guarantee that she'd *never* develop this disease, she could *assume* that her risk was probably no greater than the general risk (which is quite low). Kiyana's "scary movie" about developing neuropathy was no longer that "scary."

When you enhance situational exposures with imaginal exposure to your feared catastrophes, you weaken the bond between obsessional thoughts and anxiety. Imaginal exposure teaches you that obsessional anxiety subsides on its own, that just because you *think about* catastrophes doesn't mean they're a foregone conclusion. You'll also learn that you can live with normal everyday uncertainties.

Jonas's Devil Obsession

Another way you can use imaginal exposure is to help you directly confront repugnant, horrific, or otherwise unacceptable obsessive thoughts, words, sentences, ideas, and images that get stuck in your mind and trigger anxiety and rituals. Although you might sometimes be able to trigger these obsessions with situational exposure, doing imaginal exposure will help you more vividly confront them and keep your mind from drifting to less distressing topics.

Jonas's obsessions took the form of words such as *devil, Satan, Lucifer,* and *diablo* and images of pentagrams that he couldn't get out of his mind. These were often triggered by religious activities, such as taking Holy Communion, which Jonas felt he had to avoid. If devil thoughts came to mind, Jonas tried to think of more comforting thoughts instead (mental neutralizing rituals). He also had to repeat whatever he was doing (like tying his shoe) until the thoughts were gone (compulsive rituals). Jonas came to see me when things got so bad that simple activities like getting through doorways, turning on a light switch, and getting dressed were taking up large chunks of his day.

For situational exposure, I had Jonas perform the religious activities he had been avoiding. However, he was still having difficulty with devil obsessions. So I suggested imaginal exposure as a way of directly confronting these upsetting thoughts. Jonas resisted at first. He felt extremely guilty about purposely thinking of the devil and "contaminating his mind with ungodly thoughts." I told him that I understood and wished that there was a painless way to get rid of his obsessional problems, but that his best chance for relief was to force himself to say the words and listen to them repeatedly without any distractions, rituals, or neutralizing. After all, he was going to think these thoughts anyway—he might as well beat OCD to the punch and do it in a therapeutic way. Jonas made the courageous decision to push on with therapy even though he knew it would be a challenge!

Are you afraid to let yourself think about things that other people can freely think about?

Jonas wrote down, and then spoke out loud, the very words that provoked obsessional anxiety: "Devil . . . Lucifer . . . Satan . . . Diablo. . . ." He read these words aloud into a voice recorder and then listened to them over and over. He was frightened at first and felt very strong urges to distract, resist, and neutralize the devil thoughts. But after a week of using the voice recorder twice every day for 1 hour at a time, *without giving in to any urges to ritualize*, he noticed a substantial drop in his distress. In fact, he began to feel bored—which is a sure sign of improvement since you can't be both anxious and bored at the same time! Jonas had habituated: thinking of the devil no longer made him anxious. "Hearing my own voice speak these words over and over took all of the power out of the obsessions," he said. Now Jonas could practice his religion without fear. He knew it was normal to think of the devil from time to time. When he gave up fighting these thoughts, the thoughts left him alone.

You know you're beating OCD when you get bored during an exposure because boredom and anxiety can't coexist.

It's definitely not easy to make yourself think the very thoughts that disturb you. However, the patients I treat are usually amazed to find that when they stop fighting their obsessions—and actually *welcome* these thoughts into their mind—the thoughts begin to seem less real and less distressing. My patients are able to stop their futile struggle for control of their thoughts because it doesn't matter what thoughts, ideas, or images come to mind.

When you use imaginal exposure to confront unacceptable intrusive thoughts, you'll learn to tolerate these thoughts even if they're unwanted or intrusive. You'll put some distance between you and your obsessions, allowing you to see that they're just mental noise.

Thinking Does *Not* Make It So

The idea of imaginal exposure was frightening to Mason. He worried that purposely confronting his unwanted homosexual obsessions would make him become gay. Fern was wor-

Treatment Buddy Tip

If you find yourself shying away from imaginal exposure because you're afraid that "you are what you think," try calling on your treatment buddy for help. But rather than demanding assurances that it's okay to do imaginal exposure, share your thoughts and feelings about it. Let your treatment buddy know that you think it will be stressful. Talk about how you'll manage the feelings of anxiety and uncertainty if they intensify.

For treatment buddies: Remember that reassurance doesn't work! Instead of trying to immediately reduce your friend's or relative's distress by providing reassurance that nothing bad will come of imaginal exposure, try helping him or her by reminding him or her of the following:

- Just about everyone (whether or not they have OCD) has strange, senseless, unwanted thoughts that are similar to obsessions. Vulgar, upsetting, worrisome, shocking, violent, immoral, inappropriate, and personally unacceptable thoughts, ideas, and images that are the opposite of your personality and belief system are simply a part of life. If you haven't already, you might share some of your own with your buddy.
- Misinterpreting these thoughts leads to a vicious cycle of anxiety and obsessional problems. Doing imaginal exposure will help change these misinterpretations.
- Imaginal exposure won't take the obsessional thoughts away completely, and they'll still seem disagreeable, but confronting them repeatedly will make them seem less important or scary.

ried about confronting her blasphemous images of Jesus. "What if I become an atheist from making myself think about this too much? What if I turn against God?" she said. Bernie had avoided coming to therapy for several years because of his fear that confronting his violent obsessional thoughts would make him act out and murder members of his family.

Can repeatedly thinking a thought make a straight person become gay, a religious person turn against God, or a gentle, loving person commit heinous acts? The vast majority of people—including people with the same obsessions who use the life-savings wager technique from Step 6—say *no* (and I've never had it happen in all my experience with imaginal exposure). But I'll never be able to *completely* reassure you that nothing bad will come of thinking your obsessional thoughts, or that these thoughts don't mean anything sinister about you. When OCD gets hold of your imagination, it makes you think up reason after reason why these thoughts, doubts, images, and ideas *might* or *could* be important, dangerous, or real. So I *won't* try to convince you anymore that your obsessions are "just thoughts." Not only would that be impossible, but doing so would just be giving you short-term reassurance and feeding into

Doing imaginal exposure and thinking your obsessional thoughts over and over is worth the risk! It's not *likely* to change you into someone who enjoys having these thoughts, and it won't make you embrace or agree with your obsessions. It will, however, make these thoughts less frightening to you so that you can cope with them without needing to fight or suppress them.

OCD's plan. Instead, I'll encourage you to look uncertainty right in the eye and go forward with facing your fear.

Tips for Practicing Imaginal Exposure

Just as with situational exposure, you'll get the most out of doing imaginal exposure if you practice it correctly. So, in addition to the exposure tips I gave you in Step 7, keep the following in mind for your imaginal exposure practice:

1. **Describe your scenes in the present (or future) tense.** Your scenes should be a moment-by-moment description of the feared event in the present tense using the exact same words or pictures that appear in your mind. Don't include an analysis of the situation; just describe it as if it's happening to you right now. If you're afraid of committing harm, imagine doing the same harmful thing you're afraid to think about (for example, "I'm losing control and driving the car off the road . . ."). If you're afraid of being unsure of whether you hurt someone, imagine that you're feeling uncertain (for example, "I can't remember whether I actually *shouted* obscenities and racial slurs or just *thought* them in my mind . . .").

2. **Include details to make the scene more vivid.** Make sure you add in details about the situation to make it seem as realistic as possible. For example, if you have obsessional thoughts about your child's funeral, describe the setting. Where are you? Who else is there? What are people saying, doing, and wearing? What's their mood? Who is leading the funeral? What does the casket look like? What time of day is it, and what's the weather? Include your reactions to the situation too. How do you feel? Are you anxious? Is your heart pounding? Is your stomach upset? Are you crying?

Be careful not to go overboard with irrelevant or unimportant details such as the make and model of the hearse (funeral coach), the ages of everyone at the funeral, or the weather forecast for the next 7 days. This will distract you from the obsessional thought you're working on confronting, almost like avoidance. On a similar note, "cut to the chase" and don't spend too much time setting up or introducing the scene. Begin as abruptly as you can—for example, "I forgot to check Caroline's crib and she died in her sleep. Now I'm at her funeral. . . ."

Are the details you want to include distracting rather than specific?

3. **Focus on uncertainty.** If your obsessions concern doubts about catastrophes in the distant future or negative circumstances that can't be verified, focus your scenes on the fact that you don't know whether or not these things will happen. Purposely leave yourself in the dark about the future. Kiyana's obsession about developing a sickness many years from now (see page 208) is a good example of this. Thinking that God is upset with you is another common obsessional fear. Can humans really ever be certain of what God is thinking? If you have this obsession, I recommend focusing your script on not knowing for sure whether God is upset with you. I'll cover this later when I specifically discuss religious obsessions.

4. **Include your worst fear or image.** In addition to confronting uncertainty, you should create imaginal exposure scripts in which you visualize your worst fear coming true—your most distressing obsessional images. This can be very painful to do, but remember that

thinking about upsetting things is simply something you do in your mind—it's not the same as actually going through negative experiences. To overcome your obsessions, you'll have to learn to face even your most distressing thoughts. Think back to Gary's scene in which his parking brake failed, and Jonas's thoughts about the devil. If you obsess that God is upset with you, allow yourself to think that's really happening. If you worry about fires, burglaries, accidents, sexual experiences, violence, or injury and death, include vivid descriptions of these situations or events in your scripts.

5. **Don't include any rituals or reassurance.** At first, Farrah couldn't bring herself to face her obsessional thoughts of violently attacking her parents. She was extremely anxious and wanted to take the edge off by putting in her script that she loved her parents and that her obsessions were "just lies." But I reminded her that the purpose of imaginal exposure is to confront feared thoughts and allow the anxiety to subside on its own, without reassurance or rituals. Farrah got up the courage to try it without reassurance, and within a few practice sessions she was able to confront her violence obsessions without feeling anxiety or having to constantly reassure herself (or ask others for assurance) that she wouldn't lose control and act on her thoughts.

Do your scripts include reassurances from yourself or others that your obsessional fears are unfounded?

Farrah's story shows how important it is that you not include anything reassuring in your imaginal exposure scripts. Don't try to tell yourself that your obsessions are senseless, false, or lies. Don't imagine yourself doing rituals in your exposure scene. And don't include what other people have said about the senselessness of your fears. This will keep you from directly facing your obsessions and overcoming them. Instead, as the examples in this chapter show, include in your scenes only the distressing negative content or uncertainty about whether negative events will or won't occur. As you repeatedly confront these scenes, you'll find that you don't need to distract yourself, perform neutralizing rituals, or seek reassurance to reduce your anxiety or to make you feel safe.

Setting Up Your Imaginal Exposure Practices

Choosing Obsessional Thoughts to Confront

To get started with imaginal exposure, flip back to the imaginal hierarchy you developed in Step 4 (page 104) that contains your list of obsessional thoughts and feared consequences of not avoiding or ritualizing. Choose an item to practice in imagination. If you're conducting a situational exposure that involves a feared disaster, you should pick an imaginal hierarchy item that relates to this disaster. For example, when June (from Step 7) conducted exposure to looking at pictures of attractive men, she also confronted her obsessional doubts that she was committing adultery. Specifically, she imagined that she was an adulteress and God was very angry with her.

Some imaginal hierarchy items might not align with situational exposures—for example, unacceptable sexual or violent thoughts and images that pop into your mind without any triggers. For these types of obsessions, begin with thoughts and images that provoke

BATTLE PLAN What should you do if some of your imaginal exposure hierarchy items don't align with any situational exposures? One option is to work these items into your treatment plan depending on when you think you could confront them (that is, how easy they seem). For example, you might have some items that evoke 50 SUDs and require both types of exposures, but then use only imaginal exposure to confront a thought that triggers 60 SUDs, before switching back to situational exposure for items that evoke 70 SUDs. A second option is to finish with all items that require situational and imaginal exposure before moving onto a new hierarchy of obsessional thoughts that require only imaginal exposure.

What's most important is that you confront all the items on your hierarchy—whether you need to use imaginal exposure, situational exposure, or both—not the order in which you confront them.

less discomfort and work your way to more distressing ones, just as you would with situational exposure hierarchy items. For example, Austin had various upsetting sexual (incest) obsessions. He began by confronting images of his parents having intercourse—which triggered 50 SUDs. Then he confronted images of his grandmother's pubic hair—which triggered 60 SUDs. Next he faced his unwanted thoughts of molesting his 7-year-old niece (70 SUDs). Last, he allowed himself to imagine having sex with his sister—which was his most distressing obsession (90 SUDs).

Developing Your Scripts

The Imaginal Exposure Planning Worksheet on the facing page is a form that can help guide you through the process of writing your script. Once you've got a hierarchy item in mind, complete the worksheet, which will provide an outline for the exposure scene.

Then, using the worksheet as a guide, and keeping in mind the tips I gave you, put pen to paper and compose a script that matches the obsessional thought, idea, image, or feared consequence(s) that causes distress. The optimal length of a scenario is from 1 to 3 minutes when read aloud, although the length is not as important as the quality of what you write. Review what you've written to make sure your script contains the important details that provoke anxiety. Don't avoid distressing material. To the contrary—make sure the script vividly matches your obsessional thoughts. Also, give your script an ending where the outcome is either uncertain or tragic. You'll find suggestions and examples of imaginal exposure practices for different types of obsessional fears later in this chapter.

BATTLE PLAN Make copies of the Imaginal Exposure Planning Worksheet and have a copy of this form handy when you're ready to begin your imaginal exposure practice.

Confronting Your Obsessional Thoughts

Recording the Scene

As I've described, successful imaginal exposure entails holding the distressing scene in your mind and staying focused on it for as long as it takes your anxiety to decline without using distraction or rituals. You'll know your practice session has been successful when you can think the obsessional thought with only minimal distress, or when you start to become bored with the scene. But staying focused on a distressing thought for more than a few minutes can be difficult. Your mind will tend to wander, perhaps to less upsetting top-

Imaginal Exposure Planning Worksheet

1. Briefly describe the obsessional thought (image, feared consequence) to be confronted: ________

____

____

2. Describe the main thoughts, ideas, doubts, or images that would go through your mind if you were really in this situation: ____

____

____

____

3. Picture yourself in the feared situation and describe the following:

   - What terrible consequences are happening (or *might* happen)? (Someone or something is harmed, you're responsible, you are embarrassed, and so on) ____________________

     ____

   - Why are they happening, and what could you have done to prevent them? ____________

     ____

   - What are you feeling unsure about? ____________________
   - What are you doing? ____________________
   - What are other people doing? ____________________
   - What's going through your mind? ____________________
   - What's happening inside your body (for example, racing heart, feelings in the genitals, confusion)? ____________________
   - What are you feeling? ____________________

ics, which will hinder the exercise. Therefore, instead of just visualizing your obsessional thoughts, I suggest making a recording that you can play over and over to keep your mind on the details of the feared situation for an extended period of time.

One technique that works very well is to record your script using a digital voice recorder (DVR), available for under $100 at most office supply stores. DVRs have several advantages, including that they're transportable (most fit in the palm of your hand) so you can listen to your scene anytime, anywhere. You can also use headphones for privacy. With a DVR, you don't have to rewind any tapes; you just press a button to listen to your recording. Many DVRs also have a "loop" function that allows you to play the same recording over and over without having to reset it. This will free you from having to rewind and replay your scene during prolonged exposure and help you keep your undivided attention on the scene. Further, DVRs allow you to save and store several scripts and choose the one that you wish to listen to. You can also easily erase those you don't need anymore.

Another option is to record your script on a cassette tape. Most tapes run 30 or 60 minutes per side, so you might record your script several times to keep from having to rewind every time you want to replay the script. Endless loop tapes (which just replay themselves continuously) work particularly well since you don't need to keep stopping and rewinding them. You just have to make sure your recording is about the same length as the loop tape so that you don't record over your material.

Regardless of the technology you use to record your script, or whether you simply read it off the handwritten page, don't worry about making it *perfect*. Stumbling or stuttering on a word, making a minor mistake, or improvising a little bit won't affect the exposure. But getting too emotional will! Tracy's obsessions focused on whether or not she really had OCD—or was it something worse? She practiced imaginal exposure to the doubt that she actually had a psychotic disorder (such as schizophrenia) and was eventually going to lose her mind and need to be institutionalized. But Tracy was crying as she recorded her distressing script, and when she listened to it, she couldn't help focusing on how much distress the doubting caused her. When Tracy calmed down and recorded her scenario in a grim but serious (yet not altogether dismal) tone, she was able to concentrate on the content of the script and have success. Jokes are also something to avoid in imaginal exposures since they'll artificially reduce tension and take your mind off the obsession. The best imaginal exposure scripts allow you to keep your distressing thoughts vivid in your mind, but without so much emotion that you lose focus.

How do your obsessions sound in your head?

Confronting Your Imaginal Script

When you're ready to practice imaginal exposure, either by itself or along with situational exposure, you'll monitor your SUDs using the graph I introduced in Step 7 (I'll give you a form for doing this when we pull everything together after Step 9). You should also prepare yourself for experiencing anxiety using the same strategies I described in Step 7.

Then, begin listening to your script over and over. Close your eyes and imagine that the scene is actually happening to you. If you're confronting an unacceptable thought or image, allow it to come into your mind and remain there. You'll probably feel uncomfortable as you start, but your goal is to hang in there and remain focused on your obsession. If you need to, use the coping statements on page 183 to help you ride out the anxiety. But whatever you do, don't resort to fighting the obsessional thought or the anxiety. Don't try to analyze whether it's true or false (a mental ritual). Using rituals and other avoidance or neutralizing strategies will spoil the exposure practice and you won't benefit. Instead, just allow the unpleasant thoughts to "hang out" in your mind. Focus on the uncertainty ("Maybe you *will*, maybe you *won't*"; "Maybe it *did*, maybe it *didn't*"; and the like) or other distressing parts of the obsession. Your anxiety, distress, and the obsessions will subside when you welcome these thoughts and doubts.

Plan to spend at least 1 hour confronting the obsessional thought or image and continue each exposure until your anxiety and distress habituate—meaning that you experience only mild to moderate distress. If you stop the exercise while your SUDs are still high, you'll maintain—or perhaps intensify—your fears. Repeat the imaginal exposure exercise each time you practice the corresponding situational exposure (or every day for 1 week) until your anxiety about the specific obsessional script remains low for several practices. Then create and record other scripts corresponding to more difficult hierarchy items and situational exposure practices. Continue imaginal exposure until you've successfully confronted all the items on your imaginal exposure hierarchy and can think these unwanted thoughts with only minimal distress.

BATTLE PLAN Spend about 1 hour twice a day for a week confronting each item on your imaginal exposure hierarchy.

Imaginal Exposure for Different Types of Obsessions

BATTLE PLAN While you're planning and working on imaginal exposure, turn to the following pages to read about the types of obsessions that apply to you:

Here are some tips for how to use imaginal exposure to confront different types of obsessional thoughts. It's hard to cover every possible obsession, but I've included examples for many of the "classic" and less common ones that should help you apply imaginal exposure to any obsessions you might have.

As you read these examples and suggestions (which come from actual people I've worked with), keep in mind that you might need to confront some rather distressing, embarrassing, and vulgar thoughts and images to learn to manage your obsessions. This means forcing yourself to write down and think about intensely private and upsetting material. Remember that the guiding principle of imaginal exposure is to confront the very same obsessional thoughts and images that provoke your anxiety.

Contamination Obsessions

If you have contamination obsessions, practice imagining having the germs and illnesses that you worry about. If you obsess about contaminating others, try creating scenes in which you aren't certain whether you've made someone else sick or, depending on your particular obsessional fear, scenes in which you caused someone to get very ill because of your negligence (that is, it was *your* fault). You could use imaginal exposure along with situational exposures as follows: Suppose you're

BATTLE PLAN When you practice imaginal exposure, you don't have to think about anything worse than what you're already thinking when you have your obsessions. This technique gives you the opportunity to practice experiencing these thoughts in a more therapeutic way.

afraid of spreading traces of toxic chemicals to a family member. You might practice contact with cleaning agents and then handle something that belongs to your family member (for example, a wallet or a toothbrush). Then imagine that your loved one touches the contaminated item and becomes very sick or even dies (depending on your obsessional fear). Alternatively, you might not need situational exposure if you have spontaneous obsessional images of germs and wish to conduct imaginal exposure to thoughts of them crawling all over your body. Of course, you'll also practice resisting any washing, cleaning, or checking rituals that serve to reduce your anxiety (see Step 9).

Remember Pearl, whom I described in Step 7 (page 191)? She included imaginal exposure to getting herpes whenever she practiced situational exposures to "contaminated" items such as door handles, people, and bodily waste. Specifically, she imagined becoming ill, developing sores, being diagnosed by a doctor, and having to live with the social embarrassment of having this disease for the rest of her life. For response prevention, she refrained from washing and asking doctors for assurance. Here's one of Pearl's imaginal exposure scripts:

> *I'm beginning to feel sick and notice that I'm having headaches and fever. The lymph glands in my groin are becoming swollen and I'm having lower back pain. I notice that my skin is turning red and becoming very sensitive and blistery. I'm afraid to look at my genitals for fear that I have sores and a discharge. I'm in the doctor's office and she is examining me. As I describe my symptoms, the doctor seems to look worried that something is wrong. She tells me that it sounds like herpes, but that she'll have to check my blood and urine to be sure. She does a vaginal exam and doesn't tell me the result right away, but she looks discouraged. Then she looks at the results of the blood and urine tests. She tells me that I do have herpes. There's no cure. Now I'll have to live with this for the rest of my life. I'll never be able to date or be sexually active because no one will want to be with someone who has this disease. I'm humiliated. How will I ever manage?*

Obsessions about Responsibility for Harm or Mistakes

Imaginal exposure plays an important role in overcoming these types of obsessions, which tend to focus on disastrous consequences that you can't confront using situational exposure. Gary's parking brake obsession, which I described earlier, is a good example. If you have these types of obsessions, practice confronting your thoughts, images, and doubts (feeling uncertain) about each of the disasters you fear. You might set up your script to correspond to situational exposures you've done (as in Gary's example). If so, you should specifically include how the disaster comes about *because you failed to avoid or ritualize*. In other words, emphasize your responsibility for causing (or not doing enough to prevent) the catastrophe. For example, you paid your bill to the electric company without performing checking rituals. Now you might expose yourself in imagination to the electricity being turned off because you paid the wrong amount or put the wrong address on the envelope. Alternatively, you could confront your feared disasters in imagination without doing situational exposure. For example, you could imagine that you've hit someone with your car without realizing it and now the police are after you because you left the scene of an accident.

Recall from Step 7 that Angelo had obsessions about causing disasters such as fires, floods, and accidents. He used imaginal exposure to confront his doubts and uncertainty that were triggered by situational exposure practices. For example, when he practiced turning appliances on and off and then left the apartment without checking, he drove to his workplace (10 miles away) and sat at his desk while he exposed himself in imagination to the following scene:

> *I'm not sure I turned off all the lights in the apartment before I left. What if I left a light on? What if there's a power surge and the light catches fire? I've heard this can happen. My whole complex might burn down by the time the fire department arrives. I feel like going back to check, but I know that I can't. But my apartment could be in flames right now. We'd lose everything—clothes, furniture, financial papers, collectibles, pictures. What if we have to completely start over? It would be horrible. It would be my fault for leaving the light on and not checking carefully enough.*

For response prevention, Angelo also refrained from returning to check on his apartment. Instead of trying to analyze his doubts and figure out whether they were valid (a mental ritual), he replayed the recording of his obsessional doubt and practiced accepting the uncertainty until it lost its power to upset him. Then he imagined an actual fire.

Symmetry and Order Obsessions

If you have symmetry and order obsessions that don't involve fears of bad luck or other disasters, you might not need to use imaginal exposure in your treatment plan. Situational exposure might be sufficient to provoke anxiety. However, if you have obsessions that inexactness, imperfection, asymmetry, or odd numbers will cause something awful to occur unless you perform a ritual, you should confront these feared consequences when you practice situational exposure. For example, if you have a fear that not putting on your clothes in the correct order will lead to your mother's death, you could purposely put your clothes on incorrectly (situational exposure) and then confront thoughts of your mother dying *because you didn't dress the proper way or perform a ritual* (imaginal exposure). Of course, you would also refrain from any checking, reassurance-seeking, or repeating behaviors to make yourself feel less anxious.

Violent Obsessions

Imaginal exposure is an important weapon against violent obsessions. If you're distressed by words such as *murder, stab, death, decapitate, bullet*, and the like, you can record yourself saying these words, and then play the recording back and listen until your anxiety subsides. If your violent obsessions take the form of upsetting images or ideas (for example, of brutalizing someone you love), you must confront these thoughts exactly as they come to mind when you're obsessing. As I've said previously, this kind of exposure can be especially distressing because it may involve thinking about awful things happening to people you love. But in the long run, if you let yourself confront these images, you'll take the wind out of their sails and learn that there's no need to fight or avoid the obsession.

In Step 7, I described Paxton's problem with violent obsessions about harming and killing his newborn. For imaginal exposure practice, he allowed himself to confront awful images of acting on his unwanted thoughts. An example of one of his scripts appears below. Your scripts might need to be graphic or gruesome if your obsessions occur that way in your mind. It's important that you be honest with yourself when creating your scripts. Don't avoid the especially upsetting parts of the obsession, and don't perform any compulsive, mental, or mini-rituals to "put things right" when you confront it.

I'm taking the baby for a walk and have to cross a busy street. As I'm waiting for the light to turn so I can cross, the thought of pushing his stroller into traffic comes to mind. I decide to go with the thought and not push it out of my mind this time. I feel afraid of losing control, though. Then, all of a sudden, I can't stop myself . . . I push the stroller into the busy street and hear brakes screeching. I watch in horror as the stroller is hit by one car, then another, and another. The baby's little body is thrown out onto the street. Blood is everywhere, and his mangled little body bounces out onto the street. I'm in shock. What an awful sight. I imagine how horrified my wife will be when she finds out I killed the baby. . . .

Sexual Obsessions

Imaginal exposure is also an effective way to defeat sexual obsessions. If your obsessions concern unwanted or "forbidden" sexual words (*molest, penis, vagina, lesbian*, and the like), you can make recordings of these words and replay them until the words lose their punch. If your obsessions focus on doubts about your sexual preference, you can practice imagining that you're not sure whether you're gay or straight, and even confront images of engaging in the unwanted sexual behavior, such as images of being intimate with a member of the same sex. If you have obsessive thoughts about molesting children, you should imagine that perhaps you're a child molester. If your obsessions concern incest, you should confront sexual thoughts and images involving relatives. Again, to reclaim your imagination and defeat OCD, you have to allow yourself to confront even the most upsetting, crude, and tasteless aspects of your sexual obsessions. Don't be afraid to let yourself go and face all of the unacceptable thoughts that enter your mind as obsessions. And remember response prevention—mental rituals (for example, praying, reviewing), reassurance seeking, and checking are not allowed.

To illustrate, consider Matt from Step 7 (page 198) who had homosexual obsessions. One of his imaginal exposures involved images of having sex with his friend, Todd. The script for this exposure was as follows:

Todd and I are laughing as we embrace each other. We can't deny our love any longer. I never knew he felt the same way about me. I feel sinful, but I don't care. I'm so excited that I feel my heart racing and can hardly catch my breath. Then we look each other in the eye and I know he's thinking the same thing I am. Our lips meet and we kiss. I smell his scent and taste his saliva. We're so into each other, we can hardly catch our breaths. I'm enjoying this so much. I finally realize that I'm gay and that I love Todd. How come I denied this for so long?

If you're wondering about thinking such graphic (or even more graphic) ideas, let me remind you that your imaginal exposure scripts don't need to be any more explicit than the actual content of your obsessions—the thoughts that already pop into your mind. Matt was already having obsessions containing what he perceived as vulgar and crude images, so his imaginal exposures didn't involve thinking anything he hadn't thought of before. The exposures merely provided him with an opportunity to experience these obsessions in a different way—a way that eventually led to their decline, a way that helped him accept that they're a normal part of life. Believe it or not, when *you* do this consistently, you'll notice that the thoughts become less frequent.

Religious Obsessions

Imaginal exposure scripts for religious obsessions usually fall into two categories. The first category involves distressing blasphemous or sacrilegious words, phrases, images, and doubts—for example, anti-God phrases, images of Jesus urinating on the cross, or thoughts about having sex with the Virgin Mary or with a priest. Jonas's exposure to the word *devil*, which I described earlier in this step, is an example of this type of exercise. The second type of imaginal script involves confronting the possibility that you've committed a sin and that God is upset with you. With both types of imaginal exposure, you must also refrain from any ritualizing to reduce your distress.

Recall from Step 7 that Hattie experienced obsessional thoughts about having sex with Jesus. Therefore, she confronted these thoughts using imaginal exposure scripts that were somewhat similar to the one Matt used in the example above, although tailored to Hattie's specific images. To clarify, Hattie allowed herself to confront, over and over, her upsetting obsessional images of having sex with Jesus. But she also experienced obsessive doubts that she wasn't a good Christian and that God was upset with her. Therefore, she also confronted these obsessions using a series of scripts, an example of which appears here:

> *I'm always coming up with reasons for why I am not a good Christian woman. It feels like I don't have enough love and faith in God because of all the terrible thoughts I have all the time. I would like to know what God thinks of me. I would like to know that I'm serving Him in the most loving and faithful way possible, but I can't really be sure. My friends and my husband—even my pastor—have tried to reassure me, but they're all humans. How do they know the mind of God? Can I ever be guaranteed that God loves me? That I'm a good enough servant? Even the fact that I worry whether God loves me might make me a disbeliever and might be upsetting to God. . . .*

Although it took a great deal of courage and anxiety for Hattie to confront her sexual and scrupulous obsessions, when she allowed herself to face these thoughts and doubts head on, she found that they became less and less powerful. She also learned to accept that unwanted thoughts are a part of life. As a result, she didn't feel the need to seek constant reassurance, and she developed a deeper, stronger sense of faith.

Troubleshooting

Here are some of the most common problems you're likely to encounter when you begin practicing exposure (situational and imaginal), with solutions to help you move past them.

BATTLE PLAN If you anticipate any of the problems described in this section, try working with your treatment buddy—or with a knowledgeable professional—to help you get through these trouble spots.

What If the Exposure Exercise Doesn't Trigger Anxiety?

Kiara had obsessions that if she confronted the color black, and didn't say ritualistic prayers, bad luck would befall her loved ones. For situational exposure, she wore black clothes and refrained from her ritual prayers. She also practiced imaginal exposure to images of her family having accidents because of her failure to pray. But when Kiara kept track of her SUDs level, she found that her anxiety never became very intense. Her SUDs remained in the 20–30 range.

If you confront a situation or obsessional thought from your hierarchy and it doesn't provoke much anxiety, one of two things might be happening. The first possibility is that the situation or obsession is not actually as distressing as you had predicted when you developed your fear hierarchy. Maybe you somehow got over your fear before it came time to expose yourself to it—perhaps by learning about OCD or using cognitive therapy techniques. If this is the case, you should move on to confronting the next items on your fear hierarchies list.

Unfortunately, the second possibility—that there is a problem with how you're conducting exposure—is more likely. For example, not becoming anxious during exposure could be a sign that you're not fully facing your fear. Perhaps the exposure situation doesn't match well enough to your actual fear trigger(s). Or your imaginal exposure script might not contain the most distressing or upsetting aspects of your obsessional thoughts and images. You might be using subtle (or not-so-subtle) rituals or other strategies to take the edge off and artificially make you feel safe or protect you from the exposure. If your SUDs level increases when you begin exposure, but then rapidly decreases after only a few minutes in the feared situation, you might be using such safety cues to deal with the distress caused by exposure.

To get past this obstacle, let's analyze things more closely. You might unintentionally be doing things that interfere with your exposure. The worksheet on the facing page can help you see whether this is the case. Take a few minutes to answer the questions.

Are you fully facing your fear when you do exposure? When Kiara thought through the questions on the worksheet, she realized that she had "warned" her family and friends that she was going to wear black that particular week. By telling these people that they should be careful about having bad luck during the week, Kiara had transferred some of the responsibility for her feared consequences of wearing black to her family and friends. This subtle safety maneuver (which Kiara didn't even realize was a mistake) made her feel less frightened of conducting exposure, but it also prevented her from benefiting from the exercise. A few weeks later she again tried wearing black clothes and imag-

Are you taking precautions or doing anything to keep your anxiety in check?

1. What hierarchy item are you practicing with? ____
____

2. What are your fears about facing this situation or obsessional thought? What do you find threatening about this situation or thought? ____
____
____

3. What precautions are you taking *before you start* the exposure to make sure that your fears don't come true or to make you feel safer? ____
____
____

4. What precautions are you taking *during* the exposure to prevent something awful from happening (consider that these might be *active* or *mental* strategies)? ______________________
____
____

5. What are you doing to keep your anxiety in check during the exposure? ____________________
____
____

6. What could you do (or stop doing) to make the exposure seem more *realistic* or more *distressing*? ____
____
____

ining disasters *without* informing her friends and relatives. This time, she evoked anxiety and in the end learned that the color black was probably not going to cause bad luck.

What If the Exercise Triggers Too Much Anxiety?

Lawrence was feeling overwhelmed with fear. When he began the exposure he had planned for the week—sitting on the bathroom floor—his SUDs skyrocketed to what seemed like 101%! Even the coping statements he was using were not helping at this point. He was on the verge of giving up.

While you're supposed to feel frightened when you begin an exposure practice, there's no need to make yourself *terrified*. If you become so anxious that you feel overwhelmed, it might be a sign that you've chosen to confront a hierarchy item that you're not ready to face yet. Here are three options you can try if you find yourself in this situation:

1. Try instead to find an "intermediate" or "transitional" situation or thought to confront that's not quite as difficult as the one you're having trouble with, but that's still more challenging than your previous exposures. Remember, though, that the goal of the intermediate exposure is to help you work your way back to the initial practice you were having trouble with. Lawrence, for example, used touching the bathroom *walls* as an intermediate exposure between bathroom doorknobs (which he had previously confronted), and bathroom floors.
2. You could modify the very fear-provoking hierarchy item slightly so that it's less frightening and easier to confront. Then, when you feel comfortable in the modified situation, attempt full exposure in the originally planned way. Lawrence, for example, began by sitting on a towel on the bathroom floor. When his SUDs had decreased, he removed the towel. Then sitting on the floor seemed more doable.
3. You could try to stick it out and just remain in the exposure. Bear in mind that even high levels of anxiety won't harm you, and will also subside if you allow some time. Remember that anxiety is your response to perceived threat—your fight-or-flight system. If you embrace the anxious feelings, rather than trying to escape from them, they'll eventually return to manageable levels.

If you're having difficulty with an exposure practice that's just too anxiety-provoking, try using the worksheet on the facing page to help you decide on a troubleshooting strategy.

Moving On to Step 9

You have now learned how to use two types of exposure to defeat your problems with OCD. But as you've read, there is still another key component of treatment: response prevention. Even the most carefully planned and well-executed exposure practices will be ineffective if you continue to perform rituals. In the next step, you'll learn why response prevention is so important, and you'll begin working on a plan for reducing your rituals.

When Exposure Is Too Frightening

1. Describe the exposure practice that's provoking extremely high anxiety:

2. *Finding an intermediate exposure.* What different situation(s) or obsessional thoughts could you practice confronting that might be *more manageable* for you than #1, yet still *challenging*? This intermediate exposure(s) should provide a stepping-stone to help you work your way back to #1.

3. *Modifying the exposure.* How might you modify or adjust the exposure *temporarily* to make it less anxiety-provoking so you can resume your practice?

4. *Embracing the high anxiety.* What cognitive techniques, coping statements, and other strategies could you use to help you work through the high anxiety and remain in the exposure situation until the anxiety subsides?

5. Now, review your answers to questions 2, 3, and 4. Below, write down which strategy you will try first, second, and third.

   1. ______________________________

   2. ______________________________

   3. ______________________________

STEP 9

Defeating Your Compulsive Urges

- Read Chapters 7–9 before starting exposure practices.
- While you're learning about exposure and response prevention, you can practice the cognitive therapy techniques you learned in Chapter 6 for 45 minutes a day for 1–2 weeks.

Throughout Part III of this workbook, I've emphasized that the battle against OCD involves two strategies: (1) confronting your feared situations and (2) stopping your compulsive rituals. That's why the treatment is called *exposure* **and** response prevention—and why you need to read about both and then incorporate both into your practices. In Steps 7 and 8 you learned how to practice actual and imaginal exposure to your obsessional fears. Now, in Step 9, you'll learn the response prevention component, which means calling a halt to your overt compulsive rituals and reassurance seeking, as well as the less obvious mini- and mental rituals.

Why isn't it enough just to do exposure? If you confronted the situations that trigger obsessional fear until they didn't instill much fear anymore, wouldn't you be done? Unfortunately, as you know all too well, OCD doesn't work that way. OCD's scheme to keep control of you involves planting a false fear in your head and then convincing you that the only way to avoid the dreaded consequence is to dance to OCD's tune: to perform a ritual. OCD tells you that obeying the compulsion linked with a particular obsession is the only way to ease your anxiety and feel safe. So, exposure teaches you that you don't have to avoid your feared situations and thoughts. The trouble is, if you know that you've got a ritual waiting in the wings as a fail-safe measure *just in case*, you haven't really beaten OCD. That's why it's so important to stop ritualizing and face each feared situation armed only with the weapons of CBT, weapons that really work.

How have rituals stolen the joy from your life?

Combining response prevention with exposure practice is therefore absolutely critical to the success of your treatment program. Imagine doing an exposure practice to provoke obsessional anxiety, but then immediately yielding to OCD's demand that you ritualize to reduce the anxiety and make you feel safe again. What would happen? For one thing, you'd *never* learn that anxiety habituates on its own—even without rituals. And you'd *never* learn that you don't need rituals to keep you safe. Instead, you'd simply *strengthen* your urges to ritualize when you confront an obsession. The human brain is an amazingly quick learner, and if something works one time, your brain tells you it will work the next time too (this is why rituals develop into such strong patterns). You'd also *strengthen* the mistaken belief that ritualizing is the only way to deal with risk and uncertainty. But these are exactly the patterns that we're trying to eliminate! So exposure won't be of much help unless you also stop your rituals and discard them from your arsenal of coping strategies.

It's one of OCD's dirtiest tricks that rituals sometimes reduce your anxiety and make you feel safer temporarily, because in the long run this only feeds your obsessional fears. Rituals also lead you to become more and more dependent on ritualizing as time goes by because they seem like the only way to get relief from anxiety. Rituals keep you from developing healthier ways of managing everyday levels of risk and uncertainty, and they take time away from more productive behaviors such as working and spending time with family or friends. In other words, rituals steal the joy from your life.

How Does Response Prevention Work?

When you decrease or stop your rituals, you'll probably feel anxious and distressed at first. But if you extend your exposure practices long enough to let these feelings subside on their own, you'll weaken the urge to engage in ritualistic behaviors. When you do this repeatedly, you get used to handling these situations without ritualizing. The connection between rituals and temporarily feeling good and safe gets weaker and weaker. With time, patience, and determination, you'll reduce your dependence on rituals.

Response prevention works by giving you a chance to see that doing rituals is *not* the only way to reduce obsessional distress. Your anxiety, and your sense of uncertainty and insecurity, will subside by themselves—even as you remain exposed to your fears.

Learning to Live with Uncertainty: The Main Goal of Response Prevention

When you use response prevention and stop your rituals, you'll be giving up on obtaining a guarantee that the feared consequences you obsess over won't happen. But absolute certainty is more or less an illusion. It's hard to know in absolute terms about the things you're afraid of: Did I do enough to be safe from germs, mistakes, or bad luck? Did I hit someone with my car and not realize it? Is it really OCD that I have? Is there something seriously

Are you prepared to give up your quest for absolute certainty and accept doubt, ambiguity, and uncertainty as a part of life?

medically wrong with me? Will I lose control and kill my children one day? Am I a child molester? Will I go to hell when I die? Doing rituals might have helped you temporarily feel better about one or more of these things, but OCD always provokes more uncertainty, over and over, despite lots of facts and many assurances. So, instead of dancing to OCD's tune by ritualizing and trying to eliminate all risks of disaster, to get better you must be willing to live with reasonable uncertainty. When OCD tells you that you'd better reassure yourself, you've got to tune out these false messages and practice assuming that your best guess about the probability of danger—the one you'd bet your life savings on—is the correct one.

When you use response prevention techniques to purposely seek out uncertainty, you'll eventually get used to this feeling and move closer to putting your problems with obsessions and rituals behind you.

Getting Ready to Stop Your Rituals

Understanding that it's important to stop your rituals is one thing, but actually resisting the urge to ritualize when you're feeling very anxious is another. That's why you need to prepare carefully for response prevention.

Lucia had responsibility obsessions. She was constantly worried about making mistakes and causing (or failing to prevent) disasters—such as a house fire—to befall her family. She spent hours each day performing a variety of rituals, including checking the lights and electrical appliances to make sure she hadn't left them on or plugged in and checking and rechecking door locks and windows. Obsessions about mistakenly poisoning her family drove Lucia to wash her hands more than 20 times each day so that she could be sure no toxic substances (for example, Windex) remained on her hands. Her washing rituals had to follow certain rules that Lucia had made up. If the rule wasn't followed perfectly, or if she was interrupted, she'd have to start washing all over again. As a result, Lucia sometimes got stuck washing for up to 20 minutes at a time. She also performed repeating rituals that she believed prevented bad luck. If an obsessional thought came to mind as she was doing any ordinary behavior such as getting dressed, going through a doorway, flushing the toilet, or turning on a light switch, she had to repeat the behavior over and over until the obsession was gone.

Lucia planned to conduct situational and imaginal exposure practice, including leaving lights on and the toaster plugged in while she left her children with a babysitter and using bug repellent and sunscreen, which she avoided because of her fear of harm. She also planned to confront her distressing obsessional thoughts and images of her family getting hurt and sick as a result of her "negligence."

Monitoring: Keeping an Eye on Your Rituals

Like Lucia, you might have a number of rituals that you use in response to your obsessions and anxiety. Flip back to Step 4 (page 110), where you listed the details of your most problematic rituals. In the response prevention part of your treatment program, you'll work to stop these behaviors. To be successful, you'll need to become fully aware of when rituals are happening. *Monitoring* your rituals means taking notice of how and when you ritualize by keeping a log or diary.

I have every patient with OCD I work with monitor his or her rituals from the beginning to the end of treatment. If your rituals occur several times a day or week, you should also monitor them. Besides learning more about your rituals, self-monitoring is therapeutic and often decreases the frequency of rituals by itself. That's right—some of my patients tell me that just knowing they're keeping track motivates them to resist ritualizing. Another benefit of self-monitoring is that it gives you a way to keep track of your progress.

Monitoring your rituals can be challenging if you've never tried it before, so I've included a Ritual Monitoring Form on the next page to make it easier for you. Each time you perform a ritual, fill in the date, the time the ritual started, and a brief description of the situation or thought that triggered the need to ritualize. Then rate the intensity of your obsessional fear using the SUDs scale. Finally, write a brief description of the ritual you performed, and how many minutes it lasted. Here are some additional tips for filling out the Ritual Monitoring Form:

- Don't guess how long the ritual lasts; use a watch and try to be as accurate as you can.
- Fill out the form as soon as possible after the ritual occurs. If you wait until the end of the day, you risk forgetting important details.
- Carry your monitoring form(s) with you. If that's not possible, fill it out as soon as you can.
- At the end of each day, review your form(s) to get an idea of how much you ritualized that day.

BATTLE PLAN Make copies of the blank Ritual Monitoring Form to use throughout the time you'll be practicing exposure and response prevention. Depending on your rituals, you might need many forms.

BATTLE PLAN Begin monitoring your rituals right away so that you collect a day or two of information before you start exposure and response prevention exercises. This will give you a "baseline" or "before" picture of your rituals. When you're through with this program, you can compare this to your "after" picture and see how much less time you're spending with rituals.

Lucia's Ritual Monitoring Form from the morning of June 11th appears on page 231. You can see how she tracked the various rituals related to her fears of contamination, fires, and injuries. As soon as Lucia started self-monitoring, she realized that her rituals were more frequent than she had admitted. Through self-monitoring she became more aware of specific situations and thoughts that triggered her rituals, such as thinking about catastrophes.

Setting Your Sights

The next step is to think about exactly how you'll target your rituals. Lucia decided to begin by attacking her checking rituals because they would be triggered by the exposure practices she had planned to do during the first week of her program: leaving lights and appliances (toaster oven, computer) turned on while she left the house for a while. Next, she had planned to confront feared contaminants such as cleansers and gasoline. Since

Ritual Monitoring Form

Date	Time	Situation or thought that provoked the ritual	SUDs	Ritual	Min:sec

Lucia's Ritual Monitoring Form

Date	Time	Situation or thought that provoked the ritual	SUDs	Ritual	Min:sec
6/11	8:30 a.m.	Used bathroom, thought about germs	66	Washing	4:30
6/11	8:55	Touched garbage can	75	Washing	5:05
6/11	10:25	Thought about kids having bus accident	75	Repeat going through doorway	2:00
6/11	11:00	Leaving house, thoughts about fires	60	Checking appliances	10:00
6/11	11:30	Thought about house burning down	70	Call neighbor for assurance	3:15

doing these exposures would provoke the urge to wash her hands, Lucia decided to target her hand-washing rituals next. Lucia saved focusing on her repeating rituals for last because she knew they would be the most difficult to stop. She also hadn't planned on confronting the distressing obsessional thoughts that triggered these rituals until later in her program.

Now it's your turn. Think about the rituals that your first few exposure practices will trigger. It's a good idea to work on ending these first. Then you'll target different rituals as you confront their triggers in exposure. The Response Prevention Plan Worksheet on the next page includes places for you to write down the order in which you'll target your rituals based on which exposures you're doing. To give you a clearer idea of what you're trying to accomplish, take a look at Lucia's completed form on page 233. She described the rituals she was planning to stop, her SUDs level (how distressing it might feel to resist doing the ritual), and the corresponding exposure practices. This served as her guide for when to apply response prevention to her different types of rituals.

How to Stop Ritualizing: Response Prevention Strategies

Findings from research studies suggest that the stricter you are about stopping rituals, the better your results will be. Of course, this doesn't necessarily mean that the strictest approach—completely ending all of your rituals right off the bat when you begin your program—is the right one for you. Let me describe several useful strategies for response prevention and help you decide on the best way to proceed.

Response Prevention Plan Worksheet

Target ritual (describe response prevention plan)	SUDs	Corresponding exposure practice

Lucia's Response Prevention Plan Worksheet

Target ritual (describe response prevention plan)	SUDs	Corresponding exposure practice
Stop checking electrical outlets, on—off switches, and door and window locks. Stop calling neighbors to check on the house. Stop asking my husband to check downstairs locks in the middle of the night.	*60*	*Leaving appliances plugged in or on when I leave the house, and imagining fires. Imaginal exposure to burglaries.*
Stop hand-washing rituals.	*80*	*Have contact with feared chemicals (pesticides, oil, gasoline, etc.)*
Stop repeating everyday behaviors if I have a bad thought.	*70*	*Imaginal exposure to thoughts about the family being hurt in a fire or accident. Thoughts about death, bad luck, and the like.*

Quitting Your Rituals "Cold Turkey"

In a perfect world, you'd just abruptly stop doing all of the rituals associated with the particular obsession that you're targeting in exposure practice. The worst thing that would probably happen is that you'll feel fairly anxious at the start—although remember that this isn't dangerous and your distress will eventually subside on its own. You'd also have coping statements (page 183 in Step 7) and your treatment buddy to help you get through (but not escape from) the anxiety (I'll discuss your treatment buddy's role in response prevention later in this step). Still, quitting rituals all of a sudden isn't easy: you'll need to choose to go *toward* anxiety and uncertainty, not *away* from it.

> What's the best way to stop your rituals when you begin your program? Should you stop them all at once? Can you do it gradually? What about delaying them?

If you think you can stop all of your rituals cold turkey when you launch your CBT program, go ahead and do it. But keep in mind that resisting your rituals is almost always easier said than done. That's why, in our clinic at the University of North Carolina, we use a response prevention method that's not quite as strict. In this "modified cold turkey" approach, we ask all of our patients to do the best they can to stop their rituals, but we understand that *never* ritualizing is more a *goal* than a *requirement*. If and when patients absolutely can't resist performing a ritual (even after using the strategies for coping with anxiety and discussing it with a treatment buddy), we require that they immediately try to reexpose themselves to the feared situation that triggered the ritual (or to some other item they've already confronted in exposure practices). I recommend you consider this strategy too. It ensures that should you fall off the CBT horse, you'll be doing your best to get right back up there again.

One day, despite trying very hard to resist, Lucia just couldn't withstand the urge to go back to the kitchen and check that her toaster oven hadn't caught fire. But by checking, she undid her exposure practice. Afterward, however, Lucia had the presence of mind to leave the toaster oven plugged in, leave the kitchen, and immediately reexpose herself by doing a brief imaginal exposure to thinking about the toaster oven catching fire. This raised her anxiety level and gave Lucia a second chance to resist the urge to ritualize. On another occasion, she slipped up and washed her hands because of her fear of chemicals. Realizing that she needed to get back on the CBT horse, she immediately reexposed herself by handling a can of bug spray and, this time, was able to resist washing her hands.

If, after trying, you can't stop your rituals cold turkey, here are some other, more gradual approaches to response prevention.

Modifying the Ritual

If you've tried and tried to resist a ritual, but just can't seem to be successful, or if you're just not ready to push yourself to completely stop at this point, the next best thing is to do the ritual in "the wrong way." That is, change some aspect of the behavior so that you're doing it "incorrectly." For instance, you could change the order in which you compulsively check the locks, doors, and appliances. If you have shower rituals, you could practice washing your body parts in a different (reverse) order. If counting is part of your rituals, you could change the number you count to, or even count incorrectly (for example, 1, 4, 2, 8, 5 . . .) so that you lose track. If you have repeating rituals, you could repeat the behavior by changing something—anything: use the opposite hand, go into a different room, ritualize while standing on one foot or with your eyes closed. The object is to feel like you didn't do the ritual well enough—like you have unfinished business and need to go back and do it over again. You want to get used to feeling this way (as in habituation).

In what way can you throw OCD a curve by changing a ritual you currently find impossible to stop altogether?

By consciously manipulating a seemingly uncontrollable ritual, you'll gain some power over the behavior. You'll also teach yourself that the special rules for performing the ritual are not necessary to reduce anxiety or the chances of disaster. So, modifying a ritual is the beginning of its defeat. If you can feel comfortable ritualizing "incompletely," you're a giant leap closer to not needing the ritual at all.

This strategy is especially helpful for rituals you feel you must carry out "perfectly" or according to certain rules. When Lucia washed her hands, for example, she had to follow a specific routine to get her hands "perfectly clean": first she washed the front and back of both hands for 1 minute, then she washed between her fingers for 30 seconds, then up to a certain point on her wrists, and so on. She also had to use special heavy-duty soap. When it came time to end these rituals, she began by washing "incorrectly."

BATTLE PLAN The key to modifying a ritual is to make it feel like you didn't do a good enough job at ritualizing—like you need to do the ritual again. Once you've practiced doing the ritual "wrong" for a while, it will be easier to modify even further, or stop it altogether.

She used regular soap, washed the palms of her hands only once, and refrained from washing between her fingers. This made her feel like the ritual wasn't "good enough," which was the goal.

After a few days of modifying her washing behavior, Lucia realized that it wasn't her rule-bound ritualizing that was preventing her family from becoming ill—they were unlikely to get sick in the first place. She saw that she didn't need to wash her hands the "right way" to feel safe and comfortable. This made it easier for Lucia to gradually decrease her washing rituals.

Almost any compulsive ritual that you carry out according to a set of rules can be modified. But you can also use ritual modification with subtle or very brief (mini-) rituals. If you quickly check the rearview mirror to make sure you haven't hit anyone with your car, you could put a piece of tape on the mirror so that your view isn't perfectly clear. If you have to count to certain numbers while you ritualize, you could count incorrectly so that you aren't sure whether you lost count. If you check doors and light switches by looking at them or touching them, you could check with your eyes closed or without using your fingers. If you have ordering rituals, you can mess them up in one way or another so you get that "not just right" feeling.

This strategy also works very well with mental rituals that are difficult to stop altogether. For example, if you have prayer rituals, you can say the prayer incorrectly, pray to the wrong deity, or leave something out that seems very important. If you have to repeat certain "safe" or "lucky" words or phrases, you can also do so incorrectly, in a different language, or by visualizing the words being misspelled—anything that makes you feel like the ritual is foiled. If you have reviewing rituals, purposely remember what happened *incorrectly*. When Quinton had obsessional thoughts about the bathroom where he once found his father's pornographic magazines, he mentally ritualized by replacing the bathroom image with an image of the kitchen because it was the room in his house that was farthest from the bathroom. Quinton modified this ritual by picturing a room that was closer to the bathroom, such as the living room. Gradually he changed the room in his mental ritual to be closer to the bathroom until he was able to stop the ritual altogether and allow the bathroom thoughts to stay in his mind.

The purpose of doing rituals the wrong way is to help you see that there's nothing magical about the ritual. If you can do the ritual the wrong way, you're getting closer to not ritualizing at all.

To use this strategy effectively, you need to plan exactly how you're going to modify the ritual. The Ritual Modification Worksheet on the next page is designed to help you analyze the specific details of rituals you want to change and then figure out ways to distort or foil the rituals. First, fill in the left side of the worksheet by describing the various aspects of how you perform the ritual. Then think about what you can do differently that will spoil the ritual or make it seem ineffective. On the right side of the worksheet, jot down how you'll change different aspects of the ritual when you begin response prevention. It's not necessary to make changes to *every* aspect of the ritual—although the more you change, the better. The important thing is that you change the ritual in a way that makes it feel incomplete.

BATTLE PLAN Make copies of this worksheet so you can use it to focus on different rituals.

Ritual Modification Worksheet

Analyzing the ritual (*what you do now*)	**Modifying the ritual** (*what you'll do differently*)
Describe the actual behavior:	
Order of individual behaviors:	
Number of times you repeat the behaviors:	
Time limits (*for example, at least 3 minutes*):	
Specific items you use (*for example, special soap*):	
Location(s) where the ritual happens:	
Describe the role that other people play in the ritual (*for example, giving assurance, watching the ritual*):	
Other special rules (*for example, avoiding certain numbers of repetitions, must use right hand, someone must watch me do it*):	

Restricting Your Rituals

Another strategy is to reduce either the time you allow for the ritual or the number of times you repeat the behavior. This works best if you have rituals that last a long time (such as a ritualized showering or cleaning routine) or that need to be repeated over and over (repeating going through a doorway, for example). If your rituals don't take up much time (for example, quickly checking a door lock), ritual restriction might not be as helpful.

Lucia had trouble completely stopping her washing compulsions all at once, so she used a timer to limit how long she spent washing. She began by allowing herself to wash for a minute. After a few days, though, she reduced this to 30 seconds. From there, she went to 20 seconds, 10 seconds, and finally to no washing at all. If you use this strategy, try to push yourself as much as you can, but also be realistic in judging what you can accomplish. The goal should be to gradually reduce the ritual until it eventually doesn't occur at all.

Delaying Your Rituals

Another way to get control over your rituals is to simply postpone them. Perhaps it's only for a minute or two, or maybe several hours (or days). Of course, the longer you wait to perform the ritual, the better. Every minute you resist, you're teaching yourself that you can manage anxiety and uncertainty. So, for example, if you get the urge to say a prayer, repeat a behavior, ask for reassurance, wash, or check, try to delay for, say, 15 minutes. After that, see if you can resist for 15 more minutes, and so on for as long as you can.

How about allowing a little less time for a ritual—or fewer repetitions?

Lucia used this strategy with her repeating rituals. For one of her exposures, she walked through the doorway to her house while imagining her brother having a car accident. This provoked the urge to go back outside and walk into the house over again until the upsetting images were gone. But instead of giving in immediately, Lucia decided to postpone the ritual for 30 minutes and continue with imaginal exposure. After 30 minutes, she still felt the urge to ritualize, so she postponed for 30 *more* minutes. As it turned out, the phone rang and Lucia ended up talking with a friend for about 45 minutes, after which she forgot all about having to ritualize. She had successfully postponed her ritual until the urge decreased.

Could you thwart OCD by procrastinating?

The best thing you can do while you're delaying a ritual is to practice more exposure. Confront the trigger and use imaginal techniques to purposely think about the feared consequences you might face by not ritualizing. This is a punishing blow to OCD because you'll be proving that *you're* the boss—not OCD. Delaying a ritual also buys you time to use cognitive therapy strategies (from Step 6) and coping self-statements (from Step 7) to help you ride out your obsessional fear. You might examine the pros and cons of ritualizing or come up with more realistic interpretations of the thought or situation that triggered the urge to ritualize. This will give you a fresh perspective, and you might find you

When you postpone your rituals, you give yourself a chance to regroup and use the battle strategies you've learned in this workbook. You might find that the urge to ritualize passes sooner than you think.

no longer need to ritualize when the time to do so rolls around. Postponing is, of course, an intermediate strategy to weaken rituals. Ultimately you'll need to stop them altogether by delaying the ritual indefinitely.

Incorporating Response Prevention into Your Lifestyle

You might be able to beat your rituals using just one of the strategies described above, or you might do better with mixing and matching. Lucia combined modifying (altering and restricting her washing rituals) and delaying (postponing repeating rituals until the urge subsided). This shows how you can move from one strategy to another. It's important to think about which techniques might work best for you based on your specific rituals, daily routine, lifestyle, and where you are in your treatment program.

To be most effective, exposure and response prevention needs to become a part of your life—not something you practice for an hour or two each day.

As you confront more and more situations in exposure practice, you'll be expanding your response prevention as well. Eventually, you'll be working on trying to resist *all* of your rituals in *all* situations. Urges to ritualize can sometimes sneak up on you unexpectedly in different places and at different times. Just like it's important to practice exposure in different situations, you should also get used to consistently resisting rituals under all different circumstances. So, in addition to working on response prevention *when you practice your planned situational and imaginal exposures*, you'll eventually want to set the goal of resisting urges to ritualize *whenever and wherever they occur.* If you're not consistent with response prevention, you'll continue to feel like the best way to cope with obsessional fear is to ritualize.

BATTLE PLAN It's best to think of response prevention as a full-time job. You must always be "on call," resisting urges to perform rituals so that you can defeat OCD.

Managing High Anxiety When You Resist Rituals

Be prepared for an increase in anxiety and distress when you begin response prevention. It might feel like you're walking a tightrope and someone has taken away your safety net! But don't give in when your discomfort increases; you'll be playing right into OCD's hand. As you now know, the anxious feelings are temporary; they subside on their own if you give them time. Anxiety is not going to hurt you either. It's simply an indication that you perceive a threat—in this case, a mistaken perception that something dreadful might happen if you don't ritualize. So, as with dealing with exposure-related anxiety, the best way to manage anxiety around not ritualizing is to remind yourself that anxiety is temporary and harmless—and you can certainly cope with it. When you let your anxiety come down on its own, you'll start to feel more confident that your obsessional fears are unrealistic. In other words, you'll find that you don't need the safety net because you're a much better tightrope walker than you had thought!

When you're resisting a ritual and your anxiety mounts, that's a good time to review the coping statements you learned about in Step 7. Instead of making yourself more anxious by telling yourself how terrible it feels not to ritualize, try using the statements at the bottom of page 183. These will help you without providing an artificial escape or reassurance. Remember that coping statements are not supposed to *reduce* your anxiety, but to inspire you to ride it out. You don't have to *enjoy* being anxious (my guess is that nobody does), but you must learn to *accept* it if you're going to decrease how much it causes problems in your life.

Treatment Buddy Tip

You can also call on your treatment buddy, who has agreed to be there for you at times like these, to help you through high anxiety. Your treatment buddy might be able to temporarily distract you, help you with using coping statements or cognitive therapy techniques, or just show support and empathy. When you call on him or her, explain that you're feeling very anxious and are looking for some help with getting through it. Of course, it's not your treatment buddy's job to reassure you or to take the anxiety away, but to help you manage the discomfort until it subsides on its own.

For treatment buddies: Here are some *dos* and *don'ts* that might be helpful when your friend or relative is trying to manage intense anxiety. Watch out if your first instinct is to quell your friend's or relative's distress. While this might seem like the obvious thing to do, it's not likely to be helpful in the long run. Instead, your goal is to help your companion cope with high anxiety while resisting urges to ritualize:

Dos

- Listen attentively to what your friend or relative is concerned about.
- Remind him or her that resisting rituals is hard work and that he or she is doing a great job.
- Say that you're very glad he or she came to you instead of just going ahead and ritualizing.
- Encourage him or her to use the coping statements on page 183.
- Do something enjoyable to temporarily get away from the troubling situation—such as going for a walk, watching a movie, or playing a game.

Don'ts

- Don't ritualize for your friend or family member.
- Don't engage in any avoidance behavior for him or her.
- Avoid providing reassurance that everything will be okay.
- If your companion insists on ritualizing, it's his or her personal choice. Avoid arguing, making threats, and name calling (stress, by the way, makes OCD *worse*).
- Don't be overprotective. Let him or her be responsible for his or her own behaviors and problems.
- Never physically prevent anyone from doing rituals.

Getting Help from Family and Friends

Lucia's husband and children didn't like seeing Lucia anxious, so they had always done anything they could to help her avoid obsessional triggers and give her reassurance that everything was okay. Her husband, for example, checked all the appliances and reported their status to Lucia every night before coming to bed. Her children avoided certain parts of the house if they hadn't washed their hands. Although they *thought* they were helping Lucia, they were actually making her OCD worse.

> Do your relatives or friends "help" you carry out rituals?
>
> Do they take on your avoidance strategies?

Check off any of the following types of "assistance" that your friends or family provide or that are similar to something they do for you:

- ☐ Your roommate unplugs all of her appliances because of your fear of fires.
- ☐ At your insistence, your spouse wipes down all the mail and groceries before bringing these items into the house.
- ☐ Your kids avoid certain homes in the neighborhood because of your contamination fears.
- ☐ Your mother cuts your food for you because you're afraid of knives.
- ☐ The leader of your Bible study reassures you over and over that you're a good Christian.
- ☐ Your best friend assures you that you didn't hit anyone with your car by mistake.
- ☐ Your parents send you money to buy heavy-duty cleaning supplies and extra toilet paper.

Although these people might have the best intentions, they're inadvertently enabling OCD. So here's what you can do to get them to help you the correct way.

First, don't blame your friends and relatives. It might be hard for them to just stop what they're doing if they don't like seeing you anxious or upset. Perhaps they worry that "too much" anxiety is bad for you (although this isn't true). Maybe they're afraid that you'll be angry with them if they don't comply with your rituals and avoidance patterns (which might be true). To help them understand what treatment is all about, you should explain how response prevention works and that anxiety isn't harmful. Maybe even ask them to read Part I of this workbook.

Second, identify the ways that people in your life are involved in your problems with OCD and think about what they can do to provide the right kind of help. The success of your battle against OCD depends on your friends and relatives taking *your* side—not unwittingly helping OCD. So your friends and relatives—children and adults—should stop doing rituals at your request—and you should stop insisting that they ritualize for you. For example, your spouse or partner should stop helping you check the car for dents because of your obsessions about hitting pedestrians. Instead, the people you live with should behave as they wish from now on. No more hand washing just because you're afraid of germs, no more putting things in order for you, and no more keeping all knives locked away in certain drawers. The people you seek assurances from should also refuse to give you reassurance if you ask for it.

The Ending Others' Involvement in Your Rituals Worksheet (on page 243) provides space for writing down how significant others are involved in your ritualizing and avoidance strategies, and what they should do differently to support your response prevention plan. Lucia's completed form, which you can use as a guide, is on the next page. Completing the form helped her recognize the importance of getting her family on board with her treatment. She called a family meeting and explained how exposure and response prevention work. She told her family that anxiety isn't dangerous and that she needed to practice confronting uncertainty. She also requested that they stop doing rituals and avoiding for her. This greatly helped Lucia with her treatment.

Third, you should meet with the appropriate friends and relatives to give them specific instructions (based on your Ending Others' Involvement in Your Rituals Worksheet) for what you would like them to do (or *not* do) from now on. Ask them to refuse if you request their help with avoidance or rituals and to refuse to give you reassurance if you ask for it (for example, they can say to you, "Remember that you told me I shouldn't answer those kinds of questions anymore"). Several of my patients have come up with the idea to send people involved in their rituals a letter explaining the vicious cycle of OCD. Following is what such letters typically look like:

Dear ____________,

I've decided to work on my problems with obsessive–compulsive disorder (OCD), and I would like to ask if you would help me with my treatment. It won't require much work on your part. Actually, it will mean doing less!

Here's the problem: I have a pattern of getting very upset when I start thinking certain senseless intrusive thoughts and doubts. To cope with these *obsessions*, I also have a pattern of doing *compulsive rituals* like excessive washing, checking, praying, and asking people (like you) for reassurance that everything is okay. These rituals might make me feel a little bit better for a short while, but here's the problem: they prevent me from getting over my obsessions in the long run. When I ask you to reassure me, it prevents me from learning that my obsessive doubts are senseless. It also keeps me from learning that I can handle anxiety and normal amounts of uncertainty. This has me caught in a vicious cycle that I'm working on getting out of.

To break out of the cycle, I'm doing a treatment program where I purposely practice facing my fears and then refrain from getting reassurance. This helps me learn how to manage uncertainty and anxiety without needing so much reassurance. Although the treatment exercises make me anxious, feeling anxiety—even very intense anxiety—won't hurt me. At most, it will be uncomfortable. So the best way for me to break my OCD patterns is to confront my fears, stop fighting the anxiety, and stop getting reassurance.

Here's how you can help: I plan to try very hard to stop asking you for reassurance. But if I slip up and ask anyway, I'd like you not to answer. *That's right—I am giving you permission not to answer and to allow me to be anxious.* Instead of trying to reassure me or make me feel better, here's what I'd like you to say if I start asking you for assurances:

- It looks like you're having problems with obsessing and doubting. How can I help without reassuring you?
- Remember you sent me a letter saying I shouldn't answer these kinds of reassurance-seeking questions anymore. So I'm not going to.
- You must be pretty anxious right now. Remember that this will go away in time even if I don't answer that question.

When you say these things, there's a possibility that I will try even harder to get you to answer my questions. I will try my best not to do this, but if I do, please don't give in. I might seem very distressed, but the anxiety is not harmful. I've got to get past it myself.

As I go through this challenging time in my life, I appreciate your support and encouragement. Remember that OCD is the enemy, not me, and overcoming it is my responsibility, not yours. This letter shows that I am seriously committed to getting over OCD and that I hope you will help me in the ways I've described.

Sincerely,

____

Lucia's Ending Others' Involvement in Your Rituals Worksheet

Significant other(s)	Role in avoidance and rituals	How they can help you with response prevention
Jermaine and Jasmine (the kids)	• *Phone calls* • *Reassure me that they're okay when I ask* • *Wash, clean, and change clothes when I ask them to*	• *Don't call me to say you're okay* • *Don't answer questions about safety* • *Don't wash or change clothes during the day* • *Don't clean the kitchen table for me*
Hugh (husband)	• *Reassures me he's okay* • *Washes before touching me*	• *Don't try to reassure me that everything is okay* • *Don't wash before touching me*
Dr. Crowley	• *Gives me reassurance about chemicals when I ask*	• *Don't answer questions about chemicals or poison anymore*

Ending Others' Involvement in Your Rituals Worksheet

Significant other(s)	Role in avoidance and rituals	How they can help you with response prevention

Response Prevention for Different Types of Rituals

Here is some help for applying response prevention to different types of rituals. Although I can't address every possible ritual that you might have, you can probably adapt these suggestions and examples to most of the "classic" and the less common types of compulsive, mini-, mental, and reassurance-seeking rituals. Note that the examples in this section are the same people described in Steps 7 and 8 on exposure.

BATTLE PLAN While you're planning and working on response prevention, turn to the following pages to read about the types of rituals that apply to you:

As you read through this section, try to remember that the goal of response prevention is to weaken OCD symptoms by breaking patterns of thinking and acting. You're learning to take acceptable risks and to live with everyday levels of uncertainty. This is the only way to defeat OCD for good. But doing this means that sometimes you'll need to go above and beyond what "most people" or what "normal people" usually do. If you think about it, though, you'll find that most of what I suggest for response prevention—as was the case with exposure—is actually behavior that people do all the time without thinking about it (and without negative consequences). So, while refraining from rituals is unlikely to actually put you in any specific danger, it *will* make you feel more uncertain than if you had done the ritual. In Step 10, we'll review guidelines for ending response prevention and returning to "normal" behavior.

Treatment Buddy Tip

When you're ready to begin response prevention, let your treatment buddy know about your plan for stopping your rituals. Also, discuss how much you'd like him or her to help you. You might prefer a hands-off approach that lets you handle stopping rituals on your own. Or you might ask your buddy to keep an eye on you and let you know if he or she "catches" you ritualizing.

For treatment buddies: You might think about your role of treatment buddy as similar to that of a business consultant who is hired by a company to provide expertise. In this role, rather than constantly policing your relative or friend with OCD (for example, "Did you do any rituals today?") and giving unsolicited advice (for example, "Make sure you don't ritualize today"), you'll want to let him or her take the lead in asking *you* for help (unless otherwise discussed). In general, it's best to use gentle reminders if you see your buddy ritualizing (for example, "It looked like you were having trouble just then. I'd be glad to help you out if you'd like.").

Decontamination Rituals (Washing and Cleaning)

The goal of response prevention for decontamination rituals is to keep you feeling contaminated at all times—so that exposure to the feared contaminants never really ends. Follow the guidelines below, keeping in mind that you might have to work toward them gradually. If you choose to change or adjust these guidelines, do so using the strategies outlined earlier in this step (for example, modifying, delaying).

- Avoid washing your hands, face, and other body parts—even after using the bathroom, taking out the garbage, and before eating or handling food. It's important to brush your teeth at least twice a day, but try to shave with an electric razor to minimize contact with water. Also, avoid swimming pools during your program.

  This rule might shock you. You might be asking, "Isn't it dangerous not to wash after using the bathroom?" Actually, lots of people don't wash their hands after using the bathroom. In some cultures, this isn't done at all, and yet people live healthy lives. As for not washing before eating, people do this all the time as well; just ask anyone who goes to a ballgame or movie and buys a snack. And think about where their hands might have been! People, especially children, often touch garbage cans, floors, and other "dirty" objects without washing. Even those who claim to keep to the highest standards of cleanliness (doctors, nurses, and so on) violate their own rules—often without even thinking about it. The only difference between what happens in day-to-day life and what happens in your treatment program is that in treatment you're *purposely* confronting these situations and *deliberately* abstaining from washing.

  Will abstaining from washing increase your chances of getting sick? Maybe yes, maybe no, although *probably* not in any significant way, as you might think. Meanwhile, what's for *sure* is that the benefits of not washing (which include reducing problems with OCD) far outweigh any risks. And when you've ended your treatment program, it's perfectly fine to resume normal washing and cleaning, as I'll cover in Step 10.
- Go without using other methods to remove or prevent contamination, such as using gloves, shirtsleeves, towelettes, or tissues to touch things. Also, avoid wiping your hands on your clothes or on other objects. And don't use sanitizing gels or wipes (throw these away to avoid the temptation!). An exception is that if you are extremely fearful of urine or feces, you might wear gloves when you use the bathroom to avoid contact with these items until you're ready to do situational exposure with them.
- Don't wash or clean inanimate objects such as furniture or tools, and don't do extra loads of laundry or dishes. Wear clothes (and use dishes) at least once before washing them.
- Take one 10-minute shower each day (use a timer). This shower should be just enough to keep you hygienic and should not be turned into a ritual. The aim of showering during response prevention isn't to be *perfectly clean*, but to be *cleaner than when you started*. Use regular soap and wash each body part only once (and without ritualizing). Don't wash the shower curtain or the water faucet, and reuse the towel and washcloth until it's time to do all of the laundry. Also, once you're finished with your shower, make sure you "recontaminate" yourself with an item from your exposure list.

• Don't pressure friends or family members to participate in washing or cleaning rituals anymore—in fact, encourage them to follow the same guidelines you're following (although this is their choice). Also, don't ask others for reassurance about whether something is clean.

• Don't avoid "clean" objects or areas of your home just because you feel contaminated. Your whole environment should feel "contaminated."

• If you slip up and violate any of these guidelines, make a note of this on your Ritual Monitoring Form and immediately reexpose yourself to the contaminant that led to the slipup so that you're back to feeling contaminated, and you have another chance to habituate naturally.

Pearl (from Steps 7 and 8), who had contamination obsessions, engaged in hand-washing rituals that were triggered by contact (even imagined contact) with her feared contaminants (for example, body waste, public telephones). Because stopping all of her washing "cold turkey" from the beginning of her program would mean that she'd be exposed to her most feared contaminants (urine and feces) before she had the chance to practice exposure to them (see her exposure hierarchy on page 191), she used a selective response prevention strategy in which she gradually stopped her rituals in association with conducting exposure to her various feared contaminants. Here is what Pearl did:

• *Week 1:* Refrained from ritualizing for as long as possible after touching doorknobs and railings, but washed before eating, after using the bathroom, and after taking out the garbage. After washing, however, she immediately recontaminated with "door germs" using a paper towel she had gotten contaminated by touching it to a doorknob during an exposure practice. This way, Pearl always felt exposed to the first hierarchy item, but nothing more.

• *Week 2:* Refrained from washing as long as possible after exposure to shaking hands with people and continued to stop all washing except after contact with garbage cans and using the bathroom. She also recontaminated with "people germs" after washing.

• *Week 3:* Refrained from washing after touching garbage cans. She also recontaminated with trash can/dumpster germs after washing when using the bathroom or before eating.

• *Week 4:* Continued washing only after using the bathroom and before eating and recontaminated by touching the insides of her shoes or her dirty laundry.

• *Week 5:* After daily public bathroom exposures, practiced refraining from washing for as long as possible, but still allowed washing after urinating and defecating. Recontaminated with "public restroom germs" she had collected on a paper towel.

• *Week 6:* Ended hand washing after urinating, but still allowed it when defecating. Recontaminated with urine germs (by touching a piece of toilet paper soiled with a few drops of her own urine) after any washing.

• *Week 7:* Stopped all hand washing, including after all bathroom visits and before eating. Any washing was followed by recontamination with a piece of toilet paper containing a small stain from her feces.

Checking and Reassurance-Seeking Rituals

Most checking and reassurance-seeking rituals occur in response to obsessions about harm and mistakes, and in response to doubts about being responsible for causing (or not doing enough to prevent) feared catastrophes. But I've also worked with patients who check because of contamination and health-related fears. If you have religious obsessions, you might also have reassurance-seeking rituals. Here are some guidelines for using response prevention with these sorts of rituals:

- Stop all checking of doors, locks, windows, appliances, electrical outlets, news, the Internet, the roadside, your pockets, where you were sitting, and so on. Don't check with police or fire departments.
- If you check switches, locks, dials, outlets, or whatever by *touching* them, keep your hands off! If you check just by looking at these items, cover them with masking tape or with a large piece of paper so that you can't see them.
- Refrain from asking others—friends and relatives, doctors, clergy, sales clerks—for reassurance concerning your obsessional fears. Tell your friends and relatives not to give you assurances and instead to distract you for a little while or refer you to your treatment buddy for more help. (Read more on reassurance seeking on page 251.)
- Don't seek excessive information about the situations you're afraid of. For instance, stop searching the Internet to determine the exact likelihood of getting sick from using certain toxic substances, or the chances that you'll act on violent thoughts or become gay.
- Stop all efforts to prevent feared consequences or to assure yourself that negative outcomes won't occur. This means the following behaviors are off limits: picking up or cleaning "dangerous" objects off the ground, reporting potential hazards to others, counting, retracing steps, asking for assurances, making lists, and the like.
- If you check the rearview or side mirrors in your car, put paper or tape on the mirror to partially block your view. You'll still be able to see large objects, but you won't be able to see details or smaller objects. Don't check the outside of your car for blood or dents if you're afraid of hit-and-run accidents. Also, don't drive back to places or check the roadside where you're afraid an accident might have occurred.
- If you're afraid of making mistakes, e-mails, paperwork, and envelopes may be *briefly* proofread one time, but without the use of spelling- or grammar-checking software. Do not review mathematical calculations more than once.
- If you slip up and perform a check, try to reexpose yourself to uncertainty. The best way to do this is to use imaginal exposure to your feared consequences.

Angelo had checking rituals both at home and at work. Through the first 6 weeks of his program, he worked on eliminating the checking he performed in his apartment and in his car (selective response prevention). In fact, during his first week of exposure to leaving lights on and imagining starting a fire, he resisted the urge to go home and check for fires. He also resisted checking windows, appliances, electrical outlets, his car, and water faucets. Although he occasionally slipped up, Angelo was able to resist about 90% of his urges to check. He knew this because he used Ritual Monitoring Forms to keep track of any rituals he performed. After Angelo was able to manage without checking in his apartment, he began resisting checking rituals that he performed at work and elsewhere.

Ordering, Arranging, Counting, and Repeating Rituals

Response prevention for these rituals is straightforward: resist the urge to perform them so that you are immersed in feelings and thoughts of incompleteness, inexactness, unevenness, imbalance, or imperfection. If you perform these rituals in response to distressing obsessional thoughts or to protect you or others from disastrous consequences, you'll want to tempt fate by not ritualizing. Here are some guidelines:

- Refrain from reordering and rearranging objects. Keep your room, house, workplace, and so on, "disorderly" throughout your treatment program.
- Resist the urge to "balance things out" or achieve symmetry by counting, touching or tapping, looking or staring at things a certain way, repeating words or phrases, or retracing your steps.
- Resist the urge to reread or rewrite what you've already read or written.
- Do not repeat behaviors because you're afraid of bad luck or because you have a distressing thought in your mind. Instead, conduct imaginal exposure to bad luck or the unwanted thought.
- Do not repeat religious customs or confessions more than once just because you're afraid you didn't do them perfectly or because your mind wandered and you're afraid God will be upset. Remember to have *faith* that God understands your real intentions. (Read more on religious rituals on pages 252–253.)
- If you can't resist repeating a behavior, do it incorrectly, in a different room, or do it the wrong number of times so that it's less effective.
- Some ordering, arranging, counting, or repeating rituals are very hard to stop because they're automatic. You might feel like you can't control them. To help you gain control, start by just keeping track of when you do these rituals by self-monitoring or with the help of a handheld counter or clicker. This will make it easier to bring them under your control. Next, try modifying the ritual so that you perform it incorrectly—for example, count out of order, or distract yourself while counting, or touch or stare the "wrong" way. Once you're able to do this, it should be easier for you to stop the ritual.

Evelyn practiced gradual response prevention in which she resisted rituals that went along with the exposures she was performing. Each week, as she confronted a new exposure item, she stopped another ritual. Here's what she did:

- *Week 1:* After practicing writing letters and words imperfectly ("sloppily") she stopped rereading and rewriting—not just for the exposure, but in all of her day-to-day writing.
- *Week 2:* When she added exposure to writing sloppily in her checkbook, she also resisted her urges to go through her checkbook and rewrite and recalculate the numbers.

• *Weeks 3 and 4:* When she conducted situational exposure to moving things in her home out of order, Evelyn gave up her ordering and arranging rituals for good.

• *Week 5:* Evelyn was able to resist her left–right rituals when she conducted exposures to either *right* or *left*. However, she had trouble stopping the rituals if she came across these words unexpectedly. This was because the rituals happened automatically, before Evelyn even realized what she was doing. For example, if she saw a sign reading "No Right Turn on Red," the word *left* seemed to automatically appear in her mind. Evelyn's treatment buddy suggested that she could "undo" the ritual by practicing saying (or thinking) the opposite direction so that she'd once again have imbalance. For example, if Evelyn heard someone say, "I *left* the keys on the table," and the word *right* automatically came to mind to neutralize *left*, she then said "right" to herself to create imbalance again. This technique worked very well.

Mental Rituals

Mental rituals are much harder to notice than action rituals, and so they sometimes get forgotten in response prevention. But some of my patients' biggest breakthroughs in therapy came when they started recognizing and stopping their mental rituals. That's why I emphasized these rituals in the first part of this workbook—mental rituals are a force to be reckoned with.

Rituals that take place entirely in your mind might not seem as important or as serious as those that you actually see yourself perform (such as washing, checking, and arranging), but mental rituals are just as important to target in response prevention.

Response prevention for mental rituals targets all "safe" thoughts, words, phrases, numbers, and prayers that you repeat in your mind to neutralize unwanted thoughts, reduce anxiety, or prevent feared disasters. It also targets mental checking, analyzing, and reviewing that you do to try to achieve reassurance about your decisions or fears. But it's much harder to stop a thought than to stop an action like washing or checking. Therefore, ending mental rituals requires careful planning. Here are some tips and guidelines:

BATTLE PLAN The best form of response prevention for mental rituals is more exposure (imaginal or situational) to the obsessional thought or trigger that provoked the ritual in the first place.

• Don't intentionally repeat any words or phrases to yourself or conjure up any images that reduce anxiety, prevent feared consequences, or counteract distressing obsessional thought and doubts.

• Instead of trying *not to think* the mental ritual, try *thinking something else* instead. The "something else" should be the unwanted, distressing thought that triggered the urge to ritualize. For example, if you see the word *death*, instead of trying not to think "life" (the ritual word), deliberately think more death thoughts. You can't think the upsetting thought and do a mental ritual at the same time.

• Do not say prayers or religious phrases (for example, "God will help me") in response to obsessive fears (unless directed by a clergy member). If you're in an actual religious service, don't repeat prayers because you might have said them incorrectly or because your mind wandered. (I'll cover more on stopping religious rituals on pages 252–253 in the section on troubleshooting).

- If you perform a mental ritual automatically, go back and purposely confront the distressing obsessional thought or situation again to undo the effects of the mental ritual.
- If you can't resist doing a mental ritual, try to carry it out incorrectly so that it feels ineffective.
- Resist the urge to analyze the meaning of your unacceptable obsessional thoughts, or to try to think through or figure out where these distressing ideas come from. Instead, deliberately expose yourself to the unwanted thought and remind yourself that you have to stay uncertain about what these thoughts mean (they might or might not be important).
- If you're afraid that your obsessions mean something awful about you—for instance, that you're violent, deviant, perverted, immoral, or an otherwise awful or dangerous person—resist the urge to review your past history, monitor your body for signs of sexual arousal, "test" yourself to see if you agree with your obsessions, or do anything else to search for evidence about whether your obsessions are true.

Paxton, who had violent obsessions concerning his infant, used mental rituals to control his anxiety and reduce his fear of acting aggressively. When the upsetting thoughts came to mind, he repeated the phrase "I don't want to hurt my son" to himself over and over to help him feel better and neutralize the unwanted thoughts. He also spent time thinking about and trying to figure out (analyzing) whether he really was "the kind of person" who was capable of doing the terrible things he obsessed about.

For response prevention, Paxton stopped using the neutralizing phrase, and he stopped analyzing the meaning of his thoughts. If he did start to analyze, Paxton practiced reminding himself that he could never be sure where the thoughts came from or what they really meant. But the most useful strategy for Paxton was to simply conduct more imaginal exposure to his unwanted thoughts whenever he had the urge to ritualize. In other words, instead of thinking the safe thoughts, Paxton focused on the unwanted obsessional thoughts until his anxiety habituated.

Mini-Rituals

As with mental rituals, it's easy to overlook mini-rituals because they're often brief and very subtle. But don't let these characteristics fool you. If the mini-ritual reduces your anxiety or makes you think that you've averted a feared consequence, then you must stop using it. Becoming aware of your mini-rituals by identifying them (as you did in Step 1), understanding them (Step 2), and monitoring them (as you learned about here in Step 9) will help you anticipate when they're likely to occur and stop these behaviors. Some mini-rituals occur *during* exposure practices as you try to make the exposure situation less distressing. Of course, this will snarl the process of habituation and invalidate the exposure practice. If you find that you've performed a mini-ritual, immediately try to undo the ritual or reexpose yourself to the trigger or thought that provoked the mini-ritual.

Troubleshooting

Extreme Reassurance Seeking

If you're having problems stopping reassurance-seeking rituals, it means that you still believe you'll eventually find the "ultimate guarantee" of safety or the "definitive information" you can use to put yourself at ease about an obsession once and for all. So let me clarify this issue: If you're unable to give up your persistent reassurance-seeking, question-asking, and information-gathering behavior, the problem isn't that you haven't found the "right" or "best" information yet; the real problem is that you're demanding a kind of certainty that's simply impossible to achieve. You'd like to think that there's someone, somewhere, who can tell you *once and for all* what you need to know so that you don't have to worry anymore. But unfortunately, that person—and that information—doesn't exist. We all have to go on without a guarantee sometimes, and with only a reasonable degree of certainty. Most people are okay living with reasonable certainty about even fairly grim consequences: driving, using stairs, leaving appliances plugged in all carry *some* risk of catastrophe. But OCD makes you feel like reasonable certainty isn't enough, and so you're stuck trying—in vain—to get beyond the shadow of doubt.

If you can't stop seeking reassurance altogether, try setting some guidelines. For example, some of my patients demand to speak with authorities such as clergy, experts, or specialist doctors to get reassurance. You might wish to do the same. If so, I recommend the following:

Are you still demanding an impossible guarantee?

1. First, have you consulted with this person (or type of expert) recently? If so, what did he or she say? Are the questions you now want to ask or clarify very different from the issues you brought to this expert before? If you think you know what the expert will tell you, you're probably right, which means the only reason for the consultation is to reduce your anxiety—not to get any new information. If this is the case, you should resist talking with the expert.
2. If you can't resist speaking with an expert, arrange a fairly brief (30 minutes maximum) single meeting.
3. Prepare for your meeting by coming up with a list of broad questions or issues to address. Avoid questions about specific situations. For example, asking an infectious disease expert, "Can you explain about the risks of getting AIDS?" is more appropriate than asking "What are the chances I'll get AIDS from ____________, or from ____________, or from ____________?"
4. Stick to the questions you prepared ahead of time.
5. After the meeting, reflect on the expert's answers and try to apply them to situations that come up involving your obsessional fear. Get into the habit of asking yourself, "What would [the expert] say about this?" when you feel like you need reassurance. This will help you learn to go on your judgment and instinct, rather than having to seek assurance.

Treatment Buddy Tip

It's a great idea to ask your treatment buddy to help you come up with your list of questions if you meet with an expert. If your buddy can attend the meeting with the expert or authority, that would also be a big plus.

For treatment buddies: Help your friend or relative devise general questions, the answers to which can be applied broadly in various specific situations. By sticking to the questions you developed ahead of time, you can make sure the consultation doesn't turn into another reassurance-seeking ritual.

Dealing with Automatic Rituals

It might seem like some of your rituals happen automatically, without your awareness. For example, you might instinctively wipe your hands on your pants, count while doing things, check your pockets, or the like. If this is the case, here are a few things you can do to work on bringing these rituals under your control:

1. Make sure you understand what triggers the ritual(s). If you think it would help, go back to Step 2, where you analyzed your rituals, and work through an analysis of the automatic ritual. Understanding the context of automatic behaviors can help you assume control.
2. Carefully monitor the ritual using the Ritual Monitoring Form in this chapter. If the ritual occurs too quickly or too often to write down, purchase a handheld counter to keep track. The goal here is to teach you to pay attention to the ritual so you'll be able to stop.
3. Practice more exposure to the trigger situations and thoughts and then try to refrain from ritualizing.
4. If you notice the ritual happening outside of an exposure (in day-to-day life), try to catch it and either stop it or modify it. Add something on to the end of it if you notice the ritual after it's too late to stop or to modify it. This will make the ritual less effective.
5. Delay doing the ritual as much as you can until you're able to completely resist.

Ending Religious Rituals (Scrupulosity)

Although I've discussed religious rituals such as praying, confessing, and repeating customs in other sections of this step, you might sense that doing exposure and response prevention clashes with your religious beliefs. But as I've explained in earlier steps, there's no reason for your OCD treatment program to violate any of your religious beliefs or customs. Done correctly, CBT is perfectly compatible with religious observance. In fact, if you are a religious person suffering with OCD, I want you to use this workbook to strengthen your religious faith and bring you closer to God. I've helped many people with scrupulosity achieve these goals using the very same techniques.

I've found that the main issue is that it's not always easy to tell the difference between healthy religious behavior—which you *should not* stop during your program—and OCD behavior—which you *should* stop. This source of uncertainty provokes anxiety about violating a religious rule and triggers the need to be absolutely sure that you're not committing any violations. But, short of a miraculous revelation from God, you're stuck with having to make a judgment of whether giving up your rituals is a violation or not. You might wish to have a consultation with a clergyperson to set some guidelines (if so, use the section above on troubleshooting for reassurance seeking)—although keep in mind that when I ask my patients to tell me which of their behaviors are OCD and which are honestly part of their religion, they almost always say the same thing that a clergyperson would say. In other words, you probably know which is which—you just need to face the uncertainty.

Simply put, your "religious" behavior that is motivated by obsessional fear is not faithful. If anything, it's *untrusting*. If you have to pray several times over because your mind wandered, confess over and over because you're afraid you'll fall from God's good graces, or repeat religious customs and rituals again and again because you don't think you performed them correctly, then you don't trust that God understands that in your heart you're very devoted to your religious faith.

Imagine that your neighbor is away on a trip for a week and has asked you to take care of her dog while she's gone, but your friend keeps calling you several times each day and night to remind you again and again to feed her dog, take him for a walk, and not to give him too many treats (all things you already know since you also have a dog). What would you think? How would you feel? Certainly, your neighbor isn't showing much trust in you to take care of her dog if she's incessantly calling to remind you of these things! Ironically, when you ritualistically repeat prayers, customs, and confessions, you're treating God the same way. If God is the loving, all-knowing, and merciful being that we read about in the Bible, then He also understands what you feel in your heart and what you're doing to help yourself with OCD. He doesn't need reminders.

With this in mind, sort out what behaviors are motivated by the fear of sin and damnation, and which ones are healthy religious observance motivated by honest love and faith. When you stop fear-based rituals that only *look like* actual religious observance, you'll be growing closer to God and developing a more true sense of faith.

What If New Avoidance Patterns and Rituals Are Replacing the Old Ones?

Some traditional psychoanalytic views hold that if you stop one compulsive behavior, a brand-new one will take its place as if OCD is like a game of Whack-A-Mole. We now know that this is an overly simplistic way of thinking. Still, when you begin doing exposure and response prevention, it might seem like new rituals are emerging. There are two explanations for this. The first possibility is that your treatment program is working well, and as you eliminate the more problematic rituals, others you hadn't noticed or paid much attention to are now moving into focus. The solution here, of course, is to push on with your treatment program by focusing on these other, less noticed, rituals.

The other possibility is that as you begin stopping your rituals, you're turning to other ways to avoid or escape from anxiety. For example, you might avoid more obsessional triggers, or ritualize in more subtle ways so that things don't *seem* as bad. For example, a woman I once worked with who had severe washing rituals was able to stop them "cold turkey" within 1 week. I was in disbelief! But it turned out I had good reason for doubting her improbable instant recovery: when I asked her how she managed to stop hours of washing in only 1 week, she said that she had hired a butler so that she didn't need to touch anything that was contaminated. This elaborate (and costly) avoidance strategy was certainly not a cure for OCD.

If you develop new patterns of avoidance or ritualizing because you've made certain rituals off limits, it means your response prevention plan isn't broad enough. You should go back and make sure to end all behaviors aimed at avoiding or escaping from the fear triggers. You should probably also make sure you address your avoidance problems using situational exposure.

Now You're Ready to Go for It!

At this point you've got trustworthy intelligence about your enemy, you understand the tactics of combat, and you're armed with the best artillery available to take on OCD. Now, it's time to march confidently into battle and defeat this foe. You might not win every single clash with OCD, but don't give up. Your battle plan and weapons are proven to work. Use them carefully and correctly and you'll be victorious. In the next chapter I've included all the worksheets and tools you'll need to pull together the strategies you've learned about in Steps 6–9 to eliminate your obsessions and compulsions. In Step 10, I'll help you keep track of your progress and defend yourself from any revenge that OCD might try to take.

Putting It All Together

Now that you've learned how to use cognitive therapy, situational and imaginal exposure, and response prevention, you're just about ready to get started using these techniques together—the same way I use them in my clinical work with people who have problems with OCD. Here you'll find all the tools you need to pull together everything you've learned. I'll help you devise a timeline and schedule for your planned exposure practices. Then I'll provide you with a form to use when you practice planned exposure exercises.

Your Timeline

How Should You Schedule Your CBT Program?

I've divided the timeline for this program into weeks, which should give you enough time to learn and practice with each skill before moving on to the next one (see the timeline that begins directly below). You probably already have a good sense of the sequence from reading Steps 6–9 thoroughly, but here's a quick summary—fill in your own dates if you like so you can refer back to this as your CBT schedule:

Week 1 (Starting on: / / **)**

- Read Step 6.
- Practice cognitive therapy techniques learned in Step 6 for 45 minutes a day.

Week 2 (Starting on: / / **)**

- Continue practicing cognitive therapy techniques for 45 minutes a day.
- Read Steps 7–9.
- Look at your situational and imaginal exposure hierarchies and your response prevention plan from Step 4, and see if there's anything you need to change. Some-

times exposure items or their SUDs change when you start using cognitive techniques.

- Complete the Planned Exposure Practice Schedule on page 258 by assigning a particular situational and/or imaginal exposure hierarchy item to practice during each week and assigning target rituals to resist that correspond with your chosen exposure practices. Remember to begin with hierarchy items that provoke only moderate anxiety levels (SUDs) and gradually work up to the most distressing situational and imaginal hierarchy items.
- Begin monitoring your rituals using the worksheet on page 230 at some point during Week 2.

Week 3 (Starting on: / /)

- Begin exposure practice with the hierarchy items assigned for Week 3. Choose two times a day when you can complete 1-hour practices. At the beginning of each hour, spend 10 minutes using cognitive therapy techniques to prepare you for doing exposure. Use the Planned Exposure Practice Worksheet on page 260 to keep track of your SUDs during each exposure.
- Begin response prevention by resisting the ritual(s) that correspond to this week's exposure practice. If you perform a ritual, do a brief reexposure to the hierarchy item so that you are always feeling "exposed."
- Continue to monitor your rituals. If you're unable to resist your rituals, use the Ritual Modification Worksheet on page 236 to help you try a modified response prevention strategy until you're ready to completely stop the ritual.
- Review your Exposure Practice Worksheets and Ritual Monitoring Forms at the end of each day to help you get an idea of your progress with facing your fears and resisting rituals.
- If by the end of the week you haven't habituated to the hierarchy item(s) you're practicing, continue planned exposure until you feel that you can manage the item, even if it still provokes some anxiety. Then move on to the next item. See the box at the top of page 257 for ways to determine whether you're ready to move on.

Weeks 4–5+ (Starting on: / /)

- Practice exposure as in Week 3, but each week move on to the next exposure practice on your Planned Exposure Practice Schedule until you've confronted all of your hierarchy items. Your program should last as long as it takes to work through all the items on your hierarchy(ies), which can take as few as 5 weeks and as many as 10 or more.
- Continue resisting rituals that correspond to each week's exposure practices and all previous exposure practices.
- Continue to monitor any rituals that you're not able to resist by recording them on the Ritual Monitoring Form.
- Begin using lifestyle exposure—make opportunities in your daily life to confront the hierarchy items you've already practiced with using planned exposure.
- Continue to review your worksheets each day.

Am I Ready to Move to the Next Item on My Hierarchy?

When you're ready to move on, feeling as if you've habituated to a trigger situation or intrusive thought, and extinguished an obsessional fear, is a very personal and subjective judgment. Use any or all of the following criteria to determine whether you've conquered an item and should move to the next one:

- Do you feel generally comfortable in the exposure situation?
- Have your SUDs fallen below 20?
- Or, are your SUDs consistently in the mild range (20 or below) for 10 minutes running?
- Have your urges to ritualize decreased substantially or even disappeared?

Scheduling Your Exposure and Response Prevention Plan

The Planned Exposure Practice Schedule form on the following page represents your road map for battling OCD. This is where you'll plan out week by week which situational and imaginal exposures you'll conduct and which rituals you'll work on stopping. To do this, you'll need to go back to Step 4, where you created your initial exposure hierarchies and response prevention plan. The main difference between those hierarchies and this current treatment plan is that in this chapter you'll arrange your plan for *combining* situational and imaginal exposure and response prevention all into one place so it's easier to follow. Here's how to do it.

First, revisit your initial hierarchies and adjust any items or SUDs levels that might have changed since you read Step 4. Next, choose a situation (or intrusive thought) from the hierarchies that provokes about 30–40 SUDs and record it in the practice schedule (note that there are spaces for both situational and imaginal exposure). If your first item has a corresponding imaginal (or situational) hierarchy item, enter this in the appropriate place as well. Next, select the ritual(s) from your response prevention plan that will be provoked when you practice exposure to the hierarchy items you just wrote down. Record this ritual in the far right column of the practice schedule. Then choose the next most difficult exposure items and ritual(s) and record them in the next row of the practice schedule. The examples in Steps 7, 8, and 9 should have helped you form ideas for how to combine situational and imaginal exposure and response prevention. If necessary, read these examples again. You can also ask your treatment buddy to help you. To show you a completed Planned Exposure Practice Schedule, I've provided Angelo's (from Steps 7–9) form on page 259.

Please keep in mind that this schedule is not written in stone. In fact, I suggest you use pencil instead of pen to fill it in so that you can adjust it as needed. Many people find that once they get started, some situations are easier to confront than they'd thought, while others are more difficult and need to be put off until after exposure to other items. Feel free to make these changes as you go along, as long as they are in keeping with helping you to make ongoing progress.

Planned Exposure Practice Schedule

- When you've completed each week's practices, cross them off the list.

Week #	Exposure practice: Which hierarchy items will you practice with?	Response prevention: Which rituals will you stop?
	Situational:	
	Imaginal:	
	Situational:	
	Imaginal:	
	Situational:	
	Imaginal:	
	Situational:	
	Imaginal:	
	Situational:	
	Imaginal:	
	Situational:	
	Imaginal:	
	Situational:	
	Imaginal:	
	Situational:	
	Imaginal:	
	Situational:	
	Imaginal:	
	Situational:	
	Imaginal:	
	Situational:	
	Imaginal:	
	Situational:	
	Imaginal:	

Planned Exposure Practice Schedule: Angelo

- When you've completed each week's practices, cross them off the list.

Week #	Exposure practice: Which hierarchy items will you practice with?	Response prevention: Which rituals will you stop?
3	Situational: *Turn light switches on/off and leave the house* Imaginal: *The house catches fire and burns down*	*Checking lights*
4	Situational: *Drive past a fire station and see fire trucks* Imaginal: *The house catches fire and burns down*	*Asking for reassurance*
5	Situational: *Open and close windows in the house and then leave* Imaginal: *Someone breaks into my house because I forgot to lock the windows*	*Checking window locks*
6	Situational: *Disable and enable the parking brake of the car and leave the car* Imaginal: *The car drifts down a hill and causes an accident*	*Checking the parking brake, asking for reassurance*
7	Situational: *Turn appliances on and off and then leave the house* Imaginal: *The house catches fire and burns down*	*Checking appliances*
8	Situational: *Turn the water faucets on and off and then leave the house* Imaginal: *The house floods and I lose important things*	*Checking the faucets*

Using the Planned Exposure Practice Worksheet

The Planned Exposure Practice Worksheet on the following page is the form you should use when you conduct planned exposure exercises. It will help you through the process of conducting exposures, and you can use one copy of the worksheet for the two exposures you'll practice each day. Because you'll probably be practicing exposure for several weeks, it's a good idea to make many copies of the worksheet. We've provided one on the publisher's website (*www.guilford.com*) for you to print out. Here's how to use the worksheet when you do exposure practice. On page 263 is one of Angelo's completed worksheets.

1. *Describe the exposure practice.* Describe what the exposure practices that day will entail. What situation will you confront? What thoughts or doubts will you confront? Where will it take place? Try to make the two exposures as similar as possible, but if they differ somewhat that's okay. For example, being the last to leave your home and being the last to

Planned Exposure Practice Worksheet

Date:

1. Describe the exposure practice (what situations and/or thoughts will you confront?):

2. What ritual(s) are you resisting?

3. Which cognitive therapy strategies are you going to use?

4. What is your feared outcome of doing this exposure without ritualizing?

5. After using cognitive therapy, what is a more likely outcome?

6. Keep track of your SUDs using the graph below:

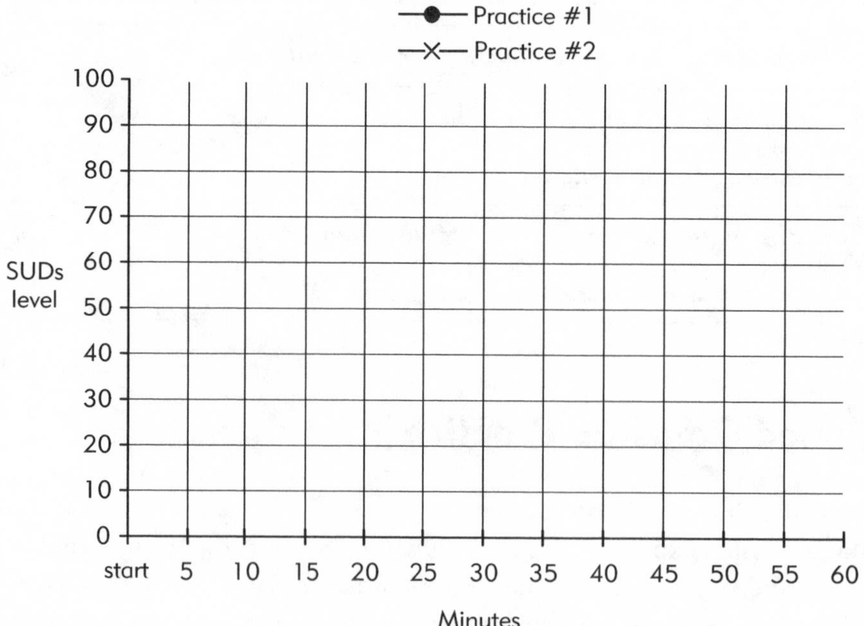

7. Describe the outcome of the exposure practice. What did you learn?

8. Examine your exposure graphs from day to day. What changes did you see?

leave your workplace might be good exposures to practice on the same day if you're working on obsessional doubts about responsibility for leaving the door unlocked (the imaginal exposures for both of these situational exposures would be similar).

2. *What rituals are you resisting?* Here, list the ritual(s) that doing this exposure practice will make you want to perform. Of course, this is the same ritual that you'll be stopping as part of response prevention.

3. *Cognitive therapy strategies.* Here, simply list the cognitive techniques that you plan to use to help set the table for these two exposure practices.

4. *Feared outcome.* Write your prediction of the feared consequences you imagine coming from facing this feared situation and thought without ritualizing. If your feared outcome is something in the distant future, indicate this on the form.

5. *Revised outcome based on cognitive therapy.* Work through the cognitive strategies you identified in Step 3 and then write down a more realistic, less threatening prediction about the outcome of doing the exposure practice. Perhaps the feared outcome is less likely than you had thought. Perhaps the risk is *acceptably low.* If you won't know whether your feared outcome will transpire until many years in the future, maybe cognitive therapy can help you better manage the inevitable uncertainty. In this case, the revised outcome might be that you'll be able to manage the inescapable uncertainty without becoming too anxious or needing to ritualize. Remember, this should not be a reassuring statement that disproves your fear but rather one that helps you take the risk and confront the uncertainty in the exposure practice. It's okay to think of this revised outcome while doing your exposure practices to help you get up the courage to confront your fears and put up with the resulting anxiety.

6. *Keep track of your SUDs.* In Step 7 I explained how to track your SUDs every 5 minutes and graph this on your worksheet. Remember to use the legend at the top of the graph to help you distinguish between your first and second exposure practices of the day. This will help you see whether repeated practice results in quicker habituation. You'll also be able to compare the results of your exposure practices from day to day and, if all goes well, see that your SUDs decrease more quickly with each time you confront the same (or similar) exposure situation.

Keep in mind, however, that not everyone finds these numeric ratings easy to use or as helpful as a more qualitative measure. If you think you'll feel bogged down by keeping track of all these numbers, don't feel like you have to do it. It's helpful to see graphically how you're doing, but if you feel like you can keep track mentally instead, that's fine. And, of course, if your obsessional fears include certain numbers, you may find it too difficult to use the SUDs and will have to rely on the consistent sense that your discomfort has reduced significantly and that you no longer feel the urge to ritualize in the target situation.

7. *What did you learn from the exposure?* After you've completed both exposure practices, describe the actual outcome of the practices. Did your SUDs go down? Was the exposure as difficult as you'd anticipated it to be? Did anything awful happen? Were you able to resist ritualizing? If your feared outcome won't take place until the distant future, were you able to feel more comfortable about the uncertainty? Did you learn that you could live with risk and doubt? Did your obsessional thoughts lose their punch?

8. *Changes in exposure graphs.* Finally, after you've finished both exposures, look over

the current and previous practice worksheets and make notes about any changes you've noticed. Is it getting easier for you to face your fears? Are your SUDs going down more quickly than they did at the beginning? Is actually *doing* exposure practices less frightening than you had thought they might be? These thoughts and comments will help keep you motivated as you work through your program. It's rewarding to see even the small steps toward your larger goals.

One of Angelo's Planned Exposure Practice Worksheets from the fifth week of his CBT program appears on the facing page. You can use this as a guide for filling out your own worksheets.

Charge!

The bugle is sounding your call to battle—full steam ahead! Armed with all the necessary information and forms, you're ready to begin your exposure and response prevention work—the heart of CBT for obsessions and rituals. This is your chance to really work hard, face your fears, and begin moving toward the goals you've set for yourself. Don't expect it to always be a piece of cake—there will be times when the going gets rough. But now you're well prepared—you can do it! Remember that you must invest anxiety now in order to have a calmer future. Your hard work *will* pay off. When you've completed your exposure practices, read Step 10 to help you with maintaining your improvement. Now, *charge*!!!

Planned Exposure Practice Worksheet: Angelo

Date: *August 6*

1. Describe the exposure practice (what situations and/or thoughts will you confront?):
   Open all the windows in the apartment, and then quickly close them all without looking closely. Then I'll leave the apartment and imagine that someone breaks in because of my negligence—maybe I left a window unlocked by mistake.
2. What ritual(s) are you resisting?
   Checking windows to make sure they're closed all the way and locked.
3. Which cognitive therapy strategies are you going to use?
   Life-saving wager technique.
4. What is your feared outcome of doing this exposure without ritualizing?
   Maybe I'll leave a window unlocked or open by mistake. I can't live with the uncertainty that someone could break in.
5. After using cognitive therapy, what is a more likely outcome?
   If I had to bet, I'd say that I won't leave anything unlocked or open. I'd also bet that I won't be broken into. It's not as likely as I sometimes think. But even still, I can't be certain.
6. Keep track of your SUDS using the graph below:

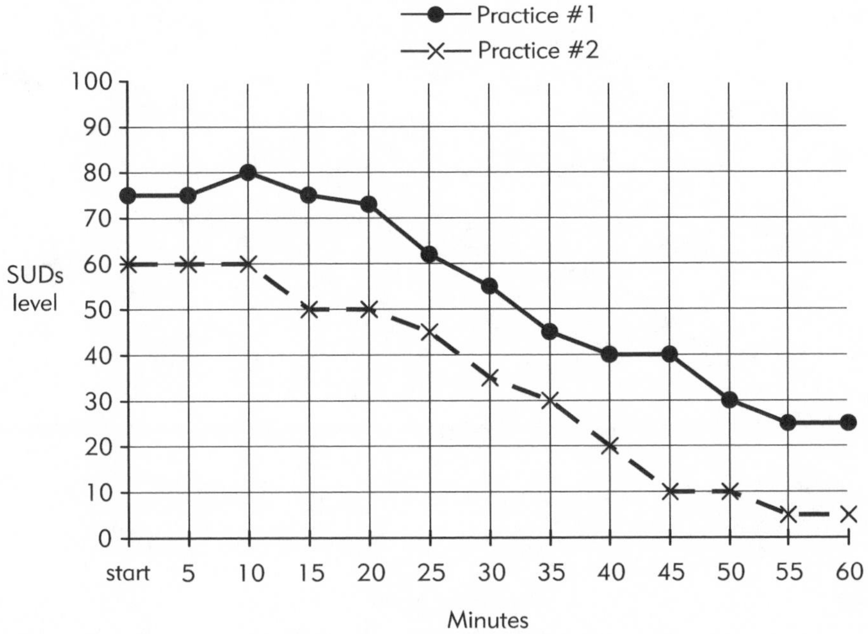

7. Describe the outcome of the exposure practice. What did you learn?
   No one broke in and I can live with uncertainty. My SUDs went down even when I didn't check.
8. Examine your exposure graphs from day to day. What changes do you see?
   My SUDs go down more and more quickly the more I practice. I'm able to resist my rituals more easily.

STEP 10

Ending Your Program and Staying Well

Over the last several weeks, you've been working on more and more challenging exposure exercises and cutting down on your avoidance and ritualizing. I hope that as a result your obsessional fears and urges to ritualize are decreasing so that you can feel more comfortable with situations and distressing thoughts that once seemed very frightening. Maybe you can now go places and do more activities you were avoiding. Perhaps freeing yourself from time-consuming rituals has given you more time for yourself and for what you really want to do with your days.

Here in Step 10, we'll shift the focus of your work from the "active phase" of treatment to the "staying well" or "maintenance" phase. We'll examine your progress and compare how you're doing now with how things were when you began your program. You'll learn how maintaining your improvement is not a single event, but rather an ongoing *process*. Lasting recovery requires you to adopt a lifestyle of practicing skills that are similar to the ones you've acquired so far. It also involves staying alert for setbacks and preventing temporary lapses from becoming full-blown relapses. If you're not already working with a qualified clinician, I'll show you how to find one, should you need one, and how to keep up to date with developments in the treatment of OCD. While it's hard for me to imagine a more powerful therapy for OCD than CBT (exposure and response prevention), research on the causes, symptoms, and treatment of OCD continues worldwide.

How do you think your life has changed since you began your program?

Ending Treatment but Living the "CBT Lifestyle"

Have you ever decided to go on a diet to lose weight? Many people who realize they're overweight and need to change their eating habits think, "I'll just go on a diet for a month or two to take off the extra pounds." But there's a problem—diets are like a light switch: *Click*, you're on a diet. *Click*, you're off a diet. As soon as the diet ends, your old eating habits return—along with the weight you'd lost. Diets can be good short-term solutions for weight loss, but they often fail in the long run.

Don't let your CBT program for OCD be like a diet! If you do, the chances are good that you'll begin slipping back into your old avoidance and ritualistic patterns before too long. Instead, think of the 10 steps in this workbook as a permanent *lifestyle change*. You've learned that the symptoms of OCD are a vicious cycle. You've learned how to plan for successful therapy and motivate yourself to face your fears. Most important, you've learned skills for reducing obsessions, avoidance, and rituals, as well as stopping the vicious cycle. Rather than leaving all of this behind once you end your program, stay well by making it a part of the way you live your life from now on. Here are some suggestions for how to integrate CBT into your lifestyle.

If staying healthy and in control of obsessions and rituals is your end goal, then your end goal really has no end. It's a lifelong goal. You have to keep confronting your fears and resisting urges to ritualize because that's what a healthy person does.

Making Exposure Part of Your Lifestyle

Just as I suggested that you *gradually* begin doing exposure practices by starting with less frightening situations, I recommend that you *gradually* taper your planned exposure practices rather than stopping abruptly. This will lower your risk of reverting to the old patterns that you've been working so hard to defeat. At first you might plan exposure practices every other day for a few weeks. Then move to a twice-weekly schedule. Then taper to once a week.

BATTLE PLAN To start the maintenance phase of your program, don't stop practices abruptly but rather taper them slowly and be prepared to return to greater frequency if your obsessions and urges to ritualize return.

Of course, if you notice that obsessional thoughts and rituals are starting to come back, you should increase your practice frequency again. If you do well with a reduced exposure schedule over a few months, then you can stop scheduling practices altogether. But that doesn't mean stopping *exposure* altogether: as I described in Step 7, you should continue to use it in all different situations in your everyday life, whenever you have the opportunity (lifestyle exposure). That is, from now on, you'll make a point of going *toward* rather than away from situations related to your obsessions—even if this doesn't provoke much distress anymore. If you're going to keep OCD from making a return, you'll need to continue experiencing the situations and distressing thoughts that you once avoided or tried to push away. Think of these postprogram practice sessions as helping you to strengthen or "overlearn" your new patterns.

Making exposure part of your lifestyle means going *toward,* instead of *away from,* the situations that have typically triggered your obsessions.

You should also continue to try out these exposures in *new* situations that are different from those you've practiced in before. For example, during the active treatment phase of her program, Natasha practiced exposure to toxic chemicals by using a certain brand of insecticide (bug spray) she had previously avoided, which became much easier for her. Next she broadened the effects of her program by purposely expanding her practice to include different types of bug sprays and similar products (for example, weed killer, fertilizer). Travis had obsessions about death that he confronted by looking at pictures of deceased relatives (for example, his grandfather). To further help himself, Travis sought out opportunities to visualize other relatives dying as well. This extended what he had learned about senseless intrusive thoughts and strengthened his new patterns.

BATTLE PLAN When you begin to practice exposure less frequently, you run the risk of forgetting to do the exercises. Don't let this happen! Create ways of reminding yourself, like marking it on your "to do" list, having your treatment buddy (or anyone you trust) remind you, or setting your computer to automatically send you reminder messages.

Another way to incorporate exposure into your lifestyle is to get into the habit of doing "mini-exposures" whenever you can. Arlene was obsessed with making mistakes in her paperwork and had largely overcome this fear by writing bank checks and addressing envelopes and then mailing these items without checking them. Using imaginal exposure, she confronted uncertainty and her feared consequences of making such mistakes. Now, even though she was finished with the active part of treatment, she conducted mini-exposures by deliberately making small mistakes in her paperwork each day (for example, misspelling a word, leaving out a punctuation mark), but without keeping close track of her SUDs. In the end, Arlene found this technique very practical since everyone makes small mistakes from time to time and she knew it was time to accept that she would too. Hugo also used mini-exposures: he purposely left some of the pictures on his walls hanging slightly crooked so that he could get used to the "not just right" feelings that this triggered.

What mini-exposures can you incorporate into your daily life to keep up your improvement?

Take a few minutes to set up five rules to help you stick with your lifestyle of confronting your fears. Here are some examples:

- Every time you leave the house, leave the iron plugged in.
- Whenever you throw something away, touch the outside of the trash can.
- Whenever you see a sharp or dangerous object, purposely think of hurting a loved one.
- Whenever you have to choose a password, make it one of the words or numbers you're uncomfortable with.
- Instead of using the bathroom before you leave the house, use a public one.

Now write *your* new mini-exposure rules in the space provided below.

MY MINI-EXPOSURE RULES

1. ____________________
2. ____________________
3. ____________________
4. ____________________
5. ____________________

Tapering Response Prevention

> **BATTLE PLAN** Post a copy of your mini-exposure rules in a place where you can easily see them (such as on the refrigerator or the bathroom mirror) until they become part of your lifestyle.

It's also time to begin relaxing your response prevention rules, and you can stop monitoring your rituals. But this doesn't mean a return to ritualizing! Rather, it means doing what most people do and acting out of *necessity* as opposed to out of *fear*. As a general rule, if you perform an action because of an obsessional fear, you should consider it a ritual and you should resist the behavior. This means that it's time to get into the habit of being aware of *why* you do each behavior that you once had difficulties with. Ask yourself questions such as "Why am I doing this?" and "Is this something that other people take for granted?" Another excellent strategy is to use the life-savings wager technique I introduced in Step 6.

After using CBT techniques for 3 months, Pavel no longer had problems with obsessional fears of unlucky numbers (13 and 666) and praying rituals. But one day he was purchasing airline tickets for his family's spring break, and the total bill came to $666.13 (no kidding!). Pavel panicked. "Both of my unlucky numbers at once! Surely God doesn't want us to go on this vacation," he thought. "Something terrible will happen to us." He felt a strong urge to pray ritualistically, but also knew this would be a step in the wrong direction. So Pavel asked himself, "If I had to bet my whole life savings that these numbers are a sign from God, or whether it's just a coincidence, where would I put my bet?" Thinking about it this way and remembering all the exposure and response prevention work he'd already completed helped Pavel see that this was probably just a coincidence. He refused to pray for safety and instead used his trip to help himself put the nail in OCD's coffin.

Adopting "normal" or common behavior patterns is a good way to extend your treatment skills to everyday life. For example, if you had covered all light switches and electrical outlets to help you refrain from checking during your program, you can uncover them now. But if you get the urge to check, do so in an ordinary way—for example, by briefly looking at the switch one time and then walking away (as opposed to touching it or poring over it). If you have decontamination rituals, you might have stopped virtually all hand washing for an extended period of time during your program. If now you have urges to wash, you can adopt a more normal pattern: it's okay to wash, but only if your hands are *noticeably dirty*. Do you have ink, grease, chemicals, or something sticky or smelly on them? If you can see, feel, or smell something unpleasant on your hands *without poring over them*, wash them *briefly*. If a quick glance or sniff doesn't reveal anything, then don't. I've italicized "without poring over them" and "briefly" because these are the keys to success! You can't afford to turn routine inspection of your hands into a compulsive ritual.

At our clinic, we encourage patients to adopt the guidelines for ordinary or "normal" behavior listed on the facing page. You might follow these guidelines as well. If you have other types of rituals not covered in this list, you'll need to come up with your own set of guidelines. On the Returning to Normal Behavior Worksheet on page 270, make a list of how you'll handle behaviors you once performed ritualistically. Ask your treatment buddy (or a trusted friend or relative) to pitch in and help if you have trouble distinguishing ordinary behavior from exaggerated or ritualized actions.

Guidelines for Returning to Normal Behavior

Washing

- Wash your hands no more than five times a day.
- Avoid using portable hand sanitizers or disinfectant gels.
- Don't take more than 20 seconds to wash your hands.
- Wash your hands only before meals, after using the bathroom, or if you can see or smell unwanted substances on your hands without close inspection.
- Use regular-strength (as opposed to heavy-duty or extra-strength) soaps.
- Don't use barriers (such as tissues, sleeves, or your foot) to open doors, touch surfaces, or flush toilets.

Showering

- Take one 10-minute shower per day.
- Take an additional 10-minute shower *only* if you have dirt, extreme perspiration, or body odors that can be noticed without close inspection.
- If you need to prepare for a formal event (for example, a date or a wedding party), an extra 10-minute shower is also okay.
- Use regular-strength (as opposed to extra-strength) soap and shampoo.

Cleaning

- Clean items in the house (showers, toilets, sinks, floors, sofas, etc.) once a month or only if you can see dust, dirt, or other unclean substances without looking closely.
- Use regular-strength (as opposed to heavy-duty or extra-strength) cleansers.
- Wash clothes only after wearing them and wash them only once with regular-strength detergent.

Checking and reassurance seeking

- In situations that provoked checking rituals, do not check more than once.
- Do not turn your car around to check for any reason (a single glance out the window or mirror is allowed).
- When doing the single check of door locks, appliances, and the like, check only visually if possible.
- Don't ask others to check for you.
- Don't ask for reassurance about an obsessional fear topic more than once (to the same person or to different people).

Praying and religious rituals

- Limit praying to worship services, before meals, and before bedtime, unless directed otherwise by a clergy member.
- Don't say prayers in response to situations related to obsessional thoughts or fears.
- Say each prayer once and do not repeat, even if your mind wanders or if you have doubts that you said the prayer perfectly (have faith that God knows you and understands your prayers).
- Perform each religious rite and ritual only once, even if you did it "imperfectly" the first time.
- Do not confess the same sin more than once.

Returning to Normal Behavior Worksheet

Now that response prevention is over, instead of performing rituals such as (list rituals):	I will substitute the following "normal" behaviors:
• ______________________	• ______________________
• ______________________	• ______________________
• ______________________	• ______________________
• ______________________	• ______________________
• ______________________	• ______________________

Troubleshooting

Keeping up with exposure and response prevention over the long term is not easy. It may seem daunting that you'll need to continue using these strategies for a while. As they become part of your lifestyle, things won't seem as difficult, but if you're having trouble staying motivated to continue, try the following suggestions:

- Make a list of the benefits of continuing to use CBT strategies in your life. How will it improve your work or school performance? Social or dating activities? How will it affect the way you view yourself? Use the worksheet on the facing page to record your answers.
- Determine your progress since you began this program (see "Measuring Your Progress" later in this step). How are things better now, compared to when you began your treatment program? Thinking about your personal progress can be very motivating.
- Choose a short-term goal and a reward for achieving this goal. Make sure you reward yourself only when you reach the goal. Use the strategies in Step 5 to help you. Record your goals and rewards on the worksheet at the bottom of the facing page.
- Make a contract with yourself in which you agree to enjoy certain activities (watching a movie, taking a trip, making a large purchase) only after you've practiced exposure to a certain feared situation, or stopped certain rituals, for an entire week. Fill in this information on the worksheet at the bottom of page 272.
- Keep track of your rituals using the monitoring form in Step 9 (page 230) and keep

What I Stand to Gain from Using CBT Strategies as Part of My Lifestyle

How will my performance improve in the areas of life I value (work, home, school, social life, volunteer work, recreation, and so on)?

____

____

____

____

How will my self-image improve?

____

____

____

____

these forms in a place where others can see them—such as on the refrigerator at home. Family members will see that you're resisting rituals and make you feel good by congratulating you on your accomplishments.

Another trouble spot to avoid is setting very rigid or absolutist goals for maintaining your improvement. Fernando completed his treatment program and hadn't performed a

Goal:

____

____

To be achieved by: / / [insert date]

Reward for reaching the goal by the deadline:

____

____

repeating or arranging ritual for several weeks. But he set an unrealistic goal for himself: he declared that he'd *never ritualize again*. This is like setting yourself up for failure. Inevitably, everyone does some ritualizing (even people without OCD!). When Fernando eventually couldn't resist an urge to arrange books on his bookshelf, he started beating up on himself: "I'm such a loser. I have no self-control." This led to other negative thoughts, such as "Now that I've broken my 'no rituals' rule, it doesn't matter if I ritualize." That's when things really started going downhill.

You can't expect perfection when it comes to battling OCD. Occasional slips, like the one Fernando had, are completely normal. And they're not caused by a lack of willpower. Usually they arise from certain situations or events or because of a lack of practice. Fortunately, all of these things are controllable—and we'll address them later in this step. The *abstinence violation effect* occurs when you set an unrealistic rule for yourself. Once you break your rule, it starts to seem like it's okay to keep breaking the rule. This leads you in the wrong direction. To avoid falling into this trap, don't be a perfectionist. Expect that from time to time you'll experience some obsessions and rituals. But remember that you know what to do about it.

Are your goals for maintaining your gains against OCD realistic?

Can you keep up the good work without being a perfectionist?

Measuring Your Progress

If you've been using your Exposure Practice Worksheets and plotting your SUDs on the graphs, you've already been watching your progress through this program. Maybe other people in your life have also told you that they've noticed changes in your mood and behavior. To get a more complete picture of where you are now, or just to cement your impressions of overall improvement, you can rate the levels of your current obsessional fear, avoidance, and rituals using the same scales you used in Step 2, before starting treatment. On page 274, you'll find the posttreatment version of the Target Symptom Rating Form. Flip back

For 1 week, starting on   /   /   [insert date], I will:

____

______________________________ [insert a specific exposure to practice every day of the week or a particular ritual to avoid doing for the week].

I will not:

____

______________________________ [insert a desirable activity, purchase, or other event that you will deny yourself at the end of the week unless you meet your week's goal].

to page 62 and enter same feared situations, thoughts, and rituals into the posttreatment version of the form. Then rate your current degree of fear, avoidance, and rituals using the 0 to 8 scale. If you need to refresh your memory for how to complete the form, read through pages 59–65 in Step 2.

If your scores are between 0 and 3, your symptoms aren't bothering you too much. If you gave yourself ratings of 4 or higher, you still have at least a moderate degree of fear or are still avoiding or ritualizing fairly often. A score of 7 or above means that you're still having significant problems that likely will require more help. But how do your ratings compare to the ones from Step 2? If they're now lower, you know you've improved. If you like, you can even figure out your percent change from pre- to posttreatment. Simply enter your scores into the following formula:

Pretreatment score – Posttreatment score ÷ Pretreatment score = Percent change

__________ – __________ ÷ __________ = __________

What about the goals you set for your program in Step 5? Refer to your Personal Goals for Battling OCD worksheet on page 131. Write the same goals you set in the space on the blank worksheet on page 275 and rate each one on the scale from 0 (no progress) to 8 (goal achieved).

What If You're Not Where You Want to Be?

Defeating an enemy as strong and as crafty as OCD is no small task. So your progress might be slower than you had hoped for. If you felt you had achieved all you could achieve in the active part of the program, but the yardsticks you just used indicate you're still struggling with OCD to some extent, don't despair. Keep up your lifestyle exposures and go back to active practices if you believe either of these two obstacles was standing in your way:

1. *You had trouble remembering to practice consistently.* Try using strategies to keep you from forgetting, such as putting reminder notes in strategic places where you'll see them (on the bathroom mirror or in the car), sending e-mails to yourself, setting an alarm clock, asking a friend or family member to remind you, or scheduling your practices at the same time each day so they become part of your routine.
2. *You sometimes avoided exposure practices due to anxiety.* Remind yourself that anxiety isn't dangerous and that it's important to allow yourself to feel anxious in the short term so you can feel better in the long run. Try using cognitive therapy strategies from Step 6 before you try your exposure practices.

If your program has stalled for other reasons, try finding a mental health professional with expertise in CBT; tips for finding a therapist who is competent to help you overcome problems with OCD are at the end of this chapter.

If you do decide to return to active practices, first take a little time to pinpoint the strategies that worked best for you over the preceding weeks. You might boost your gains if you concentrate more on those.

Target Symptom Rating Form (Posttreatment Version)

Part I. Obsessional Fears

Rate how much you are afraid of each target trigger/intrusion using the scale from 0 (no fear) to 8 (extreme fear).

0	1	2	3	4	5	6	7	8
None		Mild		Moderate		Strong		Extreme

	Feared trigger or intrusive thought	Fear rating
a.		
b.		
c.		

Part 2. Avoidance

Rate how much you avoid each item.

0	1	2	3	4	5	6	7	8
Never		Rarely		Sometimes		Often		Always
0%				50%				100%

	Feared item, situation, or intrusive thought	Rating
a.		
b.		
c.		

Part 3. Time Spent Ritualizing

Rate how much time per day you spend doing each ritual.

0	1	2	3	4	5	6	7	8
Never		Rarely		Sometimes		Often		Always

	Ritual	Rating
a.		
b.		
c.		

Achieving Personal Goals

Rate how much progress you made toward achieving the personal goals you set for your program using the scale below.

0	1	2	3	4	5	6	7	8
No progress		A little progress		Moderate progress		A great deal of progress		Goal achieved!

	Goal	Rating
1.		
2.		
3.		
4.		
5.		

What Worked Best for You?

Read through the CBT Strategies for OCD Checklist on the following page and mark those that you found most effective. In addition, think about what you've learned by using these strategies and fill out the OCD Treatment Review Worksheet on page 277.

Living without Obsessions and Rituals

Did your obsessions and rituals once take up a great deal of your time or restrict your daily activities? If so, you might have a void to fill where the OCD symptoms used to be. It's important that you learn to fill in this time with productive and rewarding activities so that you can fully and meaningfully participate in life and leave no room for obsessions and rituals to creep back into your routine. So how will you occupy the time you've won back from OCD? What will you do now that you're free from the shackles of obsessive fear?

You'll probably need to develop a new repertoire of activities, and in some cases, new skills. Social activities, hobbies, and a volunteer or paid job will be of great help in preventing a return of OCD symptoms. If your life has been seriously disrupted by OCD, or if you're especially concerned that your new endeavors will fail, seek professional help from an occupational therapist or social worker. Some examples of things my former patients have done with the time they've won back from OCD are listed at the bottom of the next page:

CBT Strategies for OCD Checklist

Place a check mark next to the strategy that you found helpful:

	Step	Strategy
1. ______	1	Learning about the symptoms, causes, and treatments of OCD
2. ______	2	Analyzing your own problems with OCD
3. ______	3	Learning about the CBT model of OCD
4. ______	4	Learning about how CBT works
5. ______	4	Creating a treatment plan for exposure and response prevention
6. ______	6	Examining the evidence
7. ______	6	Continuum technique
8. ______	6	Pie-chart technique
9. ______	6	Life-savings wager technique
10. ______	6	Double-standard technique
11. ______	6	Experimental techniques
12. ______	6	Cost–benefit analysis
13. ______	7	Situational exposure
14. ______	8	Imaginal exposure
15. ______	9	Response prevention

Activities to Do with Time Won Back from OCD

Paint
Compose music
Write a book about OCD
Join a book club
Join a dating service
Find a volunteer or paid job
Go back to school
Start/join an OCD support group
Join an exercise class
Learn how to play an instrument
Get involved in your community
Take up golf and running
Learn to play a team sport
Ride horses
Learn how to knit or do needlepoint
Go to the movies or to a play or a concert
Do crossword or jigsaw puzzles
Go out for coffee or dinner
Travel to museums all over the world
Sightsee

(*continued on page 278*)

OCD Treatment Review Worksheet

The CBT strategies that worked best for me were:

These strategies seemed to work because:

These strategies worked best for defeating which problems:

The most important things I learned in my CBT program were:

Learn to mediate and do yoga	Hike
Start collecting baseball cards or stamps	Start going to the gym
Bike	Get massages
Ski	

To get on with living life, these are the kinds of enjoyable activities you'll want to add to your life. Mickey's existence used to revolve around counting, checking, and asking for assurance. As he became less obsessed with unlucky numbers and the fear of disasters, he wondered, "Now what? I have all this free time on my hands." He tried to balance his life by engaging in enjoyable activities. One thing he did was to join a fitness club and begin training for a 5K race. He got so involved in his training program that instead of constantly obsessing about being responsible for disasters, he was having fun and feeling healthier.

If there are activities listed on page 276 and above that you've already been doing but aren't enjoying, replace them with things you'd enjoy more. If you've already got activities that you do for fun, keep them up. Keep a record of what you do for fun over the next few weeks and rate how enjoyable you find each activity. Set aside and devote time especially for these activities. Make them a priority by not allowing distractions to get in your way. Psychologists Gordon Asmundson and Steven Taylor suggest keeping track of your pleasurable activities and rating how much you enjoy them using the Activity Enjoyment Rating Form on the facing page. Make your ratings, using a 5-point scale with 0 indicating *no enjoyment* and 4 indicating *a lot of enjoyment*. Activities that you find to be so-so would be rated 2. At the end of each week, take a look at your ratings. Keep doing the activities that have ratings of 3 or 4 on average and replace the ones that are usually lower than 3 with something else. It'll take some trial and error, but eventually you'll come up with a list of things that bring you true enjoyment.

Dealing with Lapses and Preventing Relapses

It's very likely that you'll be able to maintain the gains you've made in this program, and maybe even continue to improve as time goes by. But progress toward recovery from OCD usually involves bumps in the road—even though you'll keep using CBT techniques during the maintenance phase of your program. When you hit one of these bumps, you'll need to step it up to maintain your improvement. The most important thing is that you not let these temporary setbacks turn into a full-blown return of your symptoms.

What Is a Lapse?

Simply put, a lapse is a slip—a noticeable increase in your obsessional fears after you've started making real progress in overcoming these problems. But fear and anxiety may not be the first thing you notice with a lapse; sometimes the first sign is an increase in avoidance and ritualizing. Take Judith, for example. She had made great strides in overcoming her fear

> If you find yourself avoiding a situation or seeking reassurance, is it normal behavior or a sign of increased ritualizing?

Activity Enjoyment Rating Form

Instructions: List each activity you do for enjoyment over the next few weeks. Rate how much you enjoy each activity using the following scale:

0	1	2	3	4
No enjoyment				A lot of enjoyment

Day and date	Activity	Enjoyment rating
Example	*Visited the art museum*	4
Example	*Went to the gym and worked out*	3

of working in the biochemistry lab and was much less worried about accidental exposure to toxic chemicals. But one day she realized she had called the university's Risk Management Office five times to ask for reassurance that she hadn't inhaled lethal amounts of hazardous materials. This was the first signal that Judith was experiencing a lapse.

Less obvious behaviors may also signal a lapse. P.J., for example, had worked hard to become more comfortable in areas of the city where beggars and homeless people dwelled on the street. Then, for no apparent reason, he found himself avoiding going downtown, like the time he made his wife drive alone to the train station to pick up their son who was returning home from college.

You may be thinking that I'm making a big deal out of nothing. Perhaps Judith's concerns were justified—the chemicals in the lab were, after all, potentially toxic. Maybe P.J. was just too tired to deal with driving all the way downtown. Granted, there may be a variety of explanations for Judith's and P.J.'s behavior. On the other hand, any sign of increased rituals or avoidance could also point to a lapse that needs prompt attention.

Lapse versus Relapse

Lapses are not by themselves cause for too much alarm. They're usually temporary—perhaps only a one-time occurrence—and easy to deal with if you view them as signs that you need to practice more often the CBT strategies that worked best for you (see the worksheet on page 277). However, when lapses become frequent, and more the rule than the exception, you may be headed for a *relapse*—a much more serious return to the obsessive–compulsive thinking and acting patterns of the past that are harder to control. Most all relapses can be prevented. The important thing is to try to head them off at the pass by getting to work at the first sign of a lapse. Understanding what causes lapses and relapses is the first step to keeping them in check.

It's not a matter of *if*, but *when* a lapse will occur. Lapses are inevitable and usually easy to deal with. But a relapse is a different story. It means you've missed the early warning signs that your old problems are coming back. It's critical that you recognize lapses early and do what you can to prevent them from becoming relapses.

What Causes Lapses and Relapses?

A number of factors can lead to lapses and relapses. Increased emotional or physical stress is one of the big ones. Whether it's financial difficulties, problems at work or school, relationship issues, a family tragedy/loss, personal health problems, leaving home (for example, for college), or even having a new baby, stressful events lower your resistance and sap your energy, leaving you more susceptible to unhelpful thinking and acting patterns. Incidents that coincide with your obsessional fears can also trigger lapses. Mark's obsessions about contamination from semen returned after he had a wet dream. Bonnie's obsessional thoughts about molesting children returned after she saw an advertisement for a television program about sexual predators. A lapse is understandable following coincidences like these. But it doesn't mean you're back to square one. Since you've tackled OCD once, doing it again should be even easier.

Lapses don't just occur when the going gets tough; you can have one after a period of success—when you'd least expect it. For Arnold, the worst of his problems with contamination-related OCD seemed to be behind him. Now he could open doors, use the railing, and touch other items without having to wash his hands. "It's sure nice to finally relax and be done with OCD," he said to himself. "I'm glad I don't need to do those exposures anymore." But before long, Arnold found himself starting to avoid and wash his hands more and more. This really caught him off guard. Under these circumstances, a lapse may mean that you've become too complacent. It's possible that if Arnold had continued exposure practice *even after he'd overcome his obsessions*, he might not have had the lapse.

You might also be prone to lapses if you didn't take exposure and response prevention practices far enough during treatment, that is, if you didn't face the *most fearful* triggers and thoughts on the hierarchy, if you didn't stop *all* of your rituals, if you used even subtle avoidance during exposure practice, or if you didn't confront your fears in enough different settings. Not going "all the way" with exposure and response prevention leaves the door open for OCD to creep back in.

Your Personalized Relapse Prevention Plan

Relapse prevention starts with being proactive and remaining aware of those situations likely to cause stress or trigger a lapse. You should also remain on the lookout for warning signs and approach the lapse as a temporary setback that you know how to overcome. Then you use the skills and strategies you learned throughout this workbook to turn things around. Here are the strategies I've found effective for identifying and dealing with lapses:

1. Assess Yourself from Time to Time

One of the best ways to protect against relapse is to periodically check up on how you're doing. You can simply retake the tests on page 274 to make sure you haven't unknowingly slipped back into any old obsessional, avoidance, or ritualistic patterns. You should especially monitor your symptoms during or after a particularly stressful time in your life, since these events turn out to increase the risk of lapses, as I describe next. Be careful not to go overboard and compulsively check that you're still doing okay (that is, to gain assurance). This is, itself, a ritual, and it can lead to problematic anxiety about relapsing. You're probably best off assessing your symptoms about once every 6 months.

2. Identify the "High-Risk" Situations

Since your chances of having a lapse increase when you're under stress, you can prepare for an increase in obsessions and rituals and don't have to get taken by surprise. Have you recently lost a close relative or had a close relationship come to an end? Do you have a stressful job or financial pressures? These are examples of negative stressors, but positive events that require adjustments can also produce stress. Will you be starting a new job? Having a baby? Setting out on your own for the first time? Have you recently gotten married? Any events or situations that provoke stress for you are your "high-risk" situations because they increase the odds of a lapse. When you know a stressful event is coming up, prepare yourself for a possible return of obsessions and rituals. If you're prepared, the lapse won't catch you off guard and you'll be ready to take action immediately. If the stressful event happens without warning, you still have time to act, but remember that it's important to address lapses right away. The longer you wait, the more time you're giving your obsessional fear to build.

What are some stressful high-risk situations that you anticipate in the next few months? Note these in the worksheet at the bottom of the next page and use the skills that follow to defeat potential lapses.

3. Spot the Warning Signs

Before you can prevent a relapse, you need to identify the signs that you're having a lapse. Here are some possible warning signs to look for:

- An increase in physical symptoms of anxiety when you find yourself facing an obsessional trigger
- An increase in obsessional thoughts
- An increase in rituals and avoidance behavior
- You're feeling more irritable or feeling down
- An increase in relationship stress caused by a return to avoidance and rituals

When you spot these (or other) warning signs of a return of obsessional symptoms, you know it's time to swing into relapse prevention mode and use the techniques described next to stop the lapse in its tracks.

4. Keep a Positive Attitude

You may be inclined to panic at the first sign of a lapse. But don't fall into the trap of beating up on yourself. Remember that lapses are normal and unavoidable. They occur sometimes despite your best intentions. Saying things to yourself such as "Oh no, I'm failing!" or "This is awful; I can't take this again" will only lead you into a cycle of despair and increase your stress. And remember that stress increases your obsessions and rituals. Instead of heaping criticism on yourself, simply tell yourself that something has gone wrong that you need to correct. Then take action! The following coping statements might help you deal effectively with a lapse:

"Everything's okay. This was bound to happen. Everyone has lapses."

"I'm glad I caught this before it became a relapse. I know what I have to do now."

Relapse Prevention Plan: My High-Risk Situations

1. ______________________________
2. ______________________________
3. ______________________________
4. ______________________________
5. ______________________________

"For whatever reason, I'm having some trouble with rituals. I guess it means I need to work a little harder."

"I've beaten this problem before. There's no reason I can't beat it again!"

5. Take Action

Let's start by reviewing what you've already learned about OCD from reading and working through the exercises in this book. Answer the following three questions to help you think about what you should and shouldn't do if you feel that problems with obsessions and rituals are returning. Dave had obsessional fears and doubts about causing bad luck to befall his loved ones. After completing his CBT program, he began preparing for the possibility of relapse by answering these questions. They helped remind him of what he should and shouldn't be doing to keep OCD at bay. Dave's responses are shown on the following page.

A. Write down all of the things you've learned about intrusive unwanted thoughts and how they develop into anxiety-provoking obsessions.

- ____________________
- ____________________
- ____________________
- ____________________
- ____________________
- ____________________

B. Write down the behavior patterns that might reduce anxiety, obsessions, and uncertainty in the *short term* but make your obsessional fears *worse* in the *long run*.

- ____________________
- ____________________
- ____________________
- ____________________
- ____________________
- ____________________

C. What sorts of things have you learned that help you cope with, or even overcome, your obsessional anxiety? (Hint: these could have to do with using certain techniques to change unhelpful behavior patterns.)

- ____________________
- ____________________
- ____________________
- ____________________
- ____________________
- ____________________

Dave's Answers

A. Write down all of the things you've learned about intrusive unwanted thoughts and how they develop into anxiety-provoking obsessions.

- *Everyone has negative intrusive thoughts from time to time.*
- *People without OCD treat these thoughts as senseless "mental noise."*
- *I misinterpret these thoughts as very important and meaningful.*
- *These misinterpretations make me anxious and preoccupied with the thoughts.*
- *I try to push the thought away, but that makes me have it even more.*

B. Write down your behavior patterns that might reduce anxiety, obsessions, and uncertainty in the *short term* but make you obsessional fears *worse* in the *long run*.

- *I try to analyze my obsessions and figure out whether they're true or not.*
- *I try to push bad thoughts away, but this makes them come back.*
- *I ask people for reassurance that I won't cause bad luck if I do something.*
- *I say phrases and numbers in my head (mental rituals) to prevent bad things.*
- *I avoid certain situations and items that remind me of obsessional thoughts.*

C. What sorts of things have you learned that help you cope with or even overcome your obsessional anxiety? (Hint: these could have to do with using certain techniques to change unhelpful thinking and behavior patterns.)

- *I've learned to consider evidence that calls into question whether my obsessive fears are realistic.*
- *Confronting my fears will make me anxious temporarily, but my anxiety will eventually subside and I'll learn not to be afraid.*
- *If I just go with my unpleasant thoughts, I eventually become less anxious and they bother me less and less.*
- *When I keep myself from using mental rituals, nothing awful happens to anyone.*

The next steps are for you to work through when you notice a lapse and need to take back control of your OCD symptoms:

A. Consider the evidence for and against your obsessional fears. Are there alternative ways of interpreting your intrusive thoughts? Write down more helpful interpretations and ways of thinking about your obsessions, uncertainty, and fear triggers.

- ____________________
- ____________________
- ____________________
- ____________________

B. Practice the cognitive therapy strategies you found helpful for changing unhelpful thinking patterns. List the strategies you used to control your lapse. Which were the most helpful?

- ____________________
- ____________________
- ____________________
- ____________________

C. Keep the lapse in check by not giving in to the urge to do anything that makes obsessions stronger: avoidance of situations that trigger your fear, compulsive rituals, reassurance seeking, mental rituals, thought suppression, or mini-rituals. List the things you're trying not to do. For example, "I'm not going to try to force the upsetting thoughts out of my mind" and "I'm not going to call the pastor to double-check if it's okay to have a 6 in my Social Security number."

- ____________________
- ____________________
- ____________________
- ____________________

D. If you've been avoiding fear triggers and situations, develop a step-by-step plan for practicing situational exposure to these situations. If a trigger is too frightening to confront, try an easier one first and work your way up to the more frightening situation. Make a list of the situations you're avoiding and the steps you're taking to confront them. Be sure to practice exposure in different situations. Remember that when you really push the envelope and go beyond what most people would do—such as actually touching the bottom of your shoe rather than just coming near it—this bulldozes obsessional fears to the ground so they're less likely to come back.

- ____________________
- ____________________
- ____________________
- ____________________

E. Are you having obsessive doubts and thoughts of disasters? If so, develop a plan for imaginal exposure. List the obsessional thoughts you're having problems with and describe how you will confront them using imaginal exposure techniques.

- ______________________________
- ______________________________
- ______________________________
- ______________________________

If you've been working with a treatment buddy, ask him or her to help you out. If you have a therapist, consider scheduling some "booster sessions" so that you can work together to get you back on course. Because you've already learned the necessary recovery skills once, you can probably get back on track more quickly than you'd expect. It's almost a matter of reviewing what you already know, planning the exposure practices you need to try, and cutting back on your rituals. If you carefully assess what led you to relapse and make plans for dealing with similar situations in the future, your recovery can be even stronger than before.

Seeking Professional Help

Finding a Clinician

If your problems with obsessional thoughts, avoidance, and rituals are severe, or don't respond to the self-help approach described in this workbook, consider making an appointment with a mental health treatment provider. Most likely, you'll have to look around a little before you find a qualified clinician. While we know that CBT usually works for OCD, not all therapists are familiar with, or well trained to use, these techniques. One of the best ways to find good therapists in your area is by asking the leaders or members of local OCD support groups. The Obsessive Compulsive Foundation (OCF) website (*www.ocfoundation.org*) provides a list of these groups, and even if the nearest one is some distance from you, they may know of good therapists in your area. Three organizations can also provide you with a list of professionals in your region who have indicated that they treat OCD: the OCF, the Association for Behavioral and Cognitive Therapies (*www.abct.org*), and the Anxiety Disorders Association of America (*www.adaa.org*).

You might also be able to get referral lists from your state, provincial, or region's mental health, psychological, and psychiatric associations. And if you happen to live near a major university that has a training program in psychology, or a medical school with a psychiatry department, you could call or go online and find out if they have a clinic that offers treatment from their therapists-in-training. And don't be too concerned about working with a student therapist—especially one with training or experience using CBT for anxiety and OCD: he or she will be closely supervised (and working hard to impress the supervisor!). Not only is the quality of their therapy often very good, such clinics often provide services at low cost.

If you still can't find anyone with related expertise, check out the organizations and websites listed in the Resources at the back of this book. Many of these provide information on OCD and/or can help you to find a cognitive-behavioral therapist or psychiatrist.

Checking on Qualifications

Whether or not you locate a therapist through these outlets, before agreeing to start treatment with a particular clinician, make sure he or she is licensed to practice in your state or province. Then, ask the practitioner to describe his or her qualifications and treatment approach to you (e-mail or call them on the phone rather than paying for an initial session to get this information). Here are some questions to ask a potential treatment provider and the answers you should be looking for. Don't be afraid to ask these kinds of questions—it's important that you stand up for yourself to make sure you're getting the treatment you need.

1. What kind of treatment approach do you use for OCD? (*Answer: Behavioral or cognitive behavioral. If they say anything such as "gestalt," "psychodynamic," "eclectic," "mindfulness," "psychoanalytic," "humanistic," "Rogerian," or "Jungian," this is not the person you're looking for!*)
2. Can you tell me what CBT involves? What would the therapy be like? (*Answer: The description should include facing your feared situations and thoughts [exposure] and refraining from rituals [response prevention]. If the therapist mentions "biofeedback," "EMDR," "hypnosis," "relaxation," or "thought stopping," you're not in the right place. Snapping a rubber band on your arm doesn't reduce OCD; it only leads to a sore arm.*)
3. What formal training have you had in treating OCD using CBT? (*Answer: You want a treatment provider with formal training. This means being trained in CBT in graduate school, through one-on-one training and supervision from an expert, or by attending multiple seminars or workshops. Simply reading (even a lot of reading) about CBT, or attending a few workshops or lectures, is not enough. Take it from me: you can't learn to do good CBT in a few hours. It takes months [if not years] of training.*)
4. About how many people with OCD have you worked with using CBT? (*Answer: At least 5 to 10 before you.*)
5. What kinds of results do you get with CBT? (*Answer: Research shows that most people benefit with at least a 50% reduction in their symptoms. The treatment provider should sound confident that he or she knows how to use CBT to get good results.*)
6. How long will it take me to start feeling better with CBT? How long does treatment usually last (how many sessions, weeks, or months will it take)? (*Answer: Most CBT programs work within about 20 sessions. If the provider's answer is much longer than this, it might mean he or she is using other strategies besides CBT.*)
7. Will we do exposure therapy together during the treatment sessions, or will I do it for homework? (*Answer: Look for a therapist who will help you do exposure practice in the session and also assign you more practices to conduct between sessions.*)
8. Are you able to leave your office to help me do exposure therapy? (*Answer: Yes.*)

9. Do you use imaginal exposure along with situational exposure? (*Answer: Yes.*)
10. Is it okay if I bring in some self-help materials I've been using so you can see where I'm at with working on this problem? (*Answer: Yes.*)

It's possible that you won't find a therapist who gets a "perfect score" on these questions, but answering most of them correctly is often a good sign. You should be skeptical if a potential clinician offers you a treatment you've never heard of before, such as "Thought Field Therapy" or "Rebirthing." Also, be leery of anyone who seems overly confident, claims to be able to *cure* you, or *guarantees* the treatment (anything that sounds too good to be true probably is). Finally, if the clinician can't tell you how long treatment might be expected to last, you should look for someone else.

Some therapists are knowledgeable about CBT in general, but not necessarily experienced with OCD. If this is the case, ask whether the practitioner has used CBT when working with people who have problems with phobias, social anxiety, or panic attacks. The treatment of these problems is similar to CBT for OCD. You can therefore be reasonably comfortable that this person will have a basic knowledge of what's necessary to help you with obsessions and rituals. Perhaps you might suggest using this workbook to tailor the treatment to your specific types of obsessions and rituals.

If you're thinking about using medication to help with your OCD symptoms, try to find a psychiatrist (with an MD degree) who is experienced with drug treatments for OCD. If you can't locate an OCD expert, try to find someone who is familiar with treating anxiety disorders in general. Very often, the medication treatments for OCD are the same as those for other anxiety problems.

Some Final Words

Congratulations! You've come a long way. I hope the insights, information, and CBT strategies I've included in these 10 steps have helped you overcome the problems that led you to this workbook in the first place. Besides the fact that it often works, one of the things I like most about CBT is that you practice and learn skills that are yours to keep (and use) forever. No relying on someone else's sage advice for what to do every week. No costly medication prescriptions that need refilling. You've got skills and knowledge that no one can take away from you and that won't "run out." This always reminds me of the ancient Chinese proverb "*Give* me a fish and I eat for a day. *Teach* me to fish and I eat for a lifetime." After lots of hard work, *you've* learned how to "fish" when it comes to defeating obsessions and rituals, and it's my sincere wish that you "eat" for a lifetime.

Resources

Books

Baer, Lee. *Getting Control.* New York: Plume, 2000.

Ciarrocchi, Joseph. *The Doubting Disease: Help for Religious Obsessions and Compulsions.* Mahwah, NJ: Paulist Press, 1995.

De Silva, Padmal, and Rachman, Stanley. *Obsessive–Compulsive Disorder: The Facts.* New York: Oxford University Press, 2004.

Foa, Edna, and Wilson, Reid. *Stop Obsessing: How to Overcome Your Obsessions and Compulsions.* New York: Random House, 2001.

Grayson, Jonathan. *Freedom from Obsessive–Compulsive Disorder.* New York: Berkley, 2004.

Hyman, Bruce, and Dufrene, Troy. *Coping with OCD: Practical Strategies for Living Well with Obsessive–Compulsive Disorder.* Oakland, CA: New Harbinger, 2008.

Landsman, Karen, Rupertus, Kathleen, and Pedrick, Cherry. *Loving Someone with OCD: Help for You and Your Family.* Oakland, CA: New Harbinger, 2005.

Munford, Paul. *Overcoming Compulsive Checking.* Oakland, CA: New Harbinger, 2004.

Munford, Paul. *Overcoming Compulsive Washing.* Oakland, CA: New Harbinger: 2005.

Penzel, Fred. *Obsessive–Compulsive Disorder: A Complete Guide to Getting Well and Staying Well.* New York: Oxford University Press, 2000.

Purdon, Christine, and Clark, David A. *Overcoming Obsessive Thoughts.* Oakland, CA: New Harbinger, 2005.

Organizations

United States

Organizations That Provide Resources for People with OCD, Including Information and Lists of Treatment Providers

Anxiety Disorders Association of America (ADAA)
8730 Georgia Avenue, Suite 600
Silver Spring, MD 20910
Phone: 240-485-1001
Fax: 240-485-1035
E-mail: *information@adaa.org*
Website: *www.adaa.org/AboutADAA/ContactUS.asp*

Association of Behavioral and Cognitive Therapies (ABCT)
305 7th Avenue, 16th Floor
New York, NY 10001
Phone: 212-647-1890
Fax: 212-647-1865
E-mail: *clinical.dir@abct.org*
Website: *www.abct.org* or *http://www.aabt.org*

Obsessive Compulsive Foundation (OCF)
PO Box 961029
Boston, MA 02109
Phone: 617-973-5801
E-mail: *info@ocfoundation.org*
Website: *www.ocfoundation.org*

Intensive Treatment Programs

If your problems with obsessions and rituals are particularly severe and you've tried CBT before but have not had much benefit, you might consider intensive outpatient treatment. Like our program at UNC, there are a number of clinics that offer daily (Monday through Friday) individual (one-on-one) outpatient treatment sessions for people with OCD. There are pros and cons to intensive outpatient treatment. The benefits include the fact that treatment is fairly brief, usually lasting from 3–4 weeks. Most programs also have expert therapists with lots of experience. The downside is that you might need to travel to get to one of these programs. You may also need to put your life on hold while you do the therapy. Here are some of the best-known programs offering intensive outpatient treatment for OCD:

Anxiety and OCD Treatment and Research Program
Contact: John E. Calamari, PhD
Department of Psychology
Rosalind Franklin University of Medicine and Science
3333 Green Bay Road
North Chicago, IL 60046-3095
Phone: 847-578-8747
E-mail: *john.calamari@rosalindfranklin.edu*
Website: *www.rosalindfranklin.edu*

Anxiety Disorder Center at The Institute of Living (affiliated with Yale University)
Contact: David F. Tolin, PhD
200 Retreat Avenue
Hartford, CT 06106
Phone: 800-673-2411 or 800-673-2411
Fax: 860-545-7068
Website: *www.instituteofliving.org/*

Austin Center for the Treatment of Obsessive–Compulsive Disorder
Contact: Bruce Mansbridge, PhD
Suite 300
6633 Highway 290 East
Austin, TX 78723
Phone: 512-327-9494
Fax: 512-637-5578
E-mail: *info@austinocd.com*
Website: *www.austinocd.com/*

Bio-Behavioral Institute
Contact: Fugen Neziroglu, PhD
935 Northern Boulevard, Suite 102
Great Neck, NY 11021
Phone: 516-487-7116
Fax: 516-829-1731
E-mail: *institute@bio-behavioral.com*
Website: *www.bio-behavioral.com*

Center for the Treatment and Study of Anxiety's OCD Program
Contact: Elna Yadin, PhD
Center for Treatment and Study of Anxiety
University of Pennsylvania School of Medicine
3535 Market Street, 6th Floor
Philadelphia, PA 19104
Phone: 215-746-3327
Fax: 215-746-3311
Website: *www.med.upenn.edu/ctsa/ocd.html*

Cognitive Behavior Therapy Center
Contact: Paul R. Munford, PhD
The Cognitive Behavior Therapy Center for OCD and Anxiety
990 A Street, Suite 401
San Rafael, CA 94901
Phone: 415-456-2463
Fax: 415-453-7719
E-mail: *cbtmarin@comcast.net*
Website: *www.cbtmarin.com*

Obsessive Compulsive Disorder Institute at McLean Hospital
Contact: Diane Davey, RN, MBA
115 Mill Street
Belmont, MA 02478
Phone: 617-855-3279
General information: 617-855-2000
E-mail: *davey@ocd.mclean.org*
Website: *www.mclean.harvard.edu/patient/adult/ocd.php*

Rogers Memorial Hospital
Contact: Bradley Riemann, PhD
34700 Valley Road
Oconomowoc, WI 53066
Phone: 800-767-4411, ext. 340
E-mail: *info@rogershospital.org*
Website: *www.rogershospital.org*

Saint Louis Behavioral Medicine Institute
Contact: C. Alec Pollard, PhD
1129 Macklind Avenue
St. Louis, MO 63110
Phone: 877-245-2688 or 314-534-0200
E-mail: *info@slbmi.com*

Stress and Anxiety Disorders Clinic at the University of Illinois at Chicago
Contact: Cheryl Carmin, PhD
University of Illinois at Chicago
Department of Psychiatry
Stress and Anxiety Disorders Clinic
912 South Wood Street
Chicago, IL 60612
Phone: 312-413-1225
E-mail: *Ccarmin@psych.uic.edu*
Website: *www.psych.uic.edu*

University of California Los Angeles OCD Intensive Treatment Program
Contact: Jaime Feusner, MD
300 UCLA Medical Plaza
Box 956968
Los Angeles, CA 90095-6968
Phone: 310-794-7305
E-mail: *Kmaidment@mednet.ucla.edu*

University of North Carolina at Chapel Hill Anxiety and Stress Disorders Clinic
Contact: Jonathan S. Abramowitz, PhD
Department of Psychology, UNC-CH
Campus Box 3270 (Davie Hall)
Chapel Hill, NC 27599
Phone: 919-843-8170
E-mail: *ocdprogram@unc.edu*
Website: *www.jabramowitz.com*

Western Psychiatric Institute and Clinic
Contact: Robert Hudak, MD
Western Psychiatric Institute and Clinic
3811 O'Hara Street
Pittsburgh, PA 15213
Phone: 412-586-9222
Website: *wpic.upmc.com*

Westwood Institute for Anxiety Disorders, Inc.
Contact: Eda Gorbis, PhD
921 Westwood Boulevard, Suite 223
Los Angeles, CA 90024
Phone: 323-651-1199
E-mail: *edagorbis@yahoo.com*
Website: *www.hope4ocd.com*

Hospitalization

While most psychiatric hospitals have the resources to stabilize people with OCD, usually with supportive therapy and medications, the two programs listed below are among the few that have the expertise and personnel on hand to deliver effective CBT for OCD.

Obsessive Compulsive Disorder Institute at McLean Hospital
Contact: Diane Davey, RN, MBA
115 Mill Street
Belmont, MA 02478
Phone: 617-855-3279
General Information: 617-855-2000
E-mail: *davey@ocd.mclean.org*
Website: *www.mclean.harvard.edu/patient/adult/ocd.php*

Rogers Memorial Hospital
Contact: Bradley Riemann, PhD
34700 Valley Road
Oconomowoc, WI 53066
Phone: 800-767-4411, ext. 340
E-mail: *info@rogershospital.org*
Website: *www.rogershospital.org*

Canada

L'Association/Troubles Anxieux du Québec
Information on the website is in French only.
C.P. 49018
Montréal (Québec) H1N 3T6
Phone: 514-251-0083
E-mail: *info@ataq.org*
Website: *www.ataq.org*

McMaster University Anxiety Disorders Clinic
McMaster University Medical Centre
Hamilton Health Sciences
1200 Main Street West
Hamilton, ON L8N 3Z5
Phone: 905-521-2100, ext. 73059 (for research studies information)
E-mail: *bill@macanxiety.com*
Website: *www.macanxiety.com*

OCD Centre Manitoba, Inc. (OCDC)
100-4 Fort Street
Winnipeg, MB R3C 1C4
Phone: 204-942-3331
Fax: 204-772-6706
E-mail: info@ocdmanitoba.ca
Website: *www.ocdmanitoba.ca*

Ontario Obsessive Compulsive Disorder Network
PO Box 151
Markham, Ontario
L3P 3J7
Phone: 416-410-4772
Fax: 905-472-4473
E-mail: info@ocdontario.org
Website: *www.ocdontario.org*

United Kingdom

Anxiety UK (formerly The National Phobics Society)
Zion Community Resource Centre
339 Stretford Road
Hulme, Manchester M15 4ZY
Phone: 0844 477 5774 and 0161 227 9898
Fax: 0161 226 7727
E-mail: *info@anxietyuk.org.uk* (general information)
support@anxietyuk.org.uk (support service)
media@anxietyuk.org.uk (media enquiries)

British Association for Behavioural and Cognitive Psychotherapies (BABCP)
Victoria Buildings
9-13 Silver Street
Bury BL9 0EU
Phone: 0161 797 4484
Fax: 0161 797 2670
E-mail: *babcp@babcp.com*
Website: *www.babcp.com/*

OCD Action
Davina House, Suites 506–507
137–149 Goswell Road
London EC1V 7ET
Phone: 0870 360 6232
Fax: 020 7288 0828
Help and information line: 0845 390 6232
(London local number: 020 7253 2664)
E-mail: *info@ocdaction.org.uk*
Website: *www.ocdaction.org.uk/ocdaction/index.asp*

OCD Ireland
E-mail: *info@ocdireland.org*
Website: *www.ocdireland.org/*

OCD—United Kingdom
PO Box 8955
Nottingham NG10 9AU
Phone: 0845 120 3778
E-mail: *admin@ocduk.org*
Website: *www.ocduk.org/index.htm*

Europe

Belgium
La Ligue Trouble Obsessionnel Compulsif
Website: *users.swing.be/ligue-toc*

Denmark
OCD-Foreningen
Website: *ocd-foreningen.dk*

France
AFTOC
Website: *aftoc.club.fr/index.htm*

Germany
Deutsche Gesellschaft Zwangserkrankungen
Website: *www.zwaenge.de*

Italy
Ossessioni e Compulsioni
Website: *www.ossessioniecompulsioni.it*

The Netherlands
OCD Vriendenkring
Website: *www.ocdvriendenkring.org*

Poland
ZOK
Website: *www.zok.net.pl/index.html*

Sweden
Ananke
Website: *www.ananke.org/ananke.htm*

Australia and New Zealand

Anxiety and Panic Hub
PO Box 516
Goolwa South Australia 5214
Phone: 08 8411 1106 (for callers within Australia)
61 8 8411 1106 (for callers from outside Australia)
E-mail: *aphub@bigpond.com*
Website: *www.panicattacks.com.au/*

New Zealand Centre for Rational Emotive Behavior Therapy
PO Box 2292
Stortford Lodge
Hastings, New Zealand
Phone: 64-6-870 9963
Fax: 64-6-870 9964
E-mail: *admin@rational.org.nz*
Website: *www.rational.org.nz*

The Phobic Trust of New Zealand
PO Box 41 133
77 Morningside Drive
St. Lukes, 1346
Auckland, New Zealand
Phone: +64 (0) 9 846 9776 and 0800 14 26 94 68 9 (24-hour helpline)
Fax: +64 (0) 9 849 2375
E-mail: *clinic@phobic.org.nz*
Website: *www.phobic.org.nz*

Asia

OCD Clinic, National Institute of Mental Health and Neuro Sciences, Bangalore, India
Website: *www.nimhans.kar.nic.in/ocdclinic/home.html*

Adult Psychiatrists

Venkatasubramanian Ganesan, MD
Assistant Professor of Psychiatry
Phone: +91-080-26995256
E-mail: *gvs@nimhans.kar.nic.in*

Suresh Bada Math, MD, DNB, PGDMLE
Assistant Professor of Psychiatry
Phone: +91-080-26995276
E-mail: *sbm@nimhans.kar.nic.in*

Y. C. Janardhan Reddy, DPM, MD
Additional Professor of Psychiatry
Phone: +91-080-26995278
E-mail: *jreddy@nimhans.kar.nic.in*

Child and Adolescent Psychiatrists

Shoba Srinath, DPM, MD
Professor of Child Psychiatry
Phone: + 91-080-26995265
E-mail: *shobas@nimhans.kar.nic.in*

Sathish Chandra Girimaji, MD
Professor of Child Psychiatry
Phone: +91-080-26995266
E-mail: *girimaji@nimhans.kar.nic.in*

Shekhar P. Seshadri, MD
Professor of Child Psychiatry
Phone: +91-080-26995268
E-mail: *shekhar@nimhans.kar.nic.in*

Y. P. Mukesh, MD
Assistant Professor of Child Psychiatry
Phone: +91-080-26995254
E-mail: *ypm@nimhans.kar.nic.in*

Index

D

E

S

T

U

V

W

About the Author

Jonathan S. Abramowitz, PhD, is Professor of Psychology and Director of the Anxiety and Stress Disorders Clinic at the University of North Carolina at Chapel Hill. Before moving to North Carolina, Dr. Abramowitz founded and directed the OCD and Anxiety Disorders Program at the Mayo Clinic in Rochester, Minnesota. His award-winning research on OCD has been supported by the National Institute of Mental Health, among others, and he serves on the Scientific Advisory Board of the Obsessive Compulsive Foundation. He lives in Chapel Hill with his wife and two daughters.